Immigration, Public Policy, and Health

Immigration, Public Policy, and Health

Newcomer Experiences in Developed Nations

Edited by Dennis Raphael

Canadian Scholars' Press
Toronto

Immigration, Public Policy, and Health: Newcomer Experiences in Developed Nations
Edited by Dennis Raphael

First published in 2016 by
Canadian Scholars' Press Inc.
425 Adelaide Street West, Suite 200
Toronto, Ontario
M5V 3C1

www.cspi.org

Library and Archives Canada Cataloguing in Publication

Immigration, public policy, and health : newcomer experiences in developed nations / edited by Dennis Raphael.

Includes index.
Issued in print and electronic formats.
ISBN 978-1-55130-927-9 (paperback).--ISBN 978-1-55130-928-6 (pdf).--
ISBN 978-1-55130-929-3 (epub)

1. Immigrants--Government policy--Developed countries--Textbooks. 2. Immigrants--Health and hygiene--Developed countries--Textbooks. 3. Developed countries--Emigration and immigration--Textbooks. I. Raphael, Dennis, editor

JV6271.I46 2016 325'.1 C2016-905264-8 C2016-905265-6

Text design Integra
Cover design by Em Dash Design

16 17 18 19 20 5 4 3 2 1

Printed and bound in Canada by Webcom

Canadä

MIX
Paper from responsible sources
FSC
www.fsc.org
FSC® C004071

Table of Contents

Preface

The origins of this volume are found in my experience of living in a city where over 50 percent of the population have emigrated from other nations. In the particular case of Toronto, most of this immigration over the last 30 years has come from the developing world and consists of people of colour. Despite admission requirements that immigrants be well educated and trained, these groups are struggling to make ends meet. I am intrigued that Canada has acquired a reputation for welcoming immigrants, but at the same time appears to do little to prevent this group of people from experiencing poverty and unemployment rates that are usually double those of people born in Canada. These rates not only depict a troubling image of quality of life for these new Canadians but are also portents of health problems as they are important social determinants of health. And there is evidence that the health of recent immigrants of colour to Canada shows significant declines over time. Similarly, there are concerns about their access to Canada's medicare system.

Indeed, the Toronto urban saying that the "easiest way to get a doctor is to hail a cab" has been confirmed by research that finds unemployment and underemployment—including driving a cab—is indeed the situation for many professional immigrants of colour (Xu, 2012). This situation actually led to the production of the popular film *Dr. Cabbie,* in which a physician from India resorts to driving a cab in Toronto, as he is unable to practise his profession (DeMara, 2014). While the movie's happy ending has the doctor becoming certified to practise, this is actually a rather uncommon outcome. There is some evidence of similar situations in Australia and the United Kingdom. How do these Anglo-Saxon nations fare in integrating these new waves of immigrants?

I am frequently told that immigrants of colour in the Scandinavian nations—known for their cradle-to-grave welfare states—experience discrimination and exclusion. But Sweden has been ranked best at integrating immigrants, exceeding the success of other European nations, Canada, and Australia (The Local, 2011). The quantity and quality of benefits and supports provided to citizens in Scandinavian nations far outstrips the situation in Anglo-Saxon nations. Do these benefits and supports facilitate immigrants' integration into these nations' societies? There has been, however, a rise in support for anti-immigration parties in the Scandinavian nations of Denmark, Norway, and Sweden, which does not bode well for immigration experiences. Similar to the question asked earlier, how do these Scandinavian nations fare in integrating recent immigrants, many of whom are of colour?

And finally, the mainstream media reports difficulties that Continental countries experience in integrating immigrants. I recall specifically the prime minister of Germany stating that German multiculturalism had "utterly failed" (Weaver, 2010). While there has been much in the press about the German scene, I know little about the experiences of other Continental nations such as Austria and Belgium. Similar to the Scandinavian nations,

Continental nations generally provide benefits and supports that exceed those available in the Anglo-Saxon nations. How do these Continental nations fare in integrating immigrants?

It is difficult to avoid considering how these different nations—Anglo-Saxon, Scandinavian, and Continental—are associated with Esping-Andersen's well-known typology of welfare state regimes. Anglo-Saxon nations are Liberal welfare states where the primary ideological inspiration of liberty sees the state take a backseat to the market in distributing economic and social resources among the population (Saint-Arnaud & Bernard, 2003). The Scandinavian nations are examples of the Social Democratic welfare state regime where achieving the primary ideological inspiration of equality provides the state with the primary role in allocating resources necessary for well-being. And Austria, Belgium, and Germany are examples of the Conservative welfare state regime where the ideological inspiration of solidarity dictates that the state and market acts through social insurance schemes to distribute resources to families.

While not wedded to the welfare state typology, this volume considers how these different forms of the welfare state inform our understanding of how immigrants are being integrated—or not integrated—into the social lives of these developed welfare states. It also considers how these processes are affecting the health of these immigrants. I am particularly interested in how nations that extol multiculturalism—such as Canada—have fared. Is there a consistent relationship between adoption of multiculturalism as a societal value, form of the welfare state, and integration of immigrants? Canada, for example, extols multiculturalism, but has done little to mitigate the very high poverty and unemployment rates of recent immigrants. In contrast, Sweden also extols the concept of multiculturalism, but also invests significant societal resources in immigrant integration. Little is known of how the Continental nations are faring.

The volume is organized to examine these issues. The first section considers the possibilities and challenges immigration provides to developed nations by recent patterns of immigration. It considers available broad-stroke examinations of how these nations fare in both integrating immigrants and implementing multiculturalism through public policy. It then places these issues within a political economy perspective informed by Esping-Andersen's welfare state typology. The second section contains the nine national case studies organized by welfare nation types: Anglo-Saxon (Liberal) (Australia, Canada, and the United Kingdom); Continental (Conservative) (Austria, Belgium, and Germany); and Scandinavian (Social Democratic) (Denmark, Norway, and Sweden). The third section identifies key themes and provides implications for moving forward. Hopefully, the material and analyses will provide useful directions for all nations experiencing the possibilities and challenges presented by recent patterns of immigration.

Dennis Raphael

January 2016

References

DeMara, B. (2014). *The cab ride that gave birth to* Dr. Cabbie. Retrieved from http://www.thestar.com/entertainment/movies/2014/09/18/the_cab_ride_that_gave_birth_to_dr_cabbie.html

The Local. (2011). *Sweden best at integration: Study.* Retrieved from http://www.thelocal.se/20110228/32316

Saint-Arnaud, S., & Bernard, P. (2003). Convergence or resilience? A hierarchical cluster analysis of the welfare regimes in advanced countries. *Current Sociology, 51*(5), 499–527.

Weaver, M. (2010). Angela Merkel: German multiculturalism has "utterly failed." Retrieved from http://www.theguardian.com/world/2010/oct/17/angela-merkel-german-multiculturalism-failed

Xu, L. (2012). *Who drives a taxi in Canada?* Retrieved from http://www.cic.gc.ca/english/pdf/research-stats/taxi.pdf

PART 1

Introduction and Overview

The purpose of this volume is to examine the immigration experience in nine developed nations. There is particular focus on the role that public policy plays in shaping how these immigrant experiences come to be related to health. It is informed by a welfare state analysis that considers how the operations of political and economic systems shape the making of public policy. These public policies then determine the quality and distribution of the social determinants of health that lead to specific health outcomes.

Part 1 of this volume sets the stage for our analysis and exploration of the immigration experience. Chapter 1 explores the nature of immigration in the wealthy developed nations of the Organisation for Economic Co-operation and Development. It considers why wealthy developed nations have increased the number of immigrants they take in and where these immigrants are coming from. It provides a background context for examination of the living and working conditions immigrants experience by outlining what is known about the social determinants of health and their importance in shaping health outcomes. Based on evidence from studies that rate nations on their success at integrating immigrants and implementing policies associated with multiculturalism, it provides a series of hypotheses on the living and working conditions experienced by immigrants upon their arrival and how these conditions can affect their health.

Chapter 2 considers how differing forms of the welfare state in wealthy developed nations may be approaching immigration issues and integrating immigrants into their societies. It takes as a starting point the distinctions made by Gosta Esping-Andersen between the Liberal, Social Democratic, and Conservative welfare state regimes. It outlines a series of hypotheses about the immigrant experience related to the key concepts Esping-Andersen outlined in his groundbreaking work: extent of social stratification, decommodification, and the relative role of the state, market, and family in distributing economic and social resources among the population.

It provides evidence of how the nations within this typology differ in extent of income inequality and poverty and the general quality and distribution of the social determinants of health members of each society experience. It also suggests that these nations may differ in both (1) general approaches to immigration, and (2) their willingness to provide immigrants with the resources necessary for health. The case studies provided in Part 2 of the volume provide evidence that allow assessing the validity of these hypotheses.

CHAPTER 1

Immigration: Possibilities and Challenges in the 21st Century

Abiola Sulaiman and Dennis Raphael

Chapter Objectives

This introductory chapter introduces the reader to key concepts related to immigration policy and immigrant status in various developed nations. The objectives of this chapter are:

- to examine how economic and political ideologies have historically influenced the implementation of immigration policy;
- to introduce the concept of the social determinants of health and how these shape immigrants' lived experiences and health;
- to illustrate differing forms of immigration through presentation of Canadian examples; and
- to provide some initial hypotheses of how immigrants are faring in the nations examined in this volume.

Introduction

In this chapter, we outline issues related to immigrant experiences across **developed nations**. We consider the purposes of different forms of immigration and the benefits that accrue to receiving nations and to immigrants themselves. We then outline how immigrants' lived experience in these receiving nations can impact health and quality of life through processes associated with the social determinants of health. Initial hypotheses are presented as to how immigrants fare in nine developed nations. These are based on what we know about their form of the welfare state, how these nations appear to be integrating immigrants, and their implementation of public policies that promote multiculturalism.

Historically, immigration has been an important contributor to economic and social life of developed nations. Immigration populated settler nations such as Australia and Canada and provided workers during periods of labour shortages in both settler and non-settler nations. Immigration also provides wage earners who preserve tax revenues during periods of low fertility rates. The major cities of Berlin, Brussels, Copenhagen, London, Oslo, Stockholm, Sydney, Toronto, and Vienna are now international cities, products of **globalization** and economically dependent on immigrants. These diverse cities are centres of arts, culture, education, and trade.

Debates exist regarding the purposes and goals of immigration. Immigration can be seen as primarily a means of filling employment gaps in sectors native workers either avoid or cannot fill due to low numbers. Immigration can also be seen through a different lens, as a path toward nation building through permanent settlement and family reunification. Finally, immigration can serve a humanitarian purpose, providing asylum to refugees seeking relief from war and conflict or natural disasters.

In the first economic view, immigrants should be accepted primarily to provide temporary and perhaps longer-term workers to remedy labour needs. Broadening the objectives of immigration beyond this rationale—particularly during times of fiscal imbalance and economic uncertainty—is seen as increasing the risk of national resources being drained by immigrants' use of social and other services. If not managed well, these adherents argue, immigration can reduce native workers' ability to find employment as newcomers take away jobs and do so at lower wages than native workers would accept.

Adherents to broader views of immigration point out there is sparse evidence for these arguments as immigration appears to have little effect upon employment opportunities and wages for natives. Newcomers, in their view, are less likely to be users of welfare and other services than natives. Instead there is stress upon the economic, social, and creative contributions that immigrants make to receiving nations. Supporting family reunification and safe haven to refugees are seen as actions consistent with the values and principles of the United Nations.

Despite these latter arguments, natives can come to hold anti-immigration views that lead to restrictive immigration policies that limit both immigration and family reunification and acceptance of asylum claimants. Anti-immigration policies can also create difficult living circumstances and adverse health outcomes for already arrived immigrants. These anti-immigration views can be nourished by natives experiencing economic and social insecurity associated with changing labour markets, economic globalization, and economic crises.

"Settler nations" of Australia and Canada historically provided greater settlement opportunities than European nations. Yet, in these latter nations where immigrants were primarily accepted for filling employment gaps, many immigrants choosing to remain in the host nation created integration challenges similar to those faced by settler nations. Issues of immigration as temporary employment and immigration as settlement continue to influence immigration policy and figure prominently in the national case studies that follow. The recent opening up of employment across member nations of the European Union (EU) has led to increases in both types of immigration among EU nations. There are tensions between these forms of immigration with implications for public policy.

Finally, immigration from non-EU nations constitutes an important issue for all developed nations. Many of these immigrants are fleeing war zones, ethnic-related conflicts, and economic turmoil, and in many cases all three. Many of these immigrants are of colour and members of groups with religious and ethnic traditions that are perceived as different from those of receiving nations. Where this is the case, anti-immigration political parties can gain support by fanning racist and xenophobic attitudes.

Recent History of Immigration

As the case studies will show, immigration policy in both the settler and non-settler nations in this volume has historically been restrictive, based on exclusion of particular national, racial, and ethnic groups. From Confederation in 1867 until the early 1970s, Canadian immigration policy favored those fitting the "British-French duality," that is, their cultural roots were British, American, and, to a lesser but still significant extent, Western European (Mallea & Young, 1984; Gogia & Slade, 2011). However, since the introduction of the points system in 1967 and the adoption in 1971 of a multiculturalism policy, immigration policy became less restrictive to promote "a high-immigration policy directed at nation building" and economic competitiveness by bringing in well-educated immigrants available for employment (Reitz, 2014).

It was during this mid- to late 20th-century period that this wave of Western "liberal humanitarianism"—the recognition of a moral obligation to construct an equitable and inclusive society—facilitated migrant mobility through an easing of immigration barriers based on ethnic discrimination (Shah, 2012). After the Second World War, the enactment of the British Nationality Act of 1948 gave citizens of Commonwealth nations greater access to the United Kingdom (Tomlinson, 2013). The Act coincided with nationality and citizenship acts in other Commonwealth countries. The political reasoning behind the UK Act was, however, that "immigrants would be assimilated into labour positions white workers did not want," consequently creating a new class of citizens potentially thought of as positioned beneath the working class (Tomlinson, 2013). These immigration reforms benefited developed nations and provided little for developing nations.

Canada's approach to immigration during the end of the 20th century was also aimed at strengthening domestic markets and business, filling labour shortages, and ensuring job creation (Jones, 2004). These economic considerations drove the immigration-related discourse of multiculturalism that emerged in Canada and other nations. Canada was the first nation to uphold the concept of multiculturalism as national public policy, the stated purpose of which was to promote "equitable participation of individuals and communities of all origins" (Canadian Multiculturalism Act, 1985). Later, the Immigration and Refugee Protection Act of 2001 enshrined values of family reunification and refugee protection into immigration policy (Jimenez & Crépeau, 2013). As a result, immigration increased from regions of the developing world. Canadian immigration became much more diverse through acceptance of immigrants from non-European nations.

However, in 2006, Canada's immigration policy shifted strongly toward a selective system, which, although largely racially and ethnically colour-blind, is primarily based on meeting the nation's economic needs (Gogia & Slade, 2011). The Conservative government (in power from 2006 to 2015 and replaced in November 2015 by a Liberal government) moved immigration policy away from one based on values of citizenship, family, and humanitarian concerns toward one solely concerned with meeting economic needs.

Family reunification was restricted and barriers to reduce the number of refugees entering the nation were erected. The Designated Country of Origins list of safe countries put into doubt the credibility of refugee claims from countries like Croatia, Hungary, the United States, etc. (Canadian Association of Refugee Lawyers, 2012). The restriction of various forms of immigration allowed the government to focus on entrepreneurial immigrants, a theme running through the nine case studies that follow.

Pathways to Immigration: The Canadian Scene

At the turn of the 21st century, Jones (2004) describes Canada's approach to immigration as inclusive, but primarily for those who are skilled and show entrepreneurial promise that benefits the knowledge-based economy. Immigration patterns into Canada have shifted from European nations toward the trans-Pacific region but also involve other global areas.

During the period 2010–13, China, India, and the Philippines contributed the most Canadian immigrants (see Figure 1.1) whereas the United States, the United Kingdom, and France were out of the top five. Visible minorities now make up more than 75 percent of new immigrants (Friesen, 2011). There are various streams of immigration in Canada: accepting refugees, temporary workers, and permanent residents upon entry. These are described below and find their counterparts in the other nations described in this volume.

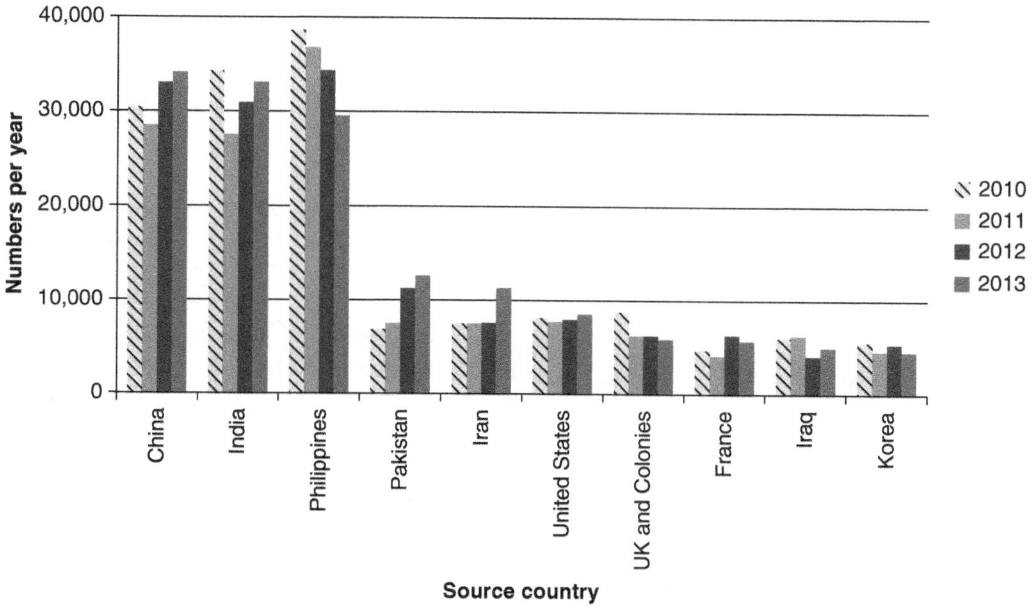

Figure 1.1: Permanent Residents in Canada by Top 10 Source Countries

Source: Government of Canada. (2015, April 23). *Facts and figures 2013—Immigration overview: Permanent residents.* Retrieved from http://www.cic.gc.ca/english/resources/statistics/facts2013/permanent/10.asp

Permanent Residency Immigration

Canada's economy-based immigration policy is what allowed Canada in 2012 to have the third highest immigrant employment rate among OECD nations (OECD, 2013b). The immigration system is primarily an economy-centric one as highlighted by its Express Entry approach, which favours skilled workers over others, including **asylum-seekers** (Mas, 2014).

This skill-based selection process was embodied in the now-defunct Canada Immigrant Investor Program (Marlow, 2014). It had few requirements and essentially was a method of buying citizenship. One needed business experience, a net worth of Can. $1.6 million, and to be ready to invest at least $800,000.

Another example of the skilled-based approach is the Express Entry program, which came into effect January 1, 2015. It is modelled after the Expression of Interest programs of Australia and New Zealand and grants entry to qualified immigrants for jobs for which there are no available Canadian workers (see Box 1.1). There is also a family reunification stream, which brings in close relatives of permanent residents in Canada. And finally, there is the class of asylum-seekers who are fleeing various forms of persecution. The Canadian Conservative government was heavily criticized in 2012 for restricting the intake of the asylum-seekers in its professed crackdown on false asylum claims and registrations. Despite their changes to the refugee system, the number of asylum-seekers registering and granted acceptance into Canada continues to rise (Keung, 2015).

Box 1.1: Express Entry Immigration Program to Launch in 2015

The Canadian Government plans to launch a new immigration system that would offer express entry to qualified immigrants for filling open jobs for which there are no available Canadian workers in 2015.

Named Express Entry—formerly referred to as Expression of Interest—this program would provide swifter entry into Canada, wherein the government and employers would select immigrants based on the skills and attributes that Canada needs. Canada's new immigration system would come into force from January 01, 2015. Under this system, prospective immigrants would apply to express their interest in coming to Canada by answering a series of questions about their professional skills, their education, languages spoken, etc.

The system would then match the skills of the prospective immigrants with the labour requirements identified by the provinces, the territories and employers. On finding a suitable match, the immigration authorities would offer Express Entry to a prospective immigrant who has applied via the:

- Federal Skilled Workers Program
- Federal Skilled Trades Program
- Canadian Experience Class Program or,
- Business Class Program

Immigration Minister Chris Alexander said that Canadian employers would be able to bring workers into Canada through the Express Entry system, with the long-term objective of making them stay behind in Canada. In a press conference, he said, "You can bring your labour market opinion, your job offer, to the Express Entry system and ensure that the person you need comes to Canada as an immigrant, not as a temporary foreign worker. Not as someone who is here with an uncertain future and likely to go back, but as a full immigrant to Canada."

Alexander said that prospective immigrants who apply via the Provincial Nominee Program could also benefit under this system as long as the concerned province and territory brought their program under the federal one. Immigration authorities would extend invitations to Express Entry candidates for applying for permanent residence if they have a valid job offer or a provincial or territorial nomination.

Other features of the Express Entry program include the fact that Canada would be able to select the best candidates, who would be able to achieve success in Canada, rather than just the next person in the queue. Immigration authorities would also have access to an improved Job Bank for matching Canadian employers with the most suitable Express Entry candidates.

The Government plans to invest $14 million over two years and $4.7 million thereafter, to ensure that Express Entry is a success.

Source: Immigration Canada. (2014). Express Entry Immigration Program to launch in 2015. Retrieved from http://www.immigration.ca/en/2014/152-canada-immigration-news-articles/2014/april/738-express-entry-immigration-program-to-launch-in-2015.html

The Canadian government's revamping of immigration policy regarding high-skilled immigrants also led to greater favorability for international students. The Canadian Experience Class (CEC) was enacted in 2008 and allows students and workers who have lived in Canada for a period of three years with one year of "skilled work experience in Canada" to apply for permanent residence (Government of Canada, 2013). The CEC currently holds the fastest-growing class of economic immigrants in Canada. This has led to an annual increase of 11.5 percent in international students in Canada at all levels from 2008 to the present (Tamburri, 2013). These various selection processes for prospective immigrants have affected the overall admittance process. It extends the skills-based criteria for most immigrants and disadvantages asylum-seeking immigrants with legitimate refugee protection claims (Laughland, 2014).

Temporary Workers

For many nations, immigrants are somewhat reluctantly accepted to meet labour shortages. Pathways to permanent residency and eventual citizenship are not assured. Issues of naturalization and settlement focus on these immigrants.

In Canada, this category of immigrants is recruited through Canada's Temporary Foreign Worker Program (TFWP) (Library of Parliament, 2014). The TFWP stream responds to labour shortages for jobs requiring lower levels of training and education. The TFWP consists of four categories of work permits: (1) higher-skilled work (i.e., managerial and professional work); (2) lower-skilled work (i.e., work requiring up to a high school diploma); (3) the primary agriculture stream; and (4) the Live-In Caregiver program (i.e., home care for children, the elderly, and those with disabilities). Each work permit is "subject to the requirement" of obtaining a positive Labour Market Impact Assessment (LMIA) (Library of Parliament, 2014). The LMIA is an application required by the federal government for employers to fill, justifying their need for hiring non-Canadians to fill the vacant jobs. Interestingly, these programs are coming under increased scrutiny as employers have used them to bring in employees at low pay even though many Canadians are available for such work.

Canada admitted 190,800 temporary foreign workers in 2011, an increase of 6.4 percent from 2010, and 98,400 foreign students in 2011, an increase of 3.3 percent over the previous year (OECD, 2013b). However, recent evidence of abuses to the temporary worker program caused the government to halt it (see Box 1.2). It is unclear how the newly elected Liberal government in Canada will reform this program.

Box 1.2: Abuses of the Temporary Worker Program in Canada

OTTAWA October 13, 2014—Prime Minister Stephen Harper, who has presided over a record increase in the use of temporary foreign labourers in Canada, has slammed the program because of "blatant" abuses and exploitation.

"I'm not saying all companies did this ... but we have seen very blatant examples of companies using this in ways that were not in the interest of Canadians," he told members of Vancouver's ethnic media.

The scathing critique was made last week. A recording of the meeting was provided this week to 24 Hours Vancouver.

Harper's criticism of the temporary foreign worker program prompted a sharp rebuke from Opposition leader Tom Mulcair. Mulcair's NDP and the labour movement have long had similar complaints about the program.

"Every single time I have raised these exact concerns with the Conservative government, the prime minister denied there were any problems with this program," Mulcair told *The Vancouver Sun*. "And now, during a secret meeting, we see him attempt to adopt NDP positions? If Stephen Harper is going to steal our ideas, he should at least do it in public.

"And, if he has truly changed his mind on temporary foreign workers, he should apologize to all those who have been hurt by this program."

The B.C. business community is one of the most aggressive users of the program, and labour groups and human rights advocates have criticized the provincial government for not adequately protecting the rights of those workers.

Harper sounded frustrated and even angry in the audio recording as he discussed how some Canadian companies and sectors have used temporary foreign workers.

He even echoed the NDP's argument that more emphasis should be placed on bringing in permanent residents who would have equal rights with Canadians, including the right to bargain collectively.

While the federal government has been conducting a review of the program, and has announced some changes, there has been no indication Ottawa plans to sharply reduce the intake of temporary migrants in favour of permanent residents.

Harper didn't name names, though he appeared to be referring to a number of high-profile instances of apparent program abuse. He told the ethnic media reporters that the temporary foreign worker program has "grown very dramatically" over the past 15 years as bureaucrats adapted to the private sector's requests.

"But what did we see?" Harper said. "We saw numerous examples of abuse of this program, outright abuse—companies importing workers for the sole purpose of paying less than the prevailing wage, companies importing workers for the purpose of permanently moving the jobs offshore to other countries, companies bringing in foreign workforces with the intention of never having them permanent, and moving the whole workforce back to another country at the end of the job."

While stressing that not all companies abuse the system, those that do are engaging in "blatant" violations, he said.

"I'm a big supporter of business, I'm a Conservative, I'm a market-oriented guy—but government was assisting these companies to work around the marketplace in a way that disadvantaged Canadian workers only for the sake of the bottom line profit."

Harper noted that "certainly" in some parts of Western Canada and particularly Alberta companies "absolutely" require temporary workers.

→

"But there must be plans for companies to transition to permanent workforces, and what I say is, if you really need temporary workers permanently then that means we need permanent workers who become Canadian and they have a right to stay here and they have a right to bargain with their employer and they have a right to be treated fairly and not just sent back to where they came from the first time they don't like something."

The federal government launched a review of the temporary foreign program after media reported in 2012 a number of controversial uses of the program, including one instance of Chinese-owned companies bringing in Chinese nationals to work in B.C. coal mines.

The number of temporary workers entering Canada has soared from 122,365 in 2005, the year before Harper became prime minister, to a record 213,573 in 2012. Combined with those still in Canada last year, the total reached 491,547, also a record.

B.C. takes a disproportionately large share of the temporary workers, with just under 50,000 arriving in 2012—or close to a quarter of the national total even though B.C. only has about 13 per cent of the national population.

A spokesman for Immigration Minister Chris Alexander said in December that the federal government's review looks at potential changes to "make sure it complements, and doesn't undercut, the recruitment of Canadian citizens and permanent residents ... while taking into account the needs of Canadian employers."

One [of] the changes the Harper government has already made is to reverse an earlier decision to allow companies to pay temporary foreign workers 15 per cent below prevailing rates in the regions where they were working.

Source: O'Neil, P. (2015, October 13). Stephen Harper takes aim at temporary foreign worker program. *Vancouver Sun*. Retrieved from http://tinyurl.com/p2n8pvc

Refugee Policy

Canada's adoption of the Multiple Borders Strategy and the United States–Canada Safe Third Country Agreement reflects its desire to deter asylum-seekers. These agreements disallow entrance from what are identified as "safe" nations such as the United States. While the United States entered into these agreements primarily to fortify its borders, Canada did so to deter asylum-seekers to Canada (Arbel & Brenner, 2013). The Canadian case study in Chapter 4 details how the Canadian government restricted asylum claims and access to health and social services by claimants.

Benefits of Immigration to Receiving Nations

Increasing economic globalization and associated immigration provide benefits to developed nations, although there is certainly debate about how these benefits are being distributed among segments of the population. Benefits stem from the added labour supply of migrants. Amidst global demographic trends of decreasing fertility rates (Figure 1.2), increasing life expectancy, and increasing numbers of seniors (Figure 1.3), the ability of the native working-age populations to sustain social and health programs in general and long-term care resources for the elderly in particular is a major concern. Immigration policy that seeks working-age immigrants is a policy response to these processes.

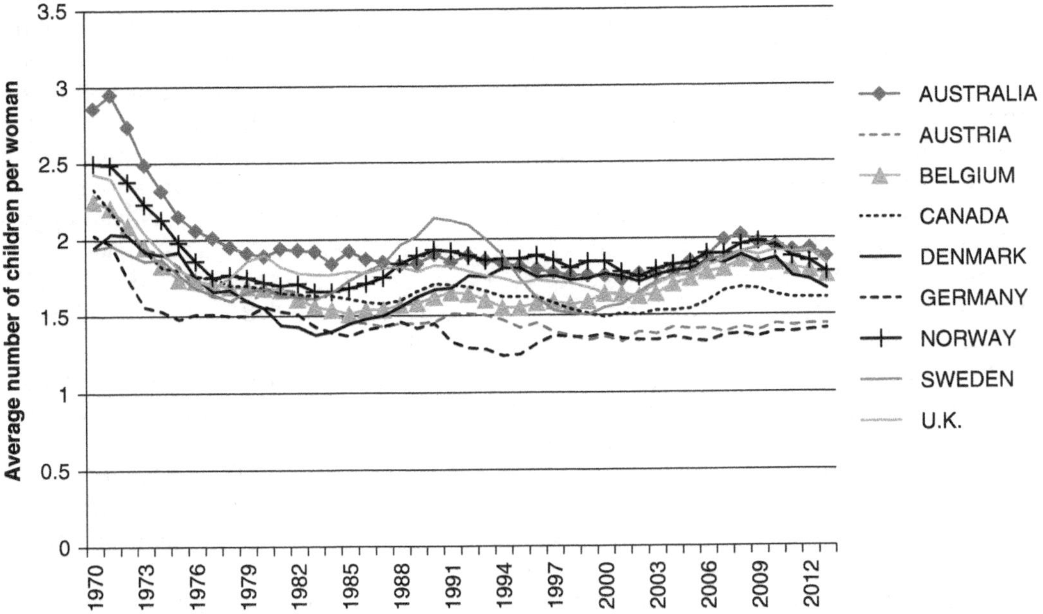

Figure 1.2: Fertility Rates as Measured by Average Number of Children Per Woman (1970–2013)

Source: https://data.oecd.org/pop/fertility-rates.htm#indicator-chart

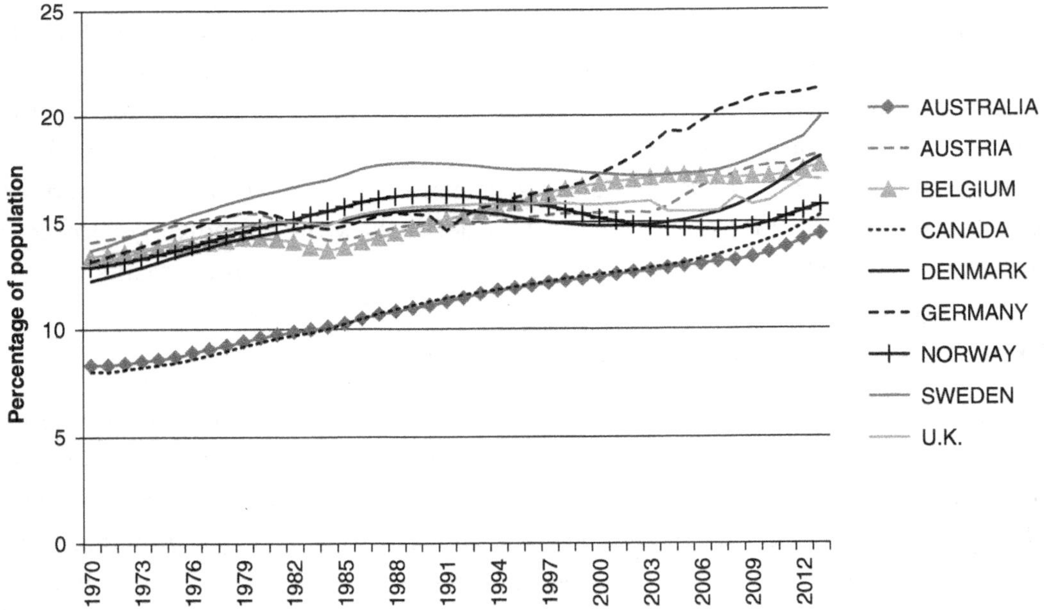

Figure 1.3: Share of the Population That Is Aged 65 and Over (1970–2013)

Source: https://data.oecd.org/pop/elderly-population.htm#indicator-chart

Policy changes have weakened barriers to economic immigration while at the same time providing opportunities for financial investment. Foreign direct investment (FDI) is the quintessential modern product of financial investment in a globalized era. FDI is described by the Organisation for Economic Co-operation and Development (OECD) as foreign-driven, privately managed "cross-border investment" for the purpose of expanding business environments (OECD, 2013a). In some cases, FDI can strengthen multilateral economic relationships. Increased foreign investment provides much-needed employment and stimulates innovation in the agriculture, engineering, and health care sectors.

Developed nations also benefit from international flows of direct foreign investment, which boosts exports and innovation (Buckley, Viechnicki, & Wigmore, 2015). This signifies the developed nations' dependency on foreign entities and ingenuity for sustainable economic development. At the macro-level then, immigration policy can align with both the interests of the global community and local economy in mind. As such, it can shape a nation's geopolitical standing and the economic and social development of both the sending country (i.e., through remittances) (World Bank Group, 2014) and the receiving country (i.e., immigrants contributing to the economy) (BAMF, 2005).

The advantages of taking in highly educated immigrants have shaped immigration policy in many nations, including Canada. For the receiving country, the advantage lies in the fact that in an age dominated by knowledge-sharing, the economy's growth depends on having a pool of human resources possessing these skills. Immigration policy fosters the sharing and flow of communication, finances, and labour among the global community. It mobilizes networks of skilled immigrants from developing nations. For developed nations, it is a chance to adopt the most skilled and talented individuals to bolster its sectors for the immediate future.

There may be benefits for the sending, developing nation in that benefits accrue through remittance-sending (the second largest source of development finance after direct foreign investment) (Waldinger, 2013). But warnings have been issued as to the costs to these developing nations' futures by developed nations poaching their most educated and talented. The loss of highly skilled and educated individuals is especially concerning considering the various economic, health, and social challenges developing nations face (Dwyer, 2007; Oberoi & Lin, 2006).

Benefits to Immigrants

The income gap between developed and developing countries is immense and creates strong incentive for people to move to the developed world. Dutt and Mukhopadhyay (2009) explain that the inequality between nations is a product of the ideological bias of the major global economic regulators. These regulators and institutions include the International Monetary Fund (IMF), the World Bank, and the World Trade Organization (WTO). The authors explain that "the basic principles governing the institutions are neoliberal in nature, and are known as the 'Washington Consensus.'"

According to Dutt and Mukhopadhyay (2009), there are fundamental consequences for less-developed nations that follow from the adoption of the Washington Consensus. First, the IMF requires developing nations to adopt forms of monetary austerity (i.e., tax increases and public spending cuts) and to devalue its currency against the dollar. This leads to a decline in purchasing power, and thus a decline in the country's standard of living. These processes drive emigration from these nations.

Second, the World Bank requires that nation's adopt deregulation practices when it comes to international trade. This encourages trade openness but also strips developing countries of leverage at the bargaining table and potentially leads to reduced revenue capacity. This puts domestic industries at a financial risk due to heightened foreign competition.

Lastly, the WTO's **Trade-Related Aspects of Intellectual Property Rights (TRIPS)** and **Trade-Related Investment Measures (TRIMs)** agreements require nations to loosen domestic "performance requirement" regulations that would inhibit the capacity of multinational corporations to fully maximize from FDI in the host country (Dutt & Mukhopadhyay, 2009). The agreements require WTO members to acknowledge and adopt intellectual property (IP) laws and policies that harmonize with "those of the major industrial countries, and imposes barriers on technology transfers." With the endless amount of patented technology, this acts as a barrier for local businesses and entrepreneurs to build upon newly patented technology to foster innovation desperately needed in developing nations. In some ways, these global economic institutions perpetuate the income gap between countries. They enforce economic policies that largely benefit economically well-off nations. This is a significant motivator for moving from a developing to a developed nation.

The benefit of immigration, of course, varies among individual immigrants. Consider an immigrant from Nigeria who, as an engineer, can make upwards of double his or her previous earnings in Canada. But also consider that this immigrant may be unable to practise his or her profession and become unemployed or underemployed. In the former preferred case, that of practising the profession, the impact for a receiving nation is also—relative to the economic impact at the national level for the sending nation—primarily positive (Scheja, 2011).

Lived Experiences of Immigrants and the Social Determinants of Health

In this volume, a primary concern is with the lived experiences of immigrants and how these experiences come to shape their health. Lived experiences are shaped by what are termed the social determinants of health, defined as the economic and social conditions that shape the health of individuals, communities, and jurisdictions as a whole (Mikkonen & Raphael, 2010). Canadian researchers have outlined 16 of these:

Indigenous status, disability status, early life, education, employment and working conditions, food security, gender, geography, health services, housing, immigration status, income and income distribution, race, social exclusion, social safety net, and unemployment and employment insecurity (Raphael, 2016). Social determinants such as Indigenous status, disability status, gender, race, and of course immigrant status can be thought of as social locations that do not by themselves lead to differing health outcomes, but interact with societal conditions to create particular health outcomes.

The emphasis upon societal conditions as determinants of health contrasts with the traditional health sciences and public health focus upon biomedical and behavioural risk factors. Since a social determinants of health approach sees the mainsprings of health as being how a society organizes and distributes economic and social resources, it directs attention to economic and social policies as a means of improving it. It also requires consideration of the political, economic, and social forces that shape their distribution among the population.

Five themes have emerged in the literature with implications for understanding immigrant experiences and their impact on health. These are:

- empirical evidence concerning the importance of the social determinants of health;
- mechanisms and pathways by which social determinants influence health;
- the importance of a life-course perspective;
- the role public policy plays in determining the quality of the social determinants of health; and
- the importance of political ideology in shaping state and societal receptivity to these concepts.

Theme 1: Empirical Evidence of the Importance of the Social Determinants of Health

Social determinants of health are about the quantity and quality of a variety of resources that a society makes available to its members. Important considerations include both their *quality* and their *distribution* among the population (Graham, 2007). These resources include, but are not limited to, conditions of childhood, access to income, education and literacy, food, housing, employment, working conditions, and health and social services.

Concern with the social determinants of health is not new. It has been known since the mid-19th century that living conditions are the primary determinants of health (Engels, 1845/1987; Virchow, 1848/1985). And since then hundreds of studies have demonstrated that the material and social circumstances to which people are exposed to in their homes, workplaces, and communities are far more important to their health (measured either subjectively or objectively) than so-called "lifestyle choices" such as using tobacco or excessive alcohol consumption, eating fruits and vegetables, or partaking in physical activity. This relationship between living and working conditions and health outcomes applies across developed and developing nations (Gordon, 2010; Nettleton, 1997; Tesh, 1990).

Much of the current volume is concerned with the present state and distribution of these and how they shape the health outcomes of immigrants. Particularly important is the question of how recent policy decisions are either improving or weakening the quality and distribution of these social determinants of health.

Theme 2: Mechanisms and Pathways That Influence Health

The British *Black* and *Health Divide* reports considered two primary mechanisms for understanding the sources of health inequalities: "cultural/behavioural" and "materialist/structuralist" and decided upon the latter as providing the most useful explanation (Townsend, Davidson, & Whitehead, 1992). The cultural/behavioural explanation sees individuals' behavioural choices (tobacco and alcohol use, diet, physical activity) as responsible for developing and dying from various diseases. The materialist/structuralist explanation sees the material conditions under which people live—access to the amenities of life, working conditions, quality of available food and housing, for example—as shaping health. Evidence and expert opinion sides with the materialist/structuralist explanation (Bartley, 2003; Graham, 2007; Raphael, 2016; World Health Organization, 2008). One widely cited model outlines how the organization of society shapes social determinants of health and health itself and lends itself to a materialist/structuralist explanation (Brunner & Marmot, 2006) (Figure 1.4).

In this model, social structure is a catch-all for the organization of society and how it distributes access to resources. Three pathways link social structure with health status. The first is a direct link between social structure, material factors, and health status. Material factors include not only positive exposures to health-enhancing environments or situations and exposures to negative health environments, but also threatening events or situations. In the second pathway, social structure shapes social and work environments to create psychological and behavioural responses that—operating through brain mechanisms—determine health status. The third pathway sees these same environments creating behavioural coping responses that directly impair bodily organs, thereby determining health. Early life, genes, and culture contribute to these processes at all levels of the model.

Theme 3: The Importance of a Life-Course Perspective

Economic and social conditions—the social determinants of health—under which individuals live their lives have a cumulative effect upon the probability of

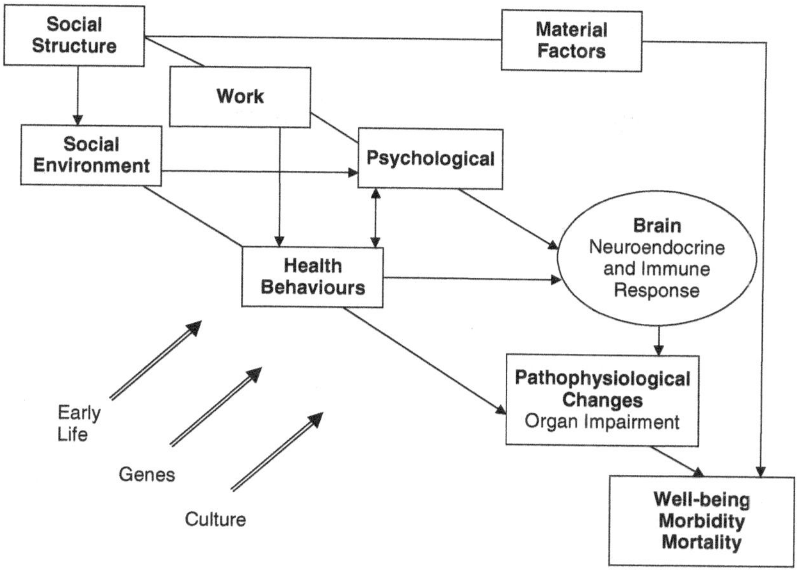

Figure 1.4: Pathways by Which the Social Determinants of Health Shape Health

The model links social structure to health and disease via material, psychosocial, and behavioural pathways. Genetics, early life, and cultural factors are further important influences upon population health.

Source: Brunner, E., & Marmot, M. G. (2006). Social organization, stress, and health. In M. G. Marmot & R. G. Wilkinson (Eds.), *Social determinants of health* (p. 9). Oxford: Oxford University Press.

developing any number of diseases. This has been repeatedly demonstrated in longitudinal studies that follow individuals across their lives (Blane, 1999) and most clearly demonstrated in the case of heart disease and stroke and adult-onset diabetes (Raphael et al., 2003; Raphael & Farrell, 2002).

Adopting a life-course perspective directs attention to how the range of social determinants of health operates at every level of development—early childhood, childhood, adolescence, and adulthood—to influence health immediately, as well as provide the basis for health or illness during later stages of the life course. Of course these circumstances are shaped and influenced by public policy.

Theme 4: The Role of Public Policy and Policy Environments

Health-threatening social determinants of health come about as a result of public policy decisions. Early life, for example, is shaped by availability of sufficient material resources to assure adequate educational opportunities, food, and housing, among others. Much of this has to do with parents' employment security, wages, and the quality of their working conditions. These factors are shaped by public policy decisions. These are not issues that usually come under individual control. A policy-oriented approach places such findings within a broader policy context and is a prime component of the case studies of immigration that follow.

Theme 5: Politics, Political Ideology, and the Social Determinants of Health

Why certain nations take up this information and apply it in the formulation of public policy while others do not can be explained in part through differing forms of the welfare state. Three distinct types of welfare states among wealthy nations have been identified: Social Democratic (e.g., Denmark, Norway and Sweden), Liberal (e.g., Australia, Canada, and the United Kingdom), and Conservative (e.g., Austria, Belgium, and Germany) (Esping-Andersen, 1990, 1999).

Social Democratic nations provide a wide range of universal and generous benefits and are proactive in developing policies that support workers, families, and gender equity. Liberal nations spend considerably less on supports and services. They offer modest universal transfers and social-insurance plans. Benefits are provided primarily through means-tested assistance, and thus are provided only to the least well-off. Health indicators such as life expectancy, premature years of life lost prior to age 70, teenage pregnancy rates, and infant mortality and low birth weight rates are better for the Social Democratic than for Liberal nations (Innocenti Research Centre, 2007, 2013; Navarro, 2004).

The questions of course are: Are these equitable distributions of the social determinants of health made available to immigrants in these differing nations? Do the more equitable distributions seen in the Social Democratic states and to a slightly lesser extent in the Conservative states accrue to immigrants as they do to the general population?

Relationship to Form of the Welfare State

As an introduction to the presentation provided in the following chapter, we present key aspects of modern welfare states and how these features may affect the immigration experience. Modern nations differ profoundly in how their economic and political systems distribute resources across the population. There are also variations in approaches toward immigration policy across these developed Western nations. A typology of Anglo-Saxon, Continental, and Nordic models has proven useful for understanding differences in public policy-making, the lived experiences of members of these societies, and health outcomes. These differences may be important to the immigrant experience.

The Anglo-Saxon Liberal Welfare State

The first model of governance is the Anglo-Saxon Liberal welfare state and includes Australia, Canada, and the United Kingdom. This model features lack of overall regulation of the economy and the labour market in particular. In conjunction with this, these nations provide modest public spending initiatives that support economic and social security despite having the capability to do so. Benefits are targeted to the least well-off and are very modest such that those not engaged in the labour market live well below the poverty line. Even full-time employment is no guarantee of not living in poverty. Their approach to social spending is marred by a "certain degree of welfare erosion" (Esping-Andersen, 1996). Not surprisingly, Canada's immigration policy centres on the needs of the economy and particularly "satisfying employers' demands for cheap, pliable labour" (Triadafilopoulos, 2010, p. 169).

The Continental Conservative Welfare State

Policies devised in Continental Conservative nations are characterized as "status oriented" and hierarchical (Rothstein & Stolle, 2003). In Continental Conservative nations, the provision of social policies is generally based on one's ability to contribute to the social insurance system through employment (Rothstein & Stolle, 2003). Austria, Belgium, and Germany are such nations. This approach sees regulation and coordination of the economy and the labour market and provision of economic and social security through rather well-developed social insurance schemes. However, these nations adhere to a "national traditions perspective" (Thomas, 2006) guided by nationalist and traditional norms and values such that conceptions of nationhood are particularist and assimilationist (Brubaker, 1990). Conservative nations are commonly perceived as the least oriented toward ideals of multiculturalism, given their reliance on *jus sanguinis*, or attribution of national citizenship on the basis of descent.

The Nordic Social Democratic Welfare State

Social Democratic nations include Denmark, Norway, and Sweden. The Nordic social model is characterized as attributing extensive social right to citizens and undertaking large public sector initiatives to support those rights. The Nordic model supports a "system of public childcare and parental leave, as well as [having an] extended gender equality legislation" (Siim, 2013, p. 617). Social rights equality is given high regard, and is evident in the redistributive nature of the welfare state ingrained in its politics and policies. Despite this general thrust there appear to be wide differences in approaches to immigration policy. Brochmann and Hagelund (2011, p. 18) argue that Danish policy had a "strong focus on integration through the labour market mixed in with a rhetoric that took a far more negative approach to cultural difference than in either Sweden or Norway." An essential goal of this volume is to examine how these differing forms of the welfare state approach immigration and whether any consistent differences among these welfare state forms are apparent.

What Is Already Known: An Overview of National Approaches toward Immigration

In preparation for the case studies that follow in Part 2, we consider existing analyses of how our nine nations differ in integrating immigrants and implementing the concept of multiculturalism. These indices provide guideposts for reading the nine case studies that follow. The case studies, however, extend beyond these broad strokes to examine the specific public policies nations implement regarding immigration and how these shape the lived experiences and social determinants of immigrants' health.

Migrant Integration

The Migrant Integration Policy Index (MIPEX) is produced as part of the Outcomes for Policy Change Project, which is co-financed by the European Fund for the Integration of Third-Country Nationals (Barcelona Centre for International Affairs, 2015). The Migrant Integration Policy Index is a tool for comparing and improving integration policy toward immigrants. Examining 31 countries in Europe and North America, it uses 148 policy indicators to provide a multi-dimensional picture of immigrants' "[o]pportunities to participate in society by assessing governments' commitment to integration."

Its policy analysis describes whether immigrants are provided with opportunities for integration through legislation in seven key areas. In the following list, we provide the components of the MIPEX and present (in italics) guiding questions for the reading of the case studies that follow.

The components of the MIPEX are:

1. Labour market mobility: Policies that provide access to employment
   How do immigrants' employment and unemployment levels compare to those native to the receiving nations? Are immigrants concentrated in lower-level occupations?
2. Family reunion: Policies that support reunification of families
   How easy is it for permanent residents to relocate family members to the host nation? Are there restrictions placed on such reunification?
3. Education: Policies that allow migrants access to education for careers, skills, and qualifications

Are immigrants able to apply their credentials and skills they acquired in their home nations? How well do their children do in school as compared to natives in the new nation?

4. Political participation: Policies that encourage participation
Are immigrants provided with opportunities to have their voices heard? Do political parties take note of their concerns?
5. Long-term residence: Policies that grant security for residents
How difficult is it to attain long-term residence?
6. Access to nationality: Policies that facilitate naturalization
How difficult is it for immigrants to acquire citizenship?
7. Anti-discrimination: Policies that protect all residents from many forms of discrimination
To what extent has racism been recognized as a barrier to immigrants' integration into their new nations? To what extent have nations implemented and enforced anti-discrimination laws?

Table 1.1 provides overall ranking (n=31) and ranking for these seven areas for the nations examined in this volume. Of particular note is the very high overall ranking of Sweden and Canada and the rather low ranking for Austria. There is also variation in rankings within nations. Canada, for example, does very well in the areas of anti-discrimination, family reunion, education, and access to nationality, less so in long-term residence and political participation. Austria scores poorly in all areas. Of note is the lack of an obvious pattern of MIPEX score and form of the welfare state, in that for overall ranking, nations from each of the welfare state clusters do rather well (top one-third) (Sweden, Canada, Australia, Belgium, and Norway) or average (mid one-third) (United Kingdom, Germany, Denmark) or poorly (Austria). We will return to these issues in Part 3 following the case studies.

Multiculturalism Index

Queen's University in Canada carries out analyses of multiculturalism policies in developed nations (Multiculturalism Policies in Contemporary Democracies, 2015). Their index consists of eight dimensions:

1. Constitutional, legislative, or parliamentary affirmation of multiculturalism at the central and/or regional and municipal levels and the existence of a government ministry, secretariat, or advisory board to implement this policy in consultation with ethnic communities

Table 1.1: Nation Scores and (Ranks) on Components and Total Scores of the MIPEX 2015 Integration Index (n=38)

	Liberal			Conservative			Social Democratic		
	Australia	Canada	United Kingdom	Austria	Belgium	Germany	Denmark	Norway	Sweden
Labour market mobility	58 (19)	81 (5)	56 (21)	64 (16)	64 (16)	86 (4)	79 (7)	90 (3)	98 (1)
Family reunion	67 (11)	79 (4)	33 (38)	50 (31)	72 (6)	57 (24)	42 (35)	63 (18)	78 (5)
Education	76 (2)	65 (4)	57 (11)	47 (16)	61 (7)	47 (16)	49 (14)	65 (4)	77 (1)
Health	67 (4)	49 (18)	64 (7)	63 (8)	53 (12)	43 (22)	53 (12)	67 (4)	62 (9)
Political participation	64 (9)	48 (20)	51 (19)	38 (21)	57 (14)	63 (11)	64 (9)	82 (1)	71 (7)
Long-term residence	54 (25)	62 (16)	51 (31)	57 (22)	85 (1)	60 (19)	74 (3)	70 (6)	79 (2)
Access to nationality	69 (5)	67 (8)	60 (13)	26 (34)	69 (5)	72 (3)	58 (15)	52 (18)	73 (2)
Anti-discrimination	74 (13)	92 (1)	85 (5)	57 (23)	78 (9)	58 (22)	50 (27)	59 (21)	85 (5)
Overall score (shaded slightly favourable; unshaded halfway favourable	66 (8)	68 (6)	57 (15)	50 (20)	67 (7)	61 (10)	59 (13)	69 (4)	78 (1)

Notes: Dark shaded: favourable (>80); medium shaded: slightly favourable (60–79); unshaded: halfway favourable (41–59); light shaded: slightly unfavourable (21–40)

Source: Adapted from MIPEX Integration Policy Index. (2015). Results infograph. Retrieved from http://www.mipex.eu/download-pdf#/add-selection

To what extent has national acceptance or rejection of the concept of multiculturalism impacted upon immigrants' lived experiences and health outcomes?

2. The adoption of multiculturalism in school curriculum
To what extent have schools adapted to the needs of immigrants and their children? Has the concept of multiculturalism been integrated into the school curriculum, therefore facilitating the integration of immigrants?
3. The inclusion of ethnic representation/sensitivity in the mandate of public media or media licensing
To what extent has the society been sensitive to the needs of ethnic and racial groups and publicizing their issues and concerns?
4. Exemptions from dress codes (either by statute or court cases)
Has there been an explicit recognition of the need to accommodate specific cultural clothing practices?
5. Allowing dual citizenship
Are citizenship processes overly restrictive, forcing immigrants to give up prior citizenships?
6. The funding of ethnic group organizations or activities
To what extent has the society recognized the need to support immigrant agencies and organizations through specific targeted funding arrangements?
7. The funding of bilingual education or mother-tongue instruction
Is there recognition of the need to support continuance of cultural heritage through education and language instruction?
8. Affirmative action for disadvantaged immigrant groups
In light of findings of lower employment and higher unemployment levels of immigrants, is there recognition of the need for affirmative action for these disadvantaged groups?

Table 1.2 provides details for the nations included in this volume. The Liberal Anglo-Saxon nations of Australia and Canada and Social Democratic Sweden score especially high. The United Kingdom and Belgium also score high while Norway and Germany score lower. Austria and Denmark score especially low.

Were we to assume that these two sets of indicators provide indicators predicting immigrants' living and working conditions that shape health, we would expect the following:

- Immigrants to Sweden and Canada do very well.
- Immigrants to Australia, Belgium, Germany, Norway, and the United Kingdom fall in the mid-range.
- Immigrants to Austria and Denmark do less well.

Table 1.2: Nation Scores on the Multiculturalism Policy Index (Potential Range: 0–8)

	Liberal			Conservative			Social Democratic		
	Australia	Canada	United Kingdom	Austria	Belgium	Germany	Denmark	Norway	Sweden
Affirmation									
School curriculum									
Media									
Exemptions									
Dual citizenship									
Funding ethnic groups									
Bilingual education									
Affirmative action									
Total score	**8**	**7.5**	5.5	*1.5*	5.5	*2.5*	*0*	3.5	**7**

Notes: Component scores: Dark = Yes (1); Shaded = Partial (.5); Unshaded = No (0).

Total scores: Strong (>6.0); Moderate (3.0–5.5); Weak (<3.0)

Source: Multiculturalism Policies in Contemporary Democracies. (2015). *Multiculturalism policies for immigrant minorities, summary scores, 1980, 2000, 2010*. Kingston, ON: Author. Retrieved from http://www.queensu.ca/mcp/immigrant-minorities/results

However, these hypotheses must be placed within the broader issue of how forms of the welfare state provide economic and social security such that it would be predicted the following:

- Immigrants to Sweden, Norway, and Denmark do very well.
- Immigrants to Austria, Belgium, and Germany fall in the mid-range.
- Immigrants to Australia, Canada, and the United Kingdom do less well.

Table 1.3 summarizes these differing sets of hypotheses.

Table 1.3: Differential Hypotheses Concerning the Situation of Immigrants in Each Nation Based on Their MIPEX and Multiculturalism Scores vs. Their Form of the Welfare State

	MIPEX and Multiculturalism Policy	Form of Welfare State
Good	Sweden and Canada	Sweden, Norway, and Denmark
Mid-range	Australia, Belgium, Germany, Norway, and the United Kingdom	Austria, Belgium, and Germany
Poor	Austria and Denmark	Australia, Canada, and the United Kingdom

The Syrian Refugee Crisis of 2015 and the Welfare State Typology

The Syrian civil war, which began in 2011 amidst other uprisings against dictatorial regimes in the surrounding regions, produced the most widely covered and unified refugee crisis of recent memory. The civil war has claimed the lives of over 200,000 Syrians and displaced over 11 million Syrians (*The Economist*, 2015), forcing many to flee to nearby Middle Eastern nations such as Lebanon with over 1 million Syrian refugees in that country, and Jordan with over 600,000.

For Syrians hoping for a better life in Europe, Turkey has been their first destination due to its geographical proximity to Syria. As of 2015, Turkey hosts the most Syrian refugees with well over 2 million (UNHCR, n.d.). To alleviate the pressures these neighbouring countries face, Canada's politically centrist Liberal government announced its resettlement plan to select and screen 25,000 Syrian refugees and provide housing over the course of 2016. In 2015, more than 160,000 asylum seekers came to Sweden. This led to a change in policy and an act was passed in 2016 restricting the possibility of asylum seekers receiving permanent residence (Swedish Migration Agency, 2016). The goal is that of the politically right-centre U.S. Democrat-led government—the U.S. federal government pledges to accommodate 10,000 Syrians—which is to exercise its responsibility to protect by alleviating the plight of millions of displaced Syrians, and to reduce the burden of the migrant crisis on European allies.

Germany's leadership in Europe to register well over 950,000 refugees as of 2015, and its call for European Union (EU) member states to apply the Union's Schengen Agreement—an open-door policy agreed upon by the 26 EU member states allowing for unfettered flow of goods and people—to the Syrian refugee crisis is an example of Germany's pivot away from its conservative-nationalist citizenship typology. The context of the Syrian refugee crisis is important to relate to the larger discussion of immigration and migrant experiences. It would appear to be conventional wisdom that the policy approaches the nations continue to choose in reaction to the crisis would be dictated by their welfare state regime disposition. This may or may not be the case. Prime Minister Merkel is now backtracking on these pledges (Karnitschnig & Eder, 2015). It is unclear as to whether leaders of Western countries will feel they have a moral obligation due to popular belief that the West's actions in the Middle East over the decades have led to the crisis.

Conclusion

This chapter has set the foundation and context appropriate for further detailed discussion of what Canadian and other immigration policies could look like in the future. As briefly touched on, the newly elected Liberal government of Canada has the opportunity in the coming decade to use the Syrian refugee crisis to shape and define what it means to ease boundaries for reasons beyond economics, at least in the short term. Our introduction of the welfare state typologies has set the framework for understanding why it is that certain countries devise the policies that they do in relation to immigration. We also introduced the concept of the social determinants of health and discussed some indicators upon which our immigrant-receiving nations have been rated.

Chapter 2 provides an overview of the concept of the welfare state and how variations in the welfare state among our nations should be related to both integration of immigrants into their respective nations as well as their exposures to health-promoting and health-threatening living and working conditions. It considers how these social determinants of health are shaped by public policy in a wide range of areas and how the nations in this volume differ in such public policy.

Critical Thinking Questions

1. What are some of the main factors that are responsible for developed nations taking in immigrants from both the developed and the developing world?
2. What do you think are some potential causes of abuses in temporary worker programs such as the Canadian one described in this chapter?

3. Based on what you read, how important do you think the form of the welfare state is in determining immigrants' living and working conditions?
4. How important do you think racism is in explaining how immigrants of colour are faring in countries such as Canada?
5. How important do you think multiculturalism is in shaping the experiences of immigrants from non-Western nations?

Glossary

Asylum-seekers are people who have fled their country of origin due to social or political oppression and arrive in neighbouring countries, typically industrialized countries, in the hopes of applying for protection as refugees.

Developed nations are typically recognized as those with relatively advanced, diverse, and free economies with high living standards, high educational attainment levels, and high income per capita levels.

Globalization is the process by which numerous nations—particularly their various economic, social, and governmental policies—conform to that of the dominant culture of free trade. This is achieved through the gradual easing of geographical borders (whether physical or virtual) leading to increased international trade and the flow of capital.

Trade-Related Aspects of Intellectual Property Rights (TRIPS) were produced out of the Uruguay international trade rounds of the General Agreement of Trades and Tariffs (GATT), which spanned from 1986 to 1994. GATT established the World Trade Organization (WTO) in 1995. TRIPS is a binding international treaty agreed upon by all members of the WTO. TRIPS served as a recognition that protecting intellectual property rights, knowledge, and information was a major international trade policy issue. TRIPS is a highly comprehensive agreement that sets standards and enforcement parameters.

Trade-Related Investment Measures (TRIMs) was produced out of the Uruguay international trade rounds of the General Agreement of Trades and Tariffs (GATT), which spanned from 1986 to 1994. TRIMs establishes rules that prohibit barriers to foreign investment within host WTO countries. Like the TRIPS agreement, TRIMS is a binding agreement that overrides all domestic trade policies and influences the shaping of future trade policies, and must conform to trade-related investment measures set out by GATT.

Recommended Readings

Chaudhuri, S., & Mukhopadhyay, U. (2014). *Foreign direct investment in developing countries: A theoretical evaluation*. New Delhi, India: Springer.

Foreign direct investment (FDI) is a major driver of economic growth from which both developed and developing nations thrive. This volume helps the reader to understand the importance of FDI in allowing developing nations to catch up technologically, and also discusses the positive and adverse socio-economic impacts stemming from FDI.

Gogia, N., & Slade, B. (2011). *About Canada: Immigration.* Winnipeg: Fernwood Publishing.

Many recent immigrants to Canada are highly trained and educated professionals, and yet few of them, contrary to the myth, find work in their area of expertise. This book provides a history of immigration in Canada and identifies key areas of concern.

Goldring, L., & Landolt, P. (2013). *Producing and negotiating non-citizenship: Precarious legal status in Canada.* Toronto: University of Toronto Press.

Producing and Negotiating Non-citizenship is a detailed discussion on what citizenship in Canada means and what it has become in reality. It goes beyond focusing simply on immigrant status, and investigates further into the social predicament of migrant workers, students, and refugee claimants in Canada.

Hirst, P., Thompson, G., & Bromley, S. (2009). *Globalization in question* (3rd ed.). Cambridge: Polity Press.

Economic globalization, which is the free flow of capital and information between borders, gave rise to international capitalism. *Globalization in Question* provides the reader the opportunity to delve deeper into the very governance model that maintains the global economy, and details the emergence of the two latest 21st-century economic powers—India and China—products of economic globalization and capitalism.

Hollifield, J., Martin, P., & Orrenius, P. (2014). *Controlling immigration: A global perspective* (3rd ed.). Stanford, CA: Stanford University Press.

In the third edition of *Controlling Immigration,* the reader is guided through a comparative study between *nations of immigrants* (e.g., Canada), *countries of immigration* (e.g., France), and *latecomers to immigration* (e.g., Spain). Their different approaches to dealing with immigration and how their migration policy goals and outcomes diverge are identified.

Related Websites

Barcelona Centre for International Affairs, MIPEX—http://www.mipex.eu/

The Migrant Integration Policy Index (MIPEX) is a unique tool that measures policies to integrate migrants in all EU member states, Australia, Canada, Iceland, Japan, South Korea, New Zealand, Norway, Switzerland, Turkey, and the United States.

International Migration Research Centre (IMRC)—http://imrc.ca/
IMRC at Wilfrid Laurier University in Waterloo, Ontario, is a research centre whose mandate is to serve as a focal point for debate, research, policy analysis, and proposal development related to international migration and mobility at the global, national, and regional scale.

Multiculturalism Policy Index (MPI)— http://www.queensu.ca/mcp/home
Based in Queen's University in Kingston, Ontario, MPI is a scholarly research project that monitors the evolution of multiculturalism policies in 21 Western democracies. The project provides information about multiculturalism policies to contribute to comparative research and the understanding of state-minority relations.

OECD International Migration—http://www.oecd.org/migration/
This website provides a wealth of reports, analyses, and data on immigration to OECD nations that include flows and labour market outcomes of immigrants.

Office of the United Nations High Commissioner for Refugees—http://www.unhcr.org/pages/4a16aa156.html
The Office of the UNHCR was established on December 14, 1950, by the United Nations General Assembly and is mandated to lead and coordinate international action to protect refugees and resolve refugee problems worldwide. Its primary purpose is to safeguard the rights and well-being of refugees.

References

Arbel, E., & Brenner, A. (2013, November). *Bordering on failure: Canada–US border policy and the politics of refugee exclusion.* Cambridge, MA: Harvard Immigration and Refugee Law Clinical Program. Retrieved from https://harvardimmigrationclinic.files.wordpress.com/2013/11/bordering-on-failure-harvard-immigration-and-refugee-law-clinical-program1.pdf

Barcelona Centre for International Affairs. (2015). *The Migrant Integration Policy Index.* Barcelona: Author. Retrieved from http://www.mipex.eu/

Bartley, M. (2003). *Understanding health inequalities.* Oxford: Polity Press.

Blane, D. (1999). The life course, the social gradiant, and health. In M. G. Marmot & R. G. Wilkinson (Eds.), *Social determinants of health* (pp. 64–80). Oxford: Oxford University Press.

Brochmann, G., & Hagelund, A. (2011). Migrants in the Scandinavian welfare state. *Nordic Journal of Migration Research, 1*(1), 13–n/a.

Brubaker, W. R. (1990). Immigration, citizenship, and the nation-state in France and Germany: A comparative historical analysis. *International Sociology, 5*(4), 379–407. Retrieved from http://www.sscnet.ucla.edu/soc/faculty/brubaker/Publications/05_Immigration_Citizenship_and_the_Nation-State_in_France_and_Germany.pdf

Brunner, E., & Marmot, M. G. (2006). Social organization, stress, and health. In M. G. Marmot & R. G. Wilkinson (Eds.), *Social determinants of health* (2nd ed.). Oxford: Oxford University Press.

Buckley, P., Viechnicki, P., & Wigmore, L. (2015). *Mapping the effects of international investment flows.* Westlake, TX: Deloitte University Press. Retrieved from http://dupress.com/articles/effects-of-foreign-direct-investment-us-infographic/

Canadian Association of Refugee Lawyers. (2012, December 14). *Designated country of origin scheme is arbitrary, unfair, and unconstitutional.* Press release. Retrieved from http://www.carl-acaadr.ca/our-work/issues/DCO#Press Release DCO

Canadian Multiculturalism Act, Revised Statutes of Canada (1985, C. 24). Retrieved from http://laws-lois.justice.gc.ca/eng/acts/C-18.7/page-1.html

Dutt, A. K., & Mukhopadhyay, K. (2009). International institutions, globalization, and the inequality among nations. *Progress in Development Studies, 9*(4), 323–37.

Dwyer, J. (2007). What's wrong with the global migration of health care professionals? Individual rights and international justice. *The Hastings Center Report, 37*(5), 36–43.

The Economist. (2015, September 30). *Syria's drained population* [Editorial]. Retrieved from http://www.economist.com/blogs/graphicdetail/2015/09/daily-chart-18

Engels, F. (1845/1987). *The condition of the working class in England.* New York: Penguin.

Esping-Andersen, G. (1990). *The three worlds of welfare capitalism.* Princeton, NJ: Princeton University Press.

Esping-Andersen, G. (Ed.). (1996). *Welfare states in transition: National adaptations in global -economies.* Newbury Park, CA: Sage.

Esping-Andersen, G. (1999). *Social foundations of post-industrial economies.* New York: Oxford University Press.

Federal Office for Migration and Refugees Migration and Integration Research Department [BAMF]. (2005, October). *The impact of immigration on Germany's society.* Retrieved from http://ec.europa.eu/dgs/home-affairs/what-we-do/networks/european_migration_network/reports/docs/emn-studies/illegally-resident/de-finalstudy-eng_en.pdf

Friesen, J. (2011, March 18). The Philippines now Canada's top source of immigrants. *The Globe and Mail.* Retrieved from http://www.theglobeandmail.com/news/national/the-philippines-now-canadas-top-source-of-immigrants/article573133/

Gogia, N., & Slade, B. (2011). *About Canada: Immigration.* Winnipeg: Fernwood Publishing.

Gordon, D. (2010). Health inequalities in developing nations. *Social Alternatives, 29*(2), 28–33.

Government of Canada. (2013, January 2). *Canadian experience class.* Retrieved from http://www.cic.gc.ca/english/immigrate/cec/

Graham, H. (2007). *Unequal lives: Health and socioeconomic inequalities.* New York: Open University Press.

Innocenti Research Centre. (2007). *An overview of child well-being in rich countries.* Florence: Innocenti Research Centre.

Innocenti Research Centre. (2013). *Child well-being in rich countries: A comparative overview.* Florence: Innocenti Research Centre.

Jimenez, E., & Crépeau, F. (2013). *The Immigration and Refugee Protection Act.* Ottawa: Policy Horizons Canada. Retrieved from http://www.horizons.gc.ca/eng/content/feature-columnist-%E2%80%93-immigration-and-refugee-protection-act

Jones, S. (2004). Canada and the globalized immigrant. *The American Behavioral Scientist, 47*(10), 1263–77.

Karnitschnig, M., & Eder, F (2015, September 15). Why Merkel changed her mind. *Politico.* Retrieved from www.politico.eu/article/merkel-changed-her-mind-migration-crisis-eu-schengen-border-control/

Keung, N. (2015, March 1). Canada's refugee acceptance rate up despite asylum restrictions. *Toronto Star.* Retrieved from http://www.thestar.com/news/immigration/2015/03/01/canadas-refugee-acceptance-rate-up-despite-asylum-restrictions.html

Laughland, O. (2014, March 31). Legal aid denied to asylum-seekers who arrive through unauthorised channels. *The Guardian.* Retrieved from http://www.theguardian.com/world/2014/mar/31/legal-aid-denied-asylum-seekers-arrive-boat

Library of Parliament. (2014, December). *Background papers: Temporary foreign workers* by S. Elgersma. Retrieved from http://www.parl.gc.ca/Content/LOP/ResearchPublications/2014-79-e.pdf

Mallea, J., & Young, J. C. (1984). *Cultural diversity and Canadian education: Issues and innovations.* Don Mills, ON: Oxford University Press.

Marlow, I. (2014, February 11). Investor road to Canada hits a dead end with immigrant program's closing. *The Globe and Mail.* Retrieved from http://www.theglobeandmail.com/news/politics/investor-road-to-canada-hits-a-dead-end-with-immigrant-programs-closure/article16821623/

Mas, S. (2014, April 22). Skilled immigrants to be offered "express entry" to Canada in 2015. *CBC News.* Retrieved from http://www.cbc.ca/news/politics/skilled-immigrants-to-be-offered-express-entry-to-canada-in-2015-1.2617961=

Mikkonen, J., & Raphael, D. (2010). *Social determinants of health: The Canadian facts.* Retrieved from http://thecanadianfacts.org

MIPEX Integration Policy Index. (2015). Retrieved from http://www.mipex.eu/download-pdf#/add-selection

Multiculturalism Policies in Contemporary Democracies. (2015). *Multiculturalism policies for immigrant minorities, summary scores, 1980, 2000, 2010.* Kingston, ON: Author. Retrieved from http://www.queensu.ca/mcp/immigrant-minorities/results

Navarro, V. (Ed.). (2004). *The political and social contexts of health.* Amityville, NY: Baywood Press.

Nettleton, S. (1997). Surveillance, health promotion, and the formation of a risk identity. In M. Sidell, L. Jones, J. Katz, & A. Peberdy (Eds.), *Debates and dilemmas in promoting health* (pp. 314–24). London: Open University Press.

Oberoi, S. S., & Lin, V. (2006). Brain drain of doctors from southern Africa: Brain gain for Australia. *Australian Health Review, 30*(1), 25–33.

OECD. (2013a). *Foreign direct investment.* Retrieved from http://www.oecd-ilibrary.org/sites/factbook-2013-en/04/02/01/index.html?itemId=/content/chapter/factbook-2013-34-en

OECD. (2013b). *International migration outlook 2013.* Paris: Author. http://dx.doi.org/10.1787/migr_outlook-2013-en

Raphael, D. (Ed.). (2016). *Social Determinants of Health: Canadian Perspectives* (3rd ed.). Toronto: Canadian Scholars' Press Inc.

Raphael, D., Anstice, S., Raine, K., McGannon, K., Rizvi, S., & Yu, V. (2003). The social determinants of the incidence and management of Type 2 Diabetes Mellitus: Are we prepared to rethink our questions and redirect our research activities? *Leadership in Health Services, 16*, 10–20.

Raphael, D., & Farrell, E. S. (2002). Beyond medicine and lifestyle: Addressing the societal determinants of cardiovascular disease in North America. *Leadership in Health Services, 15*(4), 1–5.

Reitz, J. G. (2014). *Controlling immigration: A global perspective* (3rd ed.). J. F. Hollifield, P. L. Martin, & P. M. Orrenius (Eds.). Stanford, CA: Stanford University Press.

Rothstein, B., & Stolle, D. (2003). Social capital, impartiality, and the welfare state: An institutional approach. In M. Hooghe & D. Stolle (Eds.), *Generating Social Capital: Civil Society and Institutions in Comparative Perspective*, (pp. 191–210). New York: Palgrave Macmillan.

Scheja, E. (2011, February 28). *How does migration shape economic and social development?* [Editorial]. Retrieved from http://blogs.worldbank.org/peoplemove/how-does-migration-shape-economic-and-social-development

Shah, N. (2012). *Stranger intimacy: Contesting race, sexuality, and the law in the North American West.* Oakland: University of California Press.

Siim, B. (2013). Gender, diversity, and migration—challenges to Nordic welfare, gender politics, and research. *Equality, Diversity and Inclusion: An International Journal, 32*(6), 615–28.

Swedish Migration Agency. (2016). Retrieved from http://migrationsverket.se

Tamburri, R. (2013, March 13). Changes to immigration rules are a boon to international student recruitment. *University Affairs.* Retrieved from http://www.universityaffairs.ca/changes-to-immigration-rules-are-a-boon-to-international-student_recruitment.aspx

Tesh, S. (1990). *Hidden arguments: Political ideology and disease prevention policy.* New Brunswick, NJ: Rutgers University Press.

Thomas, E. R. (2006). Immigration and changing definitions of national citizenship in France, Germany, and Britain. *French Politics, 4*(3), 237–65.

Tomlinson, S. (2013). Immigration, immigration, immigration. *Renewal: A Journal of Labour Politics, 21*(4), 66–73.

Townsend, P., Davidson, N., & Whitehead, M. (Eds.). (1992). *Inequalities in health: The Black Report and the health divide.* New York: Penguin.

Triadafilopoulos, T. (2010). Global norms, domestic institutions, and the transformation of immigration policy in Canada and the US. *Review of International Studies, 36*(1), 169–93.

UNHCR. (n.d.). *Syria regional refugee response.* Retrieved from http://data.unhcr.org/syrianrefugees/regional.php

Virchow, R. (1848/1985). Report on the typhus epidemic in Upper Silesia. In L. J. Rather (Ed.), *Collected essays by Rudolph Virchow on public health and epidemiology* (Vol. 1, pp. 205–319). Canton, MA: Science History Publications.

Waldinger, R. (2013). Immigrant transnationalism. *Current Sociology, 61*(5–6), 756.

World Bank Group. (2014, April 11). *Remittances to stay robust, despite deportations of migrant workers* [Infographic]. Retrieved from http://go.worldbank.org/KOOTCMQ2Q0

World Health Organization. (2008). *Closing the gap in a generation: Health equity through action on the social determinants of health.* Geneva: World Health Organization.

CHAPTER 2

The Political Economy of the Immigration Experience

Dennis Raphael

Chapter Objectives

This chapter outlines key concepts from a political economy approach that can illuminate the immigrant experience. The specific objectives of this chapter are:

- to outline key components of a political economy approach;
- to identify key aspects of Social Democratic, Conservative, and Liberal welfare states;
- to identify various factors that may influence the immigration experience in modern nations; and
- to identify key issues that may interact with the form of the welfare state to influence immigrants' lived experiences and the social determinants of health.

Introduction

In this chapter various hypotheses related to how differing nations have fared in meeting the challenges of immigration are outlined. The Anglo-Saxon nations with their adoption of the concept of multiculturalism appear to present a particularly positive approach to immigration issues as the concept refers to the extent to which a society takes measures to respond, value, and support the cultural and ethnic diversity of a population. This has become especially important as recent immigration patterns in developed nations involve accepting those of ethnic, racial, and religious identities that are different than those of the current population. However, the Anglo-Saxon nations are also Liberal **welfare states** where minimal attempt is made to manage the economy in the service of promoting equitable distributions of economic and social resources. Their primary organizing principle of liberty leaves these nations open to their market economies, creating the social and economic inequalities that lead to health inequalities (Saint-Arnaud & Bernard, 2003). These issues complicate integration of immigrants into the economic and social lives of societies and lead to living and working conditions that threaten health. These adverse conditions can also be heightened by exclusionary processes that include racism. In this case it is important that nations develop and implement anti-discrimination policies that respond to such processes.

The concept of multiculturalism has been more problematic in Continental nations. Yet these nations, as Conservative welfare states, make far greater efforts to manage the economy in the service of providing their members with economic and social security. Continental nations' primary organizing principle of solidarity can, if associated with ethnocentrism, lead to greater challenges in integrating immigrants, many of them of colour, into their predominantly white societies (Saint-Arnaud & Bernard, 2003). On the other hand, the concern with maintaining social solidarity and cohesion can contribute to immigrants experiencing living and working conditions that support health. Traditional concepts of solidarity and cohesion, if seen as relevant only to native-born populations, can also encourage racism toward perceived outsiders, highlighting the importance of implementing anti-discrimination policies.

Finally, the Scandinavian nations are Social Democratic welfare states whose primary organizing principle is that of equity (Saint-Arnaud & Bernard, 2003). Their long tradition of promoting equity and reducing inequalities in the economic and social spheres appears to make them best situated to respond to the challenges of immigration. They work hard to improve residents' living and working conditions, and an important question is whether this concern includes the situations experienced by recent immigrants. Like the Conservative nations, these predominantly white societies face issues in integrating immigrants from non-white nations into their societies. How these Scandinavian and other nations address these challenges is explored in the particular case studies that follow in this volume.

A key question underlying analysis of these differing approaches is the extent to which the generally greater economic and social security offered by the Social Democratic and Conservative welfare states toward their population also applies to immigrants. Nations differ in the extent to which immigrants are able to access the resources normally made available to members of that society. This issue was the focus of work by Sainsbury on immigrants' rights in settlement nations (Sainsbury, 2012). Interestingly, based on her analysis of the rights and opportunities afforded immigrants, she classified Denmark, Germany, and the United Kingdom as having a "restrictive" approach to incorporating immigrants whereby immigrants are prevented from accessing the entitlements of residency in a nation, such as universal benefits and social assistance as well as citizenship.

Sweden, France, and the United States were classified as having an "inclusionary" approach where such restrictions are less common. Australia, Austria, Belgium, and Canada were not included in her analysis.[1] In the following section I outline the key features of the differing forms of welfare states to provide a context against which the experiences—specifically with regard to living and working conditions—of immigrants can be considered.

The Political Economy of the Welfare State

A **political economy** model of society is concerned with how political ideology and power and influence operate through economic and political systems to create public policy that distributes material and social resources (Bryant, 2009). Central to this perspective is the idea that politics and economics are intrinsically related and this dynamic shapes public policy development. As applied to understanding health and the determinants of health, a political economy approach draws a direct link between these societal structures and processes; the making of public policy that shapes the social determinants of health; and the health of the overall population and specific groups classified according to social class, gender, age, and race among other characteristics (Coburn, 2010).

One of the most prominent political economy approaches is that of Esping-Andersen, who identifies three forms of modern welfare states: the Social Democratic, Conservative, and Liberal, to which some theorists have added a fourth, the Latin (Esping-Andersen, 1990, 1999, 2009).[2] These nations differ profoundly in how they address issues of resource distribution and provision of economic and social security to their residents. These approaches should impact on the experiences of immigrants, most specifically in the form of the living and working conditions they and their families experience. How these experiences translate into health outcomes is an important focus of this volume.

Three Forms of the Welfare State

The Social Democratic welfare state is associated with the Scandinavian nations of Denmark, Norway, and Sweden. It emphasizes universal welfare rights and provides generous benefits and entitlements on a generally universal basis. Their political and social history is one of political dominance by Social Democratic parties of the left, a result of political organization initiated by industrial workers and farmers that later came to include the middle class (Esping-Andersen, 1985). The labour sector is strong and has significant influence upon the making of public policy. Through universal provision of a range of benefits, these states have historically secured the loyalties of a significant proportion of the population (Esping-Andersen, 1990, 1999). The strong influence of organized labour contributes to the stability of the Social Democratic welfare state by moderating the influence of the business sector on public policy-making. A key feature of these states is the provision of universal benefits and supports across the life course.

The Conservative welfare state is associated with the Continental nations of Austria, Belgium, and Germany. It also offers generous benefits but does so through social insurance plans based on employment status (Esping-Andersen, 1990, 1999). Emphasis is on supporting the primary wage earner, usually male. Their political and social history is one of political dominance by Christian Democratic parties where traditional Church concerns with maintaining the family merges with conservative upholding of status differences among citizens. These tendencies sometimes manifest in corporatist approaches (e.g., Germany) where business interests are major influences, or statist approaches (e.g., Belgium) where the state plays an important role in providing citizen security (Pontusson, 2005). The labour sector is weaker than in the Social Democratic welfare state, but co-operation between labour and business is such that most workers are covered by collective agreements.

The Liberal welfare state is associated with the Anglo-Saxon nations of Australia, Canada, and the United Kingdom. It provides modest benefits and the state usually provides assistance only when the market fails to meet citizens' most basic needs (Esping-Andersen, 1990, 1999). The labour sector is weak, and corporate and business interests dominate the making of public policy. Their political and social history is one of dominance by business interests such that the population gives its loyalty to the employment marketplace rather than to the state as the source of economic and social security. Liberal welfare states are the least developed in terms of provision of citizen economic and social security. A key feature is their use of means-tested benefits targeted to the least well-off.

While there has been extensive debate about the value of the **worlds of welfare** typology (Arts & Gelissen, 2002; Bambra, 2007), recent analyses provide strong evidence of the distinctive aspects of the Social Democratic and Liberal welfare states with issues being raised as to placement of some of the nations identified as Conservative welfare states (Saint-Arnaud & Bernard, 2003). Most typologies agree with the placement of nations into the welfare types used in this volume. Figure 2.1 provides a summary of the key features of the different welfare states.

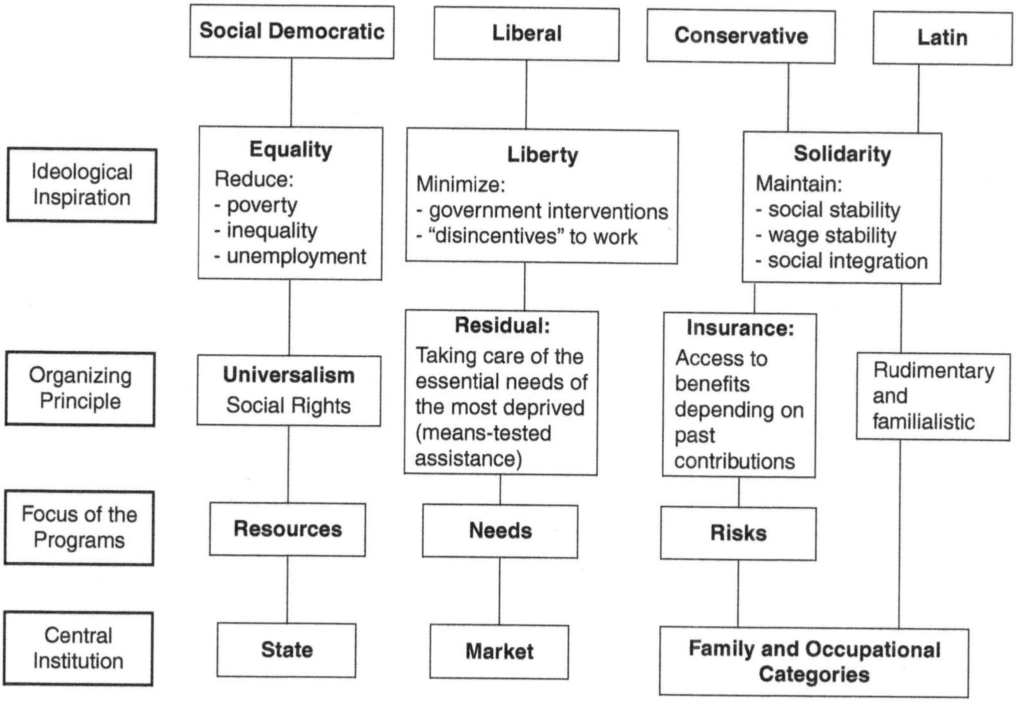

Figure 2.1: Ideological Variations in Forms of the Welfare State

Source: Saint-Arnaud, S., & Bernard, P. (2003). Convergence or resilience? A hierarchical cluster analysis of the welfare regimes in advanced countries. *Current Sociology, 51*(5), 499–527, Figure 2, 503.

Historical Traditions

An important contribution of Esping-Andersen's analysis is the identification of the historical traditions that led to—and maintain—these divergent approaches to provision of economic and social resources (Esping-Andersen, 1990). The Liberal welfare state is really the Anglo-Saxon welfare state in that it consists of the United Kingdom and its former colonies. As such it celebrates the concept of individualism, which was associated with the rise of unbridled capitalism during the Industrial Revolution.

The alternative welfare states—both Conservative and Social Democratic—arose in reaction to this governance approach by ruling and working-class circles. The Conservative welfare state grew out of a deep-rooted suspicion during the late 19th century by ruling circles of the polarizing and atomizing aspects of the Liberal approach. It has been most successful among the Western nations of Continental Europe.

The Social Democratic welfare state arose during the early 20th century through working-class opposition to societal dominance by the business sector and achieved success in the Scandinavian nations. These historical developments not only shaped their economic and political systems but the accompanying ideologies held by citizens that value equitable distribution of economic and social resources. These equitable distributions of resources are now recognized as profoundly important to health.

I have written about threats to the Social Democratic welfare state by the corrosive effects of neo-liberal retrenchment associated with economic globalization and increased immigration (Raphael, 2014b). I argue that tensions associated with such processes can fan racist and xenophobic tendencies that translate into weakened support for welfare state policies and Social Democratic parties of the left. Retrenchment reduces programs and benefits for the population in general and the vulnerable in particular. The reduction in economic and social security can lead to growing health inequalities.

The example I used was of how Sweden had undergone changes in welfare state profile associated with governance of centre-right governments while Norway had done the opposite. Since that time elections have strengthened the Left in Sweden, while in Norway the Right has been strengthened. How these changes play out in the experiences and health outcomes of immigrants will be examined in Part 2 of this volume.

In the Liberal welfare state Canada, it is argued that economic globalization and neo-liberal reorganization of the economy leads to the stoking of racism and discrimination, creating an "Economic Apartheid" by which immigrants of colour have come to occupy the most vulnerable economic and social positions in society (Galabuzi, 2005). These living conditions are likely to lead to adverse health outcomes among this group and evidence supports this hypothesis. Similar arguments have been made for the situation in Australia and the United Kingdom.

The situation in the Conservative nations is less clear. Much has been published in the popular literature about anti-immigration sentiment in Austria, Belgium, and Germany. The case studies presented in Part 2 examine how these issues may be playing out in terms of the living and working conditions immigrants experience and their health outcomes.

Relevance for Understanding the Immigrant Experience in Modern Welfare States

Clear affinities exist between key concepts in the immigration literature and the structures and processes associated with these different forms of the welfare state. There are both empirical and normative aspects to these affinities. Health researchers point to evidence of higher quality and more equitable distribution of the social determinants as well as better health outcomes and lower magnitude of health inequalities among those living in Social Democratic nations (Raphael, 2013a, 2013b). The opposite is the case for those living in Liberal nations, where greater inequities in the distribution of the social determinants of health and worse health outcomes are apparent. The Conservative nations occupy the mid-range with regard to the equitable distribution of the social determinants of health and health indicators. A key question is the extent to which these general findings concerning the distribution of the social determinants of health and health outcomes are applied to the living and working experiences as well as health outcomes of immigrants across these welfare states.

There are also normative arguments that suggest that the societal structures and processes associated with the Social Democratic welfare state should provide more favourable living and working conditions and health outcomes for immigrants. These include the Social Democratic nations' generally greater, and the Liberal nations' generally lesser, adherence to principles outlined in United Nations human rights declarations and covenants. These include issues related to the right to health, the right to health promoting living and working conditions, and the freedom from numerous forms of discrimination (Rioux, 2010).

As another example of these normative affinities, consider how member nations of the Organisation for Economic Co-operation and Development (OECD) perform on indicators of "Social Justice." This analysis applied an index consisting of indicators of poverty levels, inclusive education systems, labour market access, social cohesion, health, and intergenerational justice (Schraad-Tischler, 2011). For overall scores, the top four nations among the 31 examined include the Scandinavian Social Democratic nations in this volume: Norway ranked 2nd; Denmark, 3rd; and Sweden, 4th. The Anglo-Saxon Liberal welfare states scored lower: Canada ranked 9th; the United Kingdom, 15th; and Australia, 21st. The Continental Conservative nations' scores were mid-range in the OECD distribution: Austria ranked 13th; Germany, 14th; and Belgium, 16th.

In terms of the social determinants of health, Social Democratic welfare states, with their commitments to providing economic and social security across the lifespan, generally provide higher quality and more equitable distribution of the social determinants of health (Raphael, 2013b). These include income and wealth; employment security and working conditions; food and housing security; provision of comprehensive health and social services; and support for early childhood development, gender equity, and people with disabilities (Olsen, 2002, 2008, 2010) (details provided below).

In addition it appears—while empirical evidence is only beginning to be gathered—that the structures and processes associated with the Social Democratic welfare state minimize the vulnerabilities of those occupying specific social locations such as Indigenous descent, people of colour, unemployment, illness, disability, and working class than is the case for the Liberal welfare state (Raphael, 2012). These findings would suggest better living and working conditions for immigrants in these nations.

In terms of health outcomes, infant mortality rates as well as life expectancy favour the Social Democratic and Conservative welfare state over the Liberal (Organisation for Economic Co-operation and Development, 2013). In terms of health inequalities, evidence is less clear, but use of absolute indicators of health inequalities usually favours the Social Democratic welfare state (Bambra, 2011). The quality and distribution of the social determinants of health are clearly superior among the Social Democratic welfare states than Liberal welfare states (Raphael, 2013b). The question remains: Do these general findings apply to the health outcomes of immigrants to these differing welfare states?

Key Features of Welfare States Relevant to the Immigrants' Living and Working Conditions

In this section I consider key components of Esping-Andersen's analysis of welfare states and consider how these might impact immigrants' experience of living and working conditions. Specifically, how do welfare states address issues of stratification, decommodification, and the role of the state, the market, and the family in the distribution of economic and social resources (Esping-Andersen, 1990, 1999)? These distributions can either assure or deny immigrants' economic and social security in their new home. These concepts provide the context for understanding the sources of health outcomes.

Stratification

The Social Democratic welfare state strives to reduce social **stratification** and its effects (Esping-Andersen, 1990, 1999). Social Democratic nations have been explicitly concerned with reducing health inequalities by recognizing social inequalities as their source (Fosse, 2011). The strong redistributive effect of public policy in the Social Democratic welfare state is its key feature. Also important are its greater guarantees of employment through provision of employment security and job training and retraining when employment is lost (Raphael, 2011). Spending on active labour policy is much higher in Social Democratic than Liberal welfare states (OECD, 2011). As will be shown, income is most equitably distributed in the Social Democratic welfare state, and the least so in the Liberal.

Stratification is important to understanding the lived experiences of immigrants and how they might translate into health inequalities (Grabb, 2007). First, stratification is related to inequality in exposures to many social determinants of health. Differences in income and wealth are of special importance (McMullin & Davies, 2010). This is especially the case in Liberal nations since, as shown below, it is in these Liberal nations where more resources are commodified and need to be purchased. In addition to income and wealth differences, stratification is associated with employment insecurity and working conditions, likelihood of experiencing food and housing insecurity, and access to health and social services, all issues related to the immigrant experience (Jackson, 2009; Tremblay, 2009).

Interestingly, Social Democratic nations strive to reduce stratification through redistribution of economic resources at the same time it makes available a variety of important social determinants of health (Raphael, 2012). This is achieved through state provision of universal benefits and supports such as child care, education, employment training, family benefits, housing supplements, pensions, and comprehensive health care services. Conservative nations also fare better in these efforts compared to Liberal nations, but are not at the level seen in the Social Democratic nations (Raphael, 2013b). The main conclusion is that Social Democratic, Conservative, and Liberal welfare states represent divergent approaches to economic and social provision. In essence, extent of stratification and decommodification (see below) go hand in hand.

In addition to affecting the social determinants of health, stratification is related to the power and ability of those so stratified to influence public policy (Bambra, Fox, & Scott-Samuel, 2005; Raphael, 2014a). This is a particularly important issue with regard to the immigration experience where immigrants may lack the power to shape public policy. In terms of the established sectors of society, those at the top of the stratification ladder have more influence on elected representatives and the making of public policy (Langille, 2009).

This is especially the case in Liberal nations, where the corporate sector has worked hard to see implementation of public policies that weaken labour legislation, lower taxes on corporations and higher income earners, and reduce program spending related to the social determinants of health. In relation to the concerns of the present volume, an important question is: How much power and influence do immigrants have in influencing the public policies that shape their living and working conditions?

Decommodification

Decommodification allows for a decent quality of life independent of involvement in the paid employment market (what Esping-Andersen calls the cash nexus) (Esping-Andersen, 1990, 1999). Most measures of decommodification are focused on replacement income associated with retirement, sickness and disability, and unemployment. Using these measures, Social Democratic states are more decommodified than Conservative and Liberal welfare states (Bambra, 2005).

In addition, there are many other important aspects of day-to-day life that can be commodified or decommodified. These include child care, employment training, post-secondary education, dental care, as well as health and social services available to citizens across the lifespan as a benefit of citizenship. The availability of these supports certainly impacts the lives of those receiving them. How do differences in commodification and decommodification influence the living and working conditions that immigrants experience?

Menahem (2010) created an index of decommodified security that is relevant to this question. Menahem assessed how OECD member nations provided three types of income: (1) replacement income for the risks of old age, unemployment, sickness, and disability, plus survivors' pensions; (2) reimbursements and benefits in kind: costs of health care, family allowances, housing benefits; and (3) allowances and benefits in kind paid as a part of measures to combat social exclusion (income support, etc.). These scores are weighted to reflect poverty levels. The three Scandinavian nations examined in this volume are among the top five decommodifying nations (of 24): Sweden, ranked 1st; Denmark, 3rd; and Norway, 4th. The Anglo-Saxon nations score rather lower: Canada ranked 16th; the United Kingdom, 17th; and Australia, 19th. The Conservative nations in this volume fall near the top or middle: Germany ranked 7th; Austria, 9th; and Belgium, 12th. Do these general commodifying and decommodifying aspects of welfare states also impact the living and working conditions of immigrants, thereby affecting their health?

Role of the State, the Family, and the Market

Welfare states differ in state responsibility for economic and social security across the life course (Esping-Andersen, 1990, 1999). Such a role should be especially important to a vulnerable population such as immigrants. These differences manifest in the amount of public spending in support of the population in general and to vulnerable groups such as immigrants in particular. Indicators of such state support are provided in the following sections.

Public Policy Indicators of the Provision of the Social Determinants of Health

Nations' public policies influence the quality and distribution of the social determinants of health in a variety of ways. Public policies establish the environment within which employees negotiate their wages and benefits. Collective agreements provide means by which wages and benefits are negotiated by employees as a group rather than individuals being left to do so on their own. Swank provides evidence that such agreements are important determinants of unemployment and sickness benefits, and pension levels (Swank, 2005).

Another means by which the social determinants of health are provided involve welfare state interventions in the form of collecting revenues through taxation and fees, which are then used to provide universal or targeted benefits to the population. In essence, these transfers offer direct support to individuals as well as provide social infrastructure. Bryant points out that these benefits include: cash payments and in-kind benefits to families, public pensions, training as part of active labour market policies, and provision of early childhood, education, recreational and public health care spending (Bryant, 2010). Together these public indicators provide an overall measure of the extent of the welfare state. Elsewhere, I have provided detailed analyses of how OECD nations differ in their provision of the social determinants of health (Raphael, 2013a, 2013b). In the following sections, I summarize key findings in relation to the nations examined in this volume.

Collective Employment Agreement Coverage and Union Density

Collective employment agreements are common in the Social Democratic and Conservative welfare states. Virtually all employees are covered by collective agreements in the Conservative nations of Austria (99 percent) and Belgium (96 percent) with almost two-thirds coverage in Germany (63 percent). Figures for the Social Democratic nations are Sweden, 92 percent; Denmark, 82 percent; and Norway, 72 percent. For the Liberal nations, figures are lower: Australia, 60 percent; the United Kingdom, 35 percent; and Canada, 32 percent.

An important difference among welfare states is the source of these collective agreements. In the Social Democratic nations, union density is very high: Sweden, 68 percent; Denmark, 68 percent; and Norway, 53 percent. In the Conservative nations, figures are lower: Belgium, 52 percent; Austria, 29 percent; and Germany, 19 percent. In the Liberal nations there is also low union density: Canada, 27 percent; the United Kingdom, 27 percent; and Australia, 19 percent.

The high collective bargaining coverage of the Social Democratic welfare states is therefore associated with very high union density. Labour unions have traditionally had strong influence upon public policy in these states (Esping-Andersen, 1985). Conservative welfare states have relatively low union density, but the high collective agreement rates is a result of employers belonging to associations that negotiate collective contracts that a large majority of employers voluntarily apply to their workforce (OECD, 2004). There is what is termed an administrative extension of agreements to cover all employers in a given sector (OECD, 2004).

In Liberal political economies, such agreements do not exist. As a result, there are low proportions of their workforces operating under collective agreements. There are also low rates of union membership. Two sources of greater economic security—collective agreements and union membership—are therefore less available to immigrants in Liberal welfare states.

Overall Public Expenditure

This indicator provides a rough measure of welfare state support of individuals. Social Democratic (Sweden, 27 percent; Denmark, 25 percent; and Norway, 21 percent) and Conservative nations (Austria, 26 percent; Belgium, 26 percent; and Germany, 25 percent) collect a greater proportion of national wealth (GDP) and allocate it in the form of public expenditures than Liberal nations (the United Kingdom, 21 percent; Canada, 17 percent; and Australia, 16 percent). It is important to note that the Liberal slightly outlier, the United Kingdom, is now governed by a coalition that has implemented cuts in most government departments of between 25 percent and 40 percent (Helm, Doward, & Asthana, 2010). These differences in spending have implications for the living and working conditions of immigrants as they indicate general societal willingness to provide economic and social security. Whether these general differences affect the experiences of immigrants is a purpose of this inquiry.

Income Inequality and Poverty

There are higher levels of income inequality in the Liberal as compared to the other states (OECD, 2016a). The Gini coefficents of income inequality for the Liberal nations are: the United Kingdom, .35; Canada, .32; and Australia, .33. The Social Democratic nations show the lowest—Denmark, .25; Sweden, .27; and Norway, .25—with the Conservative nations midway: Austria, .28; Belgium, .27; and Germany, .29. There is a similar picture for extent of relative poverty. Here the Social Democratic nations lead with lower levels: Denmark, 5 percent; Sweden, 9 percent; and Norway, 8 percent; and the Liberal the highest: the United Kingdom, 10 percent; Australia, 14 percent; Canada, 12 percent; with two Conservative nations at mid levels: Austria, 10 percent; Belgium, 10 percent; and Germany at 8 percent.

Active Labour Policy

Active labour policy consists of a variety of programs that nations use to eradicate high and persistent unemployment and reduce low pay and poverty among the working-age population (OECD, 2016b). These may include formal classroom training, on-the-job training programs, subsidies to private-sector employers, job-search assistance, training programs for youth, and direct job creation for adult workers.

Denmark is a high OECD spender at 1.82 percent of GDP. Sweden spends 1.35 percent and Norway, 0.5 percent. Belgium is a mid-range spender at .72 percent, as are Germany (0.67) and Austria (0.76). Australia, Canada, and the United Kingdom are very low spenders with each at only .23 percent of GDP allocated for such programs.

Spending on Early Child Development

The quality of early child development is shaped by the economic and social resources available to parents and the extent to which governments provide a range of supports and benefits to families and their children (OECD, 2016c). Denmark, 2.0 percent; Sweden, 1.6 percent; Norway, 1.2 percent; and Belgium .7 percent are the highest spenders, while Germany, .5 percent; Austria, .5 percent; and Canada, .2 percent are the lowest. Australia allocates .6 percent and the United Kingdom allocates 1.1 percent.

Relevance for Understanding the Living and Working Conditions Experienced by Immigrants

Clear affinities *should* exist between welfare state concepts and the immigration experience. Evidence exists of more equitable distribution of the social determinants as well as better health outcomes and lower magnitude health inequalities among those living in Social Democratic nations; the opposite is the case for Liberal nations (Raphael, 2013a, 2013b). The structures and processes associated with the Social Democratic welfare state may also minimize the vulnerabilities of those occupying specific social locations such as being of Indigenous descent, a person of colour, unemployed, ill, having a disability, and working class than is the case for the Liberal welfare state (Raphael, 2012). Social locations also include being an immigrant. Are their vulnerabilities related to the form of the welfare state?

Threats to Immigrants' Living and Working Conditions and National Responses

There are a number of threats that can lead to adverse living and working conditions for immigrants. These have to do with the economic and political pressures exerted by economic globalization and neo-liberalism and how these pressures may foster xenophobia and racism toward immigrants. These issues are especially important as immigration to modern Western nations is increasingly by people of colour from the developing world.

Economic Globalization and Neo-liberalism

It is recognized that economic globalization and the resurgence of neo-liberal ideology in the past three decades—an ideology that believes that governments should withdraw from managing the economy, thereby ceding more power and influence to the business and corporate sector—is affecting the distribution of the social determinants of health in Western developed nations (Schrecker & Bambra, 2015).

Under pressure to attract investment by reducing corporate taxes and worker protections, governments come to have fewer resources for social provision and may legislate away workers' rights and benefits. These changes shape the distributions of various social determinants of health, the most important of which are the distributions of income and wealth. There is evidence that national responses to economic globalization are first and foremost made on the basis of ideology rather than economic imperatives such that to date, these effects are most apparent in Liberal welfare states such as Australia, Canada, and the United Kingdom, but can also manifest in other forms of the welfare state.

The Scandinavian nations and Canada appear to have weathered the recent recession rather well. In Sweden, however, retrenchment led to cutbacks in benefits and supports while the opposite occurred in Norway. As one example, legislation concerning temporary versus permanent employment has seen greater movement toward temporary work of lower quality in Sweden as compared to Norway and Denmark (Svalund, 2013).

Economic globalization can create economic and social conditions that weaken support for progressive public policies and political parties. During times of economic insecurity, concern for the self and family can promote individualism and weaken concern for others. This will be especially the case if these others are seen as not sharing the same backgrounds and values.

Finseraas suggests that increased immigration to Scandinavia, especially of non-Caucasian groups, presents numerous integration challenges (Finseraas, 2012). Immigration can weaken support for a well-developed welfare state through two potential pathways. The first pathway is that resentment and resistance to immigration can split traditional left-party solidarity that creates public policies that promote health. The most obvious manifestation of this is the rise of right-wing nationalist parties whose primary policy position is restricting immigration. Their strength results from citizens seeing immigration as a threat to their own economic well-being, potentially creating unemployment and driving down wages.

The danger to health-promoting public policies is that the rise of these right-wing political parties on the basis of immigration issues brings with it the excess baggage of policies inconsistent with Scandinavian and Continental principles of universalism and solidarity, respectively. These may weaken the provision of supports and benefits as well as threaten the pro-labour public policies that have shaped the form of the modern welfare state.

The second pathway is that citizens come to perceive that the greatest benefits of the welfare state accrue to immigrants such that the call for welfare state retrenchment takes on an "us–them" dimension. The "us–them" argument has been used in many discussions of why the welfare state in nations with heterogeneous populations such as Canada and the United States is undeveloped (Alesina & Glaeser, 2004; Banting, 2005). The growing strength of centre-right political parties suggests that anti-immigrant sentiments and their effects are potentially strong.

In Canada, and probably elsewhere, immigrants—especially those of colour—are especially susceptible to these effects. Government withdrawal from the provision of economic and social security results in greater commodification of the resources necessary for secure living and working conditions. This results in access to goods and services becoming subject to marketplace conditions rather than seen as entitlements provided by the state. And reliance upon the marketplace also tends to increase stratification to which immigrants are more susceptible.

Galabuzi (2005) describes this process and its interaction with issues of immigration and race in terms of growing social exclusion in Canada:

> In the late 20th and early 21st centuries, social exclusion is a by-product of a form of unbridled accumulation whose processes commodify social relations, and validate and intensify inequality along racial and gender lines.... This intensification can be traced to the restructuring of the global and national economies, which emphasized commodification of public goods, demographic shifts leading to increased global South-North migrations, changes in work arrangements towards flexible deployments and intensification of labour through longer hours, work fragmentation, multiple jobs, and increasing non-standard forms of work. Not only have these developments intensified exploitation in the labour market, but they have also engendered urban spatial segregation processes, including the gendered and racialized spatial concentration of poverty. (p. 173)

As economic issues gain dominance over issues of community and societal well-being, governments may withdraw from intervention in a wide range of public policy domains. These areas include employment and labour regulation, provision of goods and services, and provision of basic needs such as housing and shelter. The governments' withdrawal benefits those who own and control the major economic institutions. The members of classes and status groups most influenced by withdrawal of benefits and services have less influence and little power. These groups may include immigrants.

Economic conditions become more precarious and relationships among classes and status groups become more strained. Competition among groups becomes more intense, and class and status differences become heightened. Groups with less influence and power become subject to greater precariousness of employment, declining living conditions, and threatened health and quality of life. In Canada, these pressures and their effects are most apparent among recent immigrants and people of colour. Appropriately, Galabuzi's (2005) volume, which documents these effects, is entitled *Canada's Economic Apartheid: The Social Exclusion of Racialized Groups in the New Century*.

Xenophobia and Racism

As competition becomes more intense and economic and social security more precarious, xenophobia and racism can increase, with deleterious effects upon the living and working conditions of immigrants, especially those of colour. Governmental responses to such processes are necessary and differences in forms of the welfare state should be related to their activation. Determining whether this is the case is an essential component of this inquiry.

Conclusion

In this section a number of hypotheses related to how the form of the welfare state should be related to the integration of immigrants have been presented. The argument was made that the Social Democratic welfare state seen in Scandinavia seems best equipped to meet the challenges of integrating immigrants into society; the Liberal Anglo-Saxon welfare state the least able. It is unclear as to how the Conservative Continental welfare state may be doing.

Key concepts identified were those of stratification, decommodification, and social justice. For each of these concepts the Social Democratic welfare states seem to do best; the Liberals welfare states the worst. Whether these trends generalize to the experiences of immigrants and their health outcomes in these nations constitutes the focus of the chapters that follow.

Critical Thinking Questions

1. Why do you think that multiculturalism as a public policy approach has become so prominent in Liberal welfare states as opposed to other forms of the welfare state?
2. To what extent do you think that the form of the welfare state will influence how a nation deals with immigration issues and immigrant integration?
3. What form of welfare state do you live in? Do you see any obvious links between this and how immigrants are faring in your nation?
4. What role does political ideology play in the form of the welfare state? How would this political ideology play out in a nation dealing with immigration issues and immigrant integration?
5. What might be some unique aspects of nations that would lead to contradictions between their general approach to economic and social security and their approaches to immigrant integration?

Glossary

Decommodification "refers to the degree to which citizens have an alternative to complete dependence on the labour market (on working for money), in order to have an acceptable standard of living (for example, welfare, unemployment insurance, pensions, and labour market policies)" (Coburn, 2010, p. 71).

Political economy is explicitly concerned with the political and economic structures that shape the distribution of power and resources within the population. It is also specifically focused on understanding how the creation and distribution of resources influence the health and quality of life of individuals and communities. This perspective has a strong commitment to identifying how political and economic structures can be changed to promote health and well-being.

Stratification refers to the way that a society places groups at different levels of status and influence. The basis upon which this is done can be social class, gender, race, wealth and income, ethnicity, or other aspects.

Welfare state is a nation in which organized power is used to modify the play of market forces in at least three directions: first, by guaranteeing individuals and families a minimum income irrespective of the market value of their work or property; second, by narrowing the extent of insecurity by enabling individuals and families to meet certain social contingencies (e.g., sickness, old age, and unemployment) that lead otherwise to individual and family crises; and third, by ensuring that all citizens without distinction of status or class are offered the best standards available in relation to a certain agreed range of social services (Briggs, 1961).

Worlds of welfare usually refer to the welfare state typology developed by Gosta Esping-Andersen. He identified three forms: the Social Democratic, Conservative, and Liberal to which many have added a fourth, the Latin. These states differ widely in how they provide economic and social security to their members. Key aspects focus on the role of the state, the family, and the market in providing security and the extent of stratification and decommodification.

Recommended Readings

Esping-Andersen, G. (1985). *Politics against markets: The social democratic road to power.* Princeton, NJ: Princeton University Press.

Esping-Andersen, G. (1990). *The three worlds of welfare capitalism.* Princeton, NJ: Princeton University Press.

Esping-Andersen, G. (1999). *Social foundations of post-industrial economies.* New York: Oxford University Press.

Esping-Andersen, G. (2009). *The unfinished revolution: Welfare state adaptation to women's new roles.* Cambridge: Polity Press.

These volumes provide insights into the nature of modern welfare states and how their distinctive aspects emerged through particular historical traditions and influences.

Raphael, D. (2013). The political economy of health promotion: Part 1: National commitments to provision of the prerequisites of health. *Health Promotion International, 28*(1), 95–111.

Raphael, D. (2013). The political economy of health promotion: Part 2: National provision of the prerequisites of health. *Health Promotion International, 28*(1), 112–32.

These two articles relate different forms of the welfare state to their rhetorical and public policy approaches to equitably distributing the social determinants of health across the population.

Raphael, D. (2014). Challenges to promoting health in the modern welfare state: The case of the Nordic nations. *Scandinavian Journal of Public Health, 42*(1), 7–17.

This article specifically addresses some of the influences that may threaten the Nordic Social Democratic welfare state.

Sainsbury, D. (2012). *Welfare states and immigrant rights.* London: Oxford University Press.

This volume deals with the impact of welfare states on immigrants' social rights, economic well-being, and social inclusion. The author develops an analytical framework that focuses on the interplay between (1) the type of welfare state regime; (2) forms of entry, or entry categories; and (3) the incorporation regime regulating the inclusion or exclusion of immigrants. As such, it raises important issues for consideration in all nations experiencing immigration.

Saint-Arnaud, S., & Bernard, P. (2003). Convergence or resilience? A hierarchical cluster analysis of the welfare regimes in advanced countries. *Current Sociology, 51*(5), 499–527.

This article outlines the distinctive aspects of each form of the welfare state and provides empirical evidence of their validity.

Related Websites

Durham University Centre for Health and Inequalities Research (CHIR)—https://www.dur.ac.uk/chir/

CHIR is an internationally leading, interdisciplinary centre for the study of health, socio-economic, spatial, gender, and other inequalities. Through research and consultancy,

CHIR applies socio-spatial analysis to address research and policy questions in three work streams: Dimensions of Health and Inequality, Place-based Responses to Health and Inequality, and Visualizing Health and Inequality.

Indicators of Immigrant Integration 2015—http://www.oecd.org/publications/indicators-of-immigrant-integration-2015-settling-in-9789264234024-en.htm

This Organisation for Economic Co-operation and Development website provides data on the integration outcomes of immigrants and their children through 26 indicators organized around four areas: education, employment, social inclusion, and active citizenship.

Office of the United Nations High Commissioner for Refugees—http://www.unhcr.org/pages/4a16aa156.html

The Office of the UNHCR was established on December 14, 1950, by the United Nations General Assembly and is mandated to lead and coordinate international action to protect refugees and resolve refugee problems worldwide. Its primary purpose is to safeguard the rights and well-being of refugees.

Organisation for Economic Co-operation and Development (OECD)—http://www.oecd.org/

This website provides access to reports and data from the Organisation for Economic Co-operation and Development. It sees its goal as promoting policies that will improve the economic and social well-being of people around the world. The publications *Society at a Glance* and *Health at a Glance* are especially useful.

Sustainable Governance Indicators—http://www.sgi-network.org/2014/

The SGI is a platform built on a cross-national survey of governance that identifies reform needs in 41 EU and OECD countries. It brings together a broad network of experts and practitioners aiming to understand what works best in sustainable governance and offers full access to its data set to enable comparisons that generate innovation in governance.

Notes

1. Sainsbury's distinction between inclusionary and restrictive approaches has not been without criticism. It has been suggested that there has actually been convergence in approaches toward immigrants among EU nations (Cavasola, 2014).
2. Nations identified as Latin welfare states (e.g., Greece, Italy, Spain, and Portugal) are seen as less developed and even more family-oriented versions of the Conservative welfare state (Bambra, 2007; Saint-Arnaud & Bernard, 2003). Benefits are less generous and programs more fragmented than is the case for Conservative welfare states. These nations are of special contemporary interest as they are experiencing financial crises that led to adoption of severe austerity measures that have health equity implications.

References

Alesina, A., & Glaeser, E. L. (2004). *Fighting poverty in the US and Europe: A world of difference.* Toronto: Oxford University Press.

Arts, W., & Gelissen, J. (2002). Three worlds of welfare capitalism or more? A state-of-the-art report. *Journal of European Social Policy, 12*(2), 137–58.

Bambra, C. (2005). Cash versus services: Worlds of welfare and the decommodification of cash benefits and health care. *Journal of Social Policy, 34*(2), 195–213.

Bambra, C. (2007). Going beyond the three worlds of welfare capitalism: Regime theory and public health research. *Journal of Epidemiology and Community Health, 61*(12), 1098–102.

Bambra, C. (2011). Health inequalities and welfare state regimes: Theoretical insights on a public health "puzzle." *Journal of Epidemiology and Community Health, 65*(9), 740–45.

Bambra, C., Fox, D., & Scott-Samuel, A. (2005). Towards a politics of health. *Health Promotion International, 20*(2), 187–93.

Banting, K. (2005). The multicultural welfare state: International experience and North American narratives. *Social Policy and Administration, 39*(2), 98–115.

Briggs, A. (1961). The welfare state in historical perspective. *European Journal of Sociology, 2*, 251–259.

Bryant, T. (2009). *An introduction to health policy.* Toronto: Canadian Scholars' Press Inc.

Bryant, T. (2010). Politics, public policy, and health inequalities. In T. Bryant, D. Raphael, & M. Rioux (Eds.), *Staying alive: Critical perspectives on health, illness, and health care* (2nd ed.), (pp. 239–65). Toronto: Canadian Scholars' Press Inc.

Cavasola, L. (2014). Review of welfare states and immigrant rights: The politics of inclusion and exclusion. *Plurilogue: Politics and Philosophy Reviews.* Retreived from www.plurilogue.com/2014/02/welfare-states-and-immigrant-rights.html

Coburn, D. (2010). Health and health care: A political economy perspective. In T. Bryant, D. Raphael, & M. Rioux (Eds.), *Staying alive: Critical perspectives on health, illness, and health care* (2nd ed.), (pp. 65–92). Toronto: Canadian Scholars' Press Inc.

Esping-Andersen, G. (1985). *Politics against markets: The social democratic road to power.* Princeton, NJ: Princeton University Press.

Esping-Andersen, G. (1990). *The three worlds of welfare capitalism.* Princeton, NJ: Princeton University Press.

Esping-Andersen, G. (1999). *Social foundations of post-industrial economies.* New York: Oxford University Press.

Esping-Andersen, G. (2009). *The unfinished revolution: Welfare state adaptation to women's new roles.* Cambridge: Polity Press.

Finseraas, H. (2012). Anti-immigration attitudes, support for redistribution, and party choice in Europe. In J. Kvist, J. Fritzell, B. Hvinden, & O. Kangas (Eds.), *Changing social inequality: The Nordic welfare state in the 21st century* (pp. 23–44). Bristol: Policy Press.

Fosse, E. (2011). Different welfare states—different policies? An analysis of the substance of national health promotion policies in three European countries. *International Journal of Health Services, 41*(2), 255–72.

Galabuzi, G. E. (2005). *Canada's economic apartheid: The social exclusion of racialized groups in the new century.* Toronto: Canadian Scholars' Press Inc.

Grabb, E. (2007). *Theories of social inequality* (5th ed.). Toronto: Harcourt Canada.

Helm, T., Doward, J., & Asthana, A. (2010, July 3). Treasury orders cabinet ministers to brace themselves for 40% cuts. *The Guardian.*

Jackson, A. (2009). The unhealthy Canadian workplace. In D. Raphael (Ed.), *Social determinants of health: Canadian perspectives* (2nd ed.), (pp. 99–113). Toronto: Canadian Scholars' Press Inc.

Langille, D. (2009). Follow the money: How business and politics shape our health. In D. Raphael (Ed.), *Social determinants of health: Canadian perspectives* (2nd ed.), (pp. 305–17). Toronto: Canadian Scholars' Press Inc.

McMullin, J., & Davies, L. (2010). Social class and health inequalities. In T. Bryant, D. Raphael, & M. Rioux (Eds.), *Staying alive: Critical perspectives on health, illness, and care* (2nd ed.), (pp. 181–204). Toronto: Canadian Scholars' Press Inc.

Menahem, G. (2010). How can the Decommodified Security Ratio assess social protection systems? Luxembourg Income Study Working Paper no. 529. Syracuse, NY: Luxembourg Income Study.

Olsen, G. (2002). *The politics of the welfare state.* Toronto: Oxford University Press.

Olsen, G. (2008). Labour market policy in the United States, Canada, and Sweden: Addressing the issue of convergence. *Social Policy & Administration, 42*(4), 323–41.

Olsen, G. (2010). *Power and inequality: A comparative introduction.* Toronto: Oxford University Press.

Organisation for Economic Co-operation and Development. (2004). *OECD employment outlook 2004.* Paris: Organisation for Economic Co-operation and Development.

Organisation for Economic Co-operation and Development. (2011). *Social expenditure database (SOCX).* Retrieved from http://www.oecd.org/document/9/0,3746, en_2649_34637_38141385_1_1_1_1,00.html

Organisation for Economic Co-operation and Development. (2013). *Health at a glance: OECD indicators 2013 edition.* Paris: Organisation for Economic Co-operation and Development.

Organisation for Economic Co-operation and Development. (2016a). *Inequality.* Retrieved from www.oecd.org/social/inequality.htm

Organisation for Economic Co-operation and Development. (2016b). *Public expenditure and participant stocks on LMP.* Retreived from stats.oecd.org/Index.aspx?DataSetCode=LMPEXP

Organisation for Economic Co-operation and Development. (2016c). *OECD family database, PF3.1 Public spending on childcare and early education.* Retreived from www.oecd.org/social/family/database.htm

Pontusson, J. (2005). *Inequality and prosperity: Social Europe versus liberal America.* Ithaca, NY: Cornell University Press.

Raphael, D. (2011). Canadian public policy and poverty in international perspective. In D. Raphael (Ed.), *Poverty in Canada: Implications for health and quality of life* (pp. 374–405). Toronto: Canadian Scholars' Press Inc.

Raphael, D. (Ed.). (2012). *Tackling inequalities in health: Lessons from international experiences.* Toronto: Canadian Scholars' Press Inc.

Raphael, D. (2013a). The political economy of health promotion: Part 1, National commitments to provision of the prerequisites of health. *Health Promotion International, 28*(1), 95–111.

Raphael, D. (2013b). The political economy of health promotion: Part 2, National provision of the prerequisites of health. *Health Promotion International, 28*(1), 112–32.

Raphael, D. (2014a). Beyond policy analysis: The raw politics behind opposition to healthy public policy. *Health Promotion International. 30*(2), 380–96.

Raphael, D. (2014b). Challenges to promoting health in the modern welfare state: The case of the Nordic nations. *Scandinavian Journal of Public Health, 42*(1), 7–17.

Rioux, M. (2010). The right to health: Human rights approaches to health. In D. Raphael, T. Bryant, & M. Rioux (Eds.), *Staying alive: Critical perspectives on health, illness, and health care.* Toronto: Canadian Scholars' Press Inc.

Sainsbury, D. (2012). *Welfare states and immigrant rights.* London: Oxford University Press.

Saint-Arnaud, S., & Bernard, P. (2003). Convergence or resilience? A hierarchial cluster analysis of the welfare regimes in advanced countries. *Current Sociology, 51*(5), 499–527.

Schraad-Tischler, S. (2011). *Social justice in the OECD—How do the member states compare?* Gutersloh, Germany: Bertelmanns Stifung.

Schrecker, T. & Bambra, C. (2015). *How politics makes us sick: Neoliberal epidemics.* New York: Palgrave Macmillan.

Svalund, J. (2013). Labor market institutions, mobility, and dualization in the Nordic countries. *Nordic Journal of Working Life Studies, 3*(1), 123–44.

Swank, D. (2005). Globalisation, domestic politics, and welfare state retrenchment in capitalist democracies. *Social Policy and Society, 4*(2), 183–95.

Tremblay, D. G. (2009). Precarious work and the labour market. In D. Raphael (Ed.), *Social determinants of health: Canadian perspectives* (2nd ed.), (pp. 75–87). Toronto: Canadian Scholars' Press Inc.

Part 2

Case Studies of Welfare States and Immigration

In this volume, the focus is on how immigrants in different nations are faring in relation to issues of integration, health, and well-being. Informed—but not bound by—Esping-Andersen's typology of Liberal (or Anglo-Saxon), Conservative (or Continental), and Social Democratic (or Scandinavian), examination is made of how adoption of concepts such as multiculturalism, solidarity, and equity inform how they approach these issues and the consequences for immigrants of these decisions.

Part 2 contains the nine national case studies organized by welfare nation types: Anglo-Saxon (Australia, Canada, and the United Kingdom), Continental (Austria, Belgium, and Germany) and Scandinavian (Denmark, Norway, and Sweden). In each of these case studies the focus is on public policy and how it addresses, first, issues of immigration itself and second, integration of immigrants into the economic and social life of the nation.

In Canada, there is evidence that newly arrived immigrants, despite their generally higher educational credentials as compared to native-born Canadians, are experiencing living and working conditions that threaten their health. They are more likely than native-born Canadians to experience unemployment and underemployment and are more likely to live in poverty. The kind of work they take is more precarious and low paying, and they are more likely to experience housing and food insecurity. Over time they experience deterioration in health status that has come to be known in Canada as the "healthy immigrant effect." This is especially the case for immigrants from the developing world.

Particular focus is therefore on the lived experience of immigrants and how this experience is consistent with expectations of health prior to the immigration experience. Of particular concern also are health outcomes with a focus on the so-called "healthy immigrant effect." This is a situation where immigrants appear to be healthier than those born in the nation, but over time their health deteriorates to equal or fall below that of those born in the nation.

Anglo-Saxon Nations: Multiculturalism Put to the Test?

CHAPTER 3

Public Policy, Immigrant Experiences, and Health Outcomes in Australia

Hurriyet Babacan and Narayan Gopalkrishnan

Chapter Objectives

This chapter focuses on Australian immigration and multiculturalism as a case study. The specific objectives of this chapter are:

- to examine the role that immigration and multiculturalism play in the construction of the nation-state in Australia;
- to explore the role that policy plays in shaping the lived experiences of immigrants to Australia;
- to review the evidence concerning health outcomes among immigrants in Australia; and
- to analyze the interrelationship between public policy, integration, and health outcomes of immigrants and reflect on the implications for policy and program development in Australia.

Introduction

Australia is a culturally diverse society with more than 7 million immigrants arriving on its shores since the Second World War (DIAC, 2006). Immigration and cultural diversity have always featured as part of the Australian landscape since the establishment of Australia as a federated nation in 1901. Since then, governments have grappled with how to manage diversity in nation-building to secure economic and social outcomes. Developments in contemporary nation-states have necessitated a focus on pluralism and ethnic diversity. However, the national membership of the nation-state is defined through social boundaries and this often does not reflect the cultural reality and diversity within the borders of the nation-state (Ferguson & Associates, 1994). The nation-state's political and institutional approach toward culture, language, identity, and history is a crucial element in the discourse and reproduction of national identities and citizenship rights (Babacan & Herrmann, 2013; Gutmann, 2003). However, in ethnically and culturally diverse societies, belonging and inclusion have not been unproblematic. Inclusion of minorities within the nation-state has played out in paradoxical ways. It has required dual and intersecting policy agendas: one that recognizes and celebrates cultural diversity and ethnic difference, while emphasizing national common identity, unity, and social cohesion (Soroka, Johnston, & Banting, 2007). As Vasta (2007, p. 3) argues, cultural diversity policy "frequently elicits a paradox between the need for *equality* and *cultural recognition* (which is an important immigrant and ethnic minorities' position) on the one hand, and, on the other hand, the desire for *cultural assimilation*."

This chapter examines public policies of immigration and multiculturalism in Australia as noted above. It reviews the recent immigration patterns and reflects on the cultural composition of Australia. The chapter proceeds to review the settlement and integration of immigrants to Australian society and focuses on the evidence of the lived experience of immigrants. There will be a specific focus on health outcomes and determinants as a result of immigration. The final section of the paper will provide an analysis of the interrelationship between public policy and multiculturalism and immigration.

It is important to note that multicultural policies at various stages have acknowledged Indigenous Australians while tending to refer to non-Aboriginal populations. Further, many Aboriginal peoples have resisted inclusion under multicultural policies as these did not sufficiently take into account their distinctive historical experiences, undermined their claims by casting them as another ethnic group, and denied their special status as First Nations peoples (Van den Berg, 2002). Policies that address Aboriginal and Torres Strait Islander issues have accordingly developed separately in Australia and will not form part of the discussion in this chapter.

Immigration-Related Public Policy in Australia

Immigration Policy

Immigration and cultural diversity have been and still continue to be highly contentious and hotly debated issues in Australia. Since the formation of Australia as a nation-state in 1901, with the federation of independent colonies, immigration issues have been central in public policy. One of the first legislations of the newly formed Australian Parliament was the Immigration Restriction Act 1901, which restricted the entry of certain classes of people and came to form the basis of the "White Australia

Policy," which lasted until the 1970s (Hollinsworth, 2006). In the context of exclusionary measures introduced in this period, Jupp (2007, p. 9) states that "a message was sent out to the world that 'coloured' people could not settle in Australia." The non-European population was only 0.25 percent of the total. Subsequent governments have built on fear politics targeting Indonesians and other Asian populations with the slogan "populate or perish" and the "yellow peril" until the late 1930s, the Germans during the First World War, and the Japanese during the Second World War. We see more recent examples of fear politics with Muslim and Arab communities since the events of September 11, 2001 (Gopalkrishnan, 2013b; Poynting, Noble, Tabar, & Collins, 2004), and refugees and asylum-seekers (Briskman, 2011).

Paradoxically, Australia's immigration programs emphasize immigrants being allowed to settle permanently in Australia and be granted Australian citizenship. However, in recent years there is an increasing trend toward temporary migration. The key concerns in immigration policy are the size of the immigrant intake annually, how these should be selected, and the balance between permanent and temporary programs and the relative weighting in the permanent intake of the skill, business, family, and humanitarian intakes.

Contemporary Australian immigration has a number of features (Babacan & Babacan, 2009; Castles, Vasta, & Ozkul, 2012; Collins, 2013; DIBP, 2014b; Gopalkrishnan, 2006; Hugo, 2014; Jupp, 2007; Marginson, Nyland, Sawir, & Forbes-Mewett, 2010):

- A non-discriminatory immigration policy has been adopted from the early 1970s with the abandonment of the White Australia Policy, allowing for immigration from a diverse number of source countries.
- The size of the immigration intake has increased, although this has varied with economic recessions.
- The balance of the Migration Program has shifted toward the skill stream from the mid-1990s with a reduction in family migration.
- The humanitarian intake is separated from immigrant intake and the proportion of the humanitarian intake is declining as a percentage of the total intake.
- There has been a major policy change toward asylum-seekers (also called boat people and now called illegal maritime entrants) with mandatory detention and offshore processing of boat arrivals. Immigration policy in the 2000s focuses strongly on unauthorized boat arrivals and border protection. The Australian government has attracted negative criticism from different quarters for different action against asylum-seekers such as refusal to allow disembarkation of asylum-seekers, demonization of asylum-seekers as a strategy used for election purposes, passing of legislation to excise parts of Australia from migration zones, and mandatory detention centres in Pacific Island countries.

- There is a dramatic increase in temporary immigration with the creation of a range of visa classes.
- Australia has had a large influx of international students and has the fourth largest population of foreign students in the world. DIAC (2013) estimated 485,342 international students in Australia in 2008–9, but the numbers have declined to about 250,000 due to violent attacks on international students.

The direction of immigration policies has continued to be dynamic and changing with economic conditions of decline in manufacturing in Australia, integration into the global economy, deregulation of finance, and the shift to a global knowledge economy. Although the United Kingdom and New Zealand immigrants make up the largest ethnic groups in Australia, the remainder of the recent arrivals are mainly from Asia, Africa, and the Middle East. Commenting on the changing nature of immigration, Collins (2013, p. 162) states that "we have seen a fundamental transformation in Australian immigration policy from a predominantly settler immigration model for half a century to an increasingly guest worker immigration model in the last decade, a change largely unnoticed because of the popular and bipartisan political preoccupation with a few thousand boat arrivals annually."

An additional change in immigration has been the spatial location and settlement of immigrants in Australia. In the past, the majority of immigrant settlement has been in large cities or towns with sizable employment opportunities. Over the last decade the Australian government has introduced policies that have redirected immigrants to regional areas. Regional settlement in Australia increased from 771,574 to 1,001,645 (Hugo, 2014). The result is a spatially dispersed cultural diversity in Australia. However, this is not a simple process of relocation but raises significant issues of integration, particularly in relation to a lack of support infrastructure, access to services, and prejudicial attitudes toward immigrants (Jordan, Krivokapic-Skoko, & Collins, 2011; Missingham, Dibden, & Cocklin, 2006).

Multiculturalism and Settlement Policies

The policies of **multiculturalism** have provided the policy framework for immigrant settlement in Australia since the 1970s. Multicultural policies have undergone different phases. The first is the *assimilationism* phase during which immigrants were expected to learn English, adopt Australian cultural practices, and become indistinguishable from the Australian-born population as quickly as possible. This phase lasted from around 1900 to 1965 and linked up with the infamous White Australia Policy. The second phase was *integration*, from 1966 to the 1970s, when it was recognized that difficulties immigrants faced could be addressed if they could integrate successfully in Australian society without losing their national identities.

The focus was on addressing deficiencies that immigrants had, providing equal access to opportunities, and allowing individuals to maintain their own culture without prejudice or disadvantage (Jupp, 2007).

The next phase of *egalitarian multiculturalism* (Jayasuriya, 1997) began with the election of the Whitlam Labour government in 1973 with a focus on cultural pluralism. There was bipartisan support for multiculturalism regardless of political persuasion. A major immigrant settlement review was conducted, and the Galbally Report (1978) became the foundational document linking multiculturalism with immigrant settlement and welfare and began the process of committing the government to addressing social inequality and assuming responsibility and support for immigrant settlement and welfare (Jayasuriya, 1997).

The following phase (1983–96) focused on *social justice and economic benefits* to the multicultural mosaic. Also, this era was characterized by deregulation, opening of financial markets, attempts at efficient use of human resources, and the greater engagement of Australia with the Asia-Pacific region. There was a major shift toward accepting into Australia more skilled immigrants with high levels of qualifications. This era was characterized by notions of "productive diversity," which advocated in policy the benefits of cultural diversity to economic development, in growing in trade and business via the cultural and language skills, global business networks, and market knowledge of immigrants (Babacan, 2006).

An important policy initiative was the launch of the National Agenda for Multicultural Australia in 1988 by the prime minister. The new policy contained three dimensions: cultural identity, social justice, and economic efficiency (OMA, 1989). The National Agenda marked a shift away from an "ethnic group" model toward a "citizenship" model. As a public policy measure, it incorporated ethnic diversity as being central to contemporary Australian society. It recognized that the state had the duty to take measures to ensure equal opportunity and prevent marginalization of minority groups. This period was marked by an institutionalization of multiculturalism. All Commonwealth government departments were expected to report annually against "access and equity" statements, or benchmarks. This new approach was facilitated by a number of government departments, including the Office of Multicultural Affairs (OMA) in the Department of Prime Minister and Cabinet and other key institutions. These institutional mechanisms provided research and service infrastructure for multiculturalism at the state and federal levels (Babacan, 2006; Ho, 2013).

The Conservative government of John Howard (1996–2007) refined the definition of multiculturalism and was a low point for official support for multiculturalism. This era is referred to as the *social cohesion* phase with a focus on *unity in diversity*. Unlike the earlier policy, this policy was not couched in citizenship terms but expressed in terms of "civic duties" and introduced the demand for mutual obligations and emphasized unified national identity, Australian values, and community harmony with an outline of the "limits" to cultural diversity (Levey, 2012, p. 7). The term "multicultural affairs" was removed from the name of the ministry and "multiculturalism" was largely removed from official discourses (Ho, 2013). The deinstitutionalization of multiculturalism began with many key agencies being de-funded.

After this period, questioning of immigration and multiculturalism began to re-emerge. Discourses surrounding counterterrorism became conjoined with asylum policy and law-and-order issues (e.g., Lebanese gang rapes, the Cronulla riots) (Babacan & Babacan, 2007; Poynting & Noble, 2004) and served as justification for a retreat from multiculturalism. Under national security and counterterrorism measures, a series of initiatives were introduced that eroded civil liberties, freedoms, and human rights. There was an attempt to define Australian values and defend the "Australian way of life" as a response to cultural diversity. The election of a Labour government in 2007 brought about new agendas. The key policy framework was *social inclusion* and addressing inequality. This paid lip service to issues of disadvantage based on cultural diversity. The important consideration was the establishment of the National Anti-Racism Strategy, which was welcome in the face of the denial of racism in the public discourse on cultural diversity (Babacan & Gopalkrishnan, 2008; Nelson, 2013). However, despite the series of initiatives on anti-racism, this period witnessed racially motivated attacks on international students, particularly Indian students (Dunn & Nelson, 2011; Pyke, Bertone, Gill, & Grossman, 2011).

The election of the current Abbott government in 2013 marked another decline in multicultural policy. Multiculturalism was moved from the immigration portfolio to social security, suggesting a narrowed focus, and put under the stewardship of the minister for social security who, as immigration minister in the Howard government, was responsible for cutting the intake of humanitarian entrants from African countries on the grounds that they had trouble integrating into Australian society (Harrison, 2007). The department was renamed the Department of Immigration and Border Protection, emphasizing the focus on security issues. The use of the word "protection" in the department's name implies a threat and yet it is widely accepted that this is a political stance rather than any real threat of being swamped by boat people. A new round of security legislation was introduced and passed despite outcries from human rights and civil society agencies. The Abbott government's policy paradigms about multiculturalism are still evolving. The general thrust of debates is negative and is reminiscent of the Howard years.

In each of these phases of multicultural policy, the essential Anglo institutional frameworks remained unaltered. Migrants are accepted as citizens and given rights that were conditional upon accepting the common structures of society (the basic legal and political institutions, administrative systems, and rule of law) and with English as the official language. These requirements have remained unaltered over time in the evolution of multicultural policy in Australia (Babacan, 2006; Jupp, 2007). The importance of multicultural policy, however, is that it has been a nation-state intervention to facilitate immigrant settlement in Australia via the systems of the state. Multicultural policies continue to evolve in Australia, although, at the federal government level, the responses have been lukewarm since the late 1990s. The momentum for multiculturalism continues to be maintained by state governments where multicultural policies and programs have remained strong and intact (Babacan & Ben-Moshe, 2009; Levey, 2012). While the recent public discourses negate particular aspects of multiculturalism, the Australian populations support a multicultural way of life, if not the policy. Various studies indicate support for cultural diversity in the general population and many lead multicultural cosmopolitan lives (Collins, 2013; Dunn & Nelson, 2011). The question remains: What is the alternative for a culturally diverse Australia if multiculturalism is abandoned? Levey (2012, p. 12) points out that the alternative is much worse and warns: "abolish Australian multiculturalism and the strong cultural nationalist impulse in this country would go unchecked. Liberty and equality in Australia would be the first casualties."

Recent Immigration Patterns

Sustained immigration has been a central feature of Australia's nation building history. The 2011 National Census of the population revealed that 26 percent of Australians were born overseas, and an additional 20 percent have either one or both parents born overseas, implying that 46 percent of the population are either immigrants or the children of immigrants (ABS, 2013). Over 260 languages, including Indigenous languages, are spoken in Australia. Markus, Jupp, and McDonald (2009, p. 152) point out that "Australia is one of the few nations to be built by planned immigration," with immigrants coming from over 200 source countries (DIBP, 2014b).

About 1 million migrants arrived in each decade following 1950: 1.6 million between 1945 and 1960; about 1.3 million in the 1960s; about 960,000 in the 1970s; about 1.1 million in the 1980s; and 900,000 in the 1990s (DIMA, 2001, pp. 18–19). From the late 1960s onward, Australia opened immigration to non-European immigrants with large intakes from Southeast Asia.

There were a number of reasons for the changing composition of immigrants, including post-colonial reordering globally and the influence of civil and human rights, Australia's opening trade and political relationship with Asia, the rise of the Cold War and anti-Communist refugees such as those from Vietnam and Cambodia, and skill shortages in the face of declining fertility (Castles et al., 2012). This shift in immigration policy has resulted in one of the most culturally diverse populations in the world. The proportion of the Australian population born overseas increased from 23 percent in 2000 to 26.5 percent in 2009 (OECD, 2011, p. 261), and Australia was among the top three OECD countries to have permanent immigration inflows (after New Zealand and Switzerland) (OECD, 2011, p. 43). Jakubowicz and Ho (2013, p. 27) note that despite residues of racism, Australia has undergone a significant transformation in the last 50 years from being against the admittance of non-white immigrants to a country with one of the largest cultural mixes. They attribute this to two shared goals: (1) that Australians have a preference toward migration rather than being against it, although arguments persist as to which groups are preferred; and (2) Australians now generally agree that public policy should not enshrine racial discrimination, particularly since Australia has become signatory to key international conventions.

Table 3.1 presents the top 10 countries of birth for the overseas-born population in Australia in 2011.

Table 3.1: Top 10 Countries of Birth of Immigrants in Australia

Country of Birth	% of Overseas-Born
United Kingdom	20.8
New Zealand	9.1
China	6.0
India	5.6
Italy	3.5
Vietnam	3.5
Philippines	3.2
South Africa	2.8
Malaysia	2.2
Germany	2.0

Source: ABS. (2012). *Cultural diversity in Australia: Reflecting nation-stories from the 2011 census.* Canberra: Australian Bureau of Statistics. Retrieved from http://www.abs.gov.au/ausstats/abs@.nsf/lookup/2071.0main+features902012-2013

Immigrants from the United Kingdom have been the top category since the beginning of colonial settlement of Australia. Europeans in general have largely dominated the source countries, but this is a declining trend. For example, European immigrants made up 52 percent of the overseas-born in 2001, but this has decreased to 40 percent in 2011 (ABS, 2012). Asian-born immigrants, on the other hand, increased from 24 percent of the overseas-born population in 2001 to 33 percent in 2011. This is visible in the profiles of recent immigrants. Recent arrivals accounted for 47 percent of the total Indian-born population in Australia and 35 percent of the total Chinese-born population. In contrast, only 11 percent of the total United Kingdom–born population were recent arrivals (ABS, 2012).

Australia's immigration intake comprises different categories: the annual migration intake program (skill and family streams), the humanitarian entrant program, and New Zealand entrants based on a bilateral agreement between Australia and New Zealand. In 2013, the skill stream accounted for 53 percent of immigration; the family stream, 27 percent; the humanitarian program, 8 percent; and New Zealand citizens, 11 percent of total entrants (DIBP, 2014b). There is also a temporary visa category enabling people to stay for different periods of time for a range of reasons that includes international students, temporary skilled (457 visa) workers, bridging visa holders, and working holidaymakers. The number of temporary visa holders in Australia has increased drastically and is around 1.1 million (around 5.1 percent of Australia's population) (DIBP, 2014b).

Recent immigration intakes reflect the preoccupation of the Australian government on economic development with some gestures toward family and humanitarian concerns. The immigration policies exhibit selectivity in age, occupation, and background. This "bias" extends implicitly into humanitarian and family migration. The constitution of who has good settlement potential and the economic cost of an immigrant to Australia are highly debated. The critics of current approaches to immigration argue that there is a limit to rational economic policy determining social relationships with problems with establishing systems of migration based on occupations and the ability to predict industry demands accurately. In the process, there is loss of important human considerations such as family relationships and human rights of asylum-seekers (Jupp, 2007).

Lived Experience: Integration, Disadvantage, and Discrimination

Immigration and multicultural policies in Australia use the term "settlement" in describing the integration of immigrants. Thus, the debates about integration have been couched in terms relating to how well immigrants to Australia settle (Jupp, McRobbie, & York, 1991). The National Population Council of Australia (NPC, 1988, p. 3) defined "settlement" as "the process by which an immigrant establishes economic viability and social networks following immigration in order to contribute to, and make full use of, opportunities generally available in the receiving society." While settlement is about adjustment, self-determination, and support systems in a new environment and institutional supports, it is also a lived social experience with complex dimensions at both the subjective and objective levels (Collins, 2013). Moreover, Adelman, Borowski, Burstein, and Foster (1994) argue that settlement needs to be seen from the perspective of promoting long-term equality of outcomes in relation to resources and power in society. Successful immigrant integration would result in immigrants—regardless of cultural, linguistic, or religious background—having equal life chances and equitable outcomes in the economic, educational, political, and social realms, and where immigrant disadvantage and discrimination would be minimal or declining over the settlement period and over generations (Collins, 2013).

The settlement outcomes for skilled immigrants are generally better than family and humanitarian entrants (DIAC, 2011). The success of integration is measured on a range of outcomes such as employment, income, housing, and social inclusion measures. The studies of immigrant integration in Australia have been patchy, particularly with the dismantling of institutions of multiculturalism such as the Office for Multicultural Australia and the Bureau of Immigration and Population Research, both of which provided extensive and reliable research data. The Joint Standing Committee on Migration has recommended the collection of disaggregated data and the establishment of a research agency to collect data and undertake research on immigration and multiculturalism (APH, 2013). The patchy nature of the evidence does not enable consistency of data, or longitudinal collection, and leaves major gaps in many areas. Notwithstanding this, some indicators of the lived experience of immigrants are as follows.

Labour Market Outcomes

In the postwar years there were clear patterns of labour market segmentation as immigrants from a non-English-speaking background had generally inferior labour market positions and rewards (Collins, 1991). Even with a shift to more skilled immigration, the labour market outcomes for immigrants are not very satisfactory. At the time of the 2011 Census, immigrants made up 31 percent of the total labour force. The proportion of the immigrant population not in the labour force was higher in comparison to the Australian-born population at 39.6 percent as opposed to 32.8 percent. Further, the immigrant population has a slightly higher unemployment rate (6.5 percent as opposed to 5.3 percent) (DIBP, 2014a). Looking at recent migrants from 2002, there is continual decline in those who are employed full-time. In fact, those with the highest rates of unemployment and non-participation in the labour force are those who arrived in 2011 (13.5 percent unemployed and 45.4 percent non-participation) (DIBP, 2014a).

Unemployment levels vary for different groups. In 2011, skilled immigrants sponsored by a relative (rather than employer) had unemployment rates of 13 percent, higher than the national average, and family migrants had 29 percent unemployment (DIAC, 2011, pp. 4–5). Humanitarian immigrants had the worst labour market outcomes. Hugo (2014) has identified that humanitarian entrants have the highest levels of unemployment; for example, the rate for those from Somalia was 30.7 percent and for those from Sudan was 28.2 percent, compared to the Australian average of less than 6 percent. Colic-Peisker and Tilbury (2005) also point out that people from refugee backgrounds have been found to be allocated the lowest-level jobs regardless of their formal qualifications, skills, and experience.

The labour market outcomes differ for immigrant men and women on all visa categories. Overall, men were more likely to be employed full-time than women. In 2013, 92 percent of employed male migrants with Australian citizenship were employed full-time compared with 57 percent of females; 86 percent of employed males on a permanent visa were employed full-time compared with 58 percent of females; and 72 percent of employed male temporary residents were employed full-time compared with 54 percent of females (ABS, 2014).

The industries that immigrants work in are predominantly in the lower skill end of the labour market. There are three sectors in which migrant workers outnumber those born in Australia. These are taxi and road transport (62 percent), clothing manufacturing (53.7 percent), and poultry processing (50.5 percent). Although there are a number of high-level occupations in this mix, the majority of migrants are employed in low-skilled occupations. The skill level also varies with the different migration streams. The humanitarian stream has only 11 percent in "highest skill level" occupation and 36.6 percent in the "lowest skill level" occupations. The family stream has 26.7 percent in "highest skill level" and 22.2 percent in "lowest skill level," and the skill stream has 43.9 percent in "highest skill level" occupations with only 13.2 percent in "lowest skill level" (DIBP, 2014a).

Immigrants to Australia tend to have higher levels of education than do Australian-born people. More than half of all those (54.9 percent) who hold postgraduate degrees were born outside Australia (9 percent of all immigrants compared to less than 5 percent of Australian-born). The children of parents born overseas also attain higher levels of education. For example, of those with both parents born overseas, 60 percent completed year 12 compared to 53 percent with one Australian-born parent and 45 percent with both Australian-born parents (DIBP, 2014a).

Poverty and Income

The Australian Council of Social Services conducted a major poverty study in 2010 and the "profile of poverty" from this study revealed that 26.2 percent of all adults living in households below the 50 percent poverty line in Australia are from a non-English-speaking country (ACOSS, 2012). The "risk of poverty" analysis showed that adults born in countries where English is not the main language faced a much higher risk of poverty (15.8 percent using the <50 percent of average income poverty line) than those born in Australia (10.6 percent) or in an English-speaking country (11.7 percent).

This is likely to reflect the difficulties that migrants from non-English-speaking countries face in securing well-paid employment in Australia (ACOSS, 2012). Other studies have indicated similar results. For example, Borooah and Mangan (2007) concluded that Lebanese, North African, and Vietnamese migrants have lower household income, employment status, and housing conditions than "white" new arrivals from Europe, Great Britain, and New Zealand with the same length of settlement time in Australia. For many refugee and humanitarian entrants, the poverty levels are higher as they arrive in Australia with few or no financial resources (Beer & Foley, 2003). The Refugee Council of Australia (RCOA, 2013, p. 4) points out that humanitarian entrants may be in significant debt to people overseas as well as people in Australia, and they may face significant challenges in securing employment during the early stages of settlement and may consequently have very limited income. Additionally, many refugee entrants send remittances to family members living in dire situations overseas, often giving a significant portion of their limited income.

Housing and Homelessness

In a recent study, housing availability and affordability were nominated as the highest priorities in need of attention by people living in poverty and by human services agencies (ACOSS, 2013). In a survey of approximately 9,000 recently arrived immigrants in 2010, it was found that around half of all family-stream migrants and three-quarters of skill-stream migrants were in rented accommodation. Almost one in four family-stream migrants lived with other family members. Approximately 25 percent reported difficulties finding housing due to the high cost of housing, competition for housing, and problems getting references and background checks (DIAC, 2010).

Immigrants also are at risk of homelessness. At the time of the 2011 Census over one-third of all homeless people were recorded as being born overseas (36 percent). There was also evidence of changes in the circumstances of people born overseas since the 2006 Census because about three-quarters of the increase in estimated numbers of homeless between 2006 and 2011 was accounted for by people born overseas. Homelessness Australia conducted a survey of specialist homelessness services in 2013 and it was reported that more than half of the services were supporting clients from culturally diverse backgrounds (AIHW, 2013) and identified that clients born overseas required longer period of support (96 days for overseas-born compared to 78 days for Australian-born). Dawes and Gopalkrishnan (2014) found that the majority of homelessness experienced by members of culturally and linguistically diverse communities was hidden and secondary homelessness, involving people frequently moving from one temporary shelter to another, including friends' homes. Because of the hidden nature of secondary homelessness, much of the homelessness experienced by culturally diverse communities is not easily quantifiable.

In a recent study on housing for refugees, Forrest, Hermes, Johnston, and Poulsen (2012) concluded that refugees face challenges in securing appropriate, affordable, and stable accommodation. These barriers include financial hardship, lack of appropriate accommodation, difficulties navigating the private rental market, a lack of social and community capital, and the impact of family separation and breakdown. Other authors have pointed to discrimination by landlords and real estate agents (Dawes & Gopalkrishnan, 2014). Forrest et al. (2012, p. 202), argue that these barriers faced by refugees have "implications beyond just satisfactory and affordable housing: they also involve successful adjustment ... into the wider socio-economic structure of ... society."

Racism and Discrimination

Racism and discrimination are part of daily life for many ethnic communities in many Western countries, impacting adversely on different spheres of their lives, and adversely affecting their life chances (Hollinsworth, 2006). The nature and extent of this issue is also often hidden, as most racist incidents are not reported for a range of reasons (Dunn, Forrest, Burnley, & McDonald, 2004). As an example, in one study conducted over three years in Queensland, up to 70 percent of racist incidents were not reported (Babacan & Hollinsworth, 2009, p. 5).

A number of studies have been conducted that demonstrate the reality of racism. Dunn et al. (2004) (in a research project on racism to which one of the authors is also principal researcher), in a large national study, demonstrated that 78 percent of Australians believe humankind is made up of separate races; 41 percent believe that there are cultural groups that do not fit into Australian society; 85 percent believe there is racial prejudice in Australia, although, paradoxically, 87 percent believed that it is a good thing for society to be made up of different cultures. Experiences of racism were also identified in this national study with 18 percent of these in the workplace, 17 percent in educational settings, 18 percent in a shop or restaurant, and 16 percent at public or sporting events. Significantly, 23 percent identified as being treated less respectfully, 27 percent identified as being called names or insulted, and 16 percent identified as not being trusted due to "ethnicity, culture or race" (Dunn et al., 2004, p. 156).

Babacan and Hollinsworth (2009) found similar outcomes in their study. They identified 12 types of racist incidents that people experienced, including physical violence, threat of physical violence, property damage, verbal harassment, written harassment, racist graffiti, offensive media content, social exclusion (e.g., in work, school, or social events), discrimination and unfair treatment, and institutional racism (Babacan & Hollinsworth, 2009, pp. 22–24).

Research indicates that experiences of racism are not "one-off" events that can be dismissed as coincidence or unfortunate circumstance. It constitutes part of "everyday racism" (Essed, 2002), of the lived reality in the lives of people, and connects structural forces of racism with routine situations of everyday life. It is noted that racial stressors have multifarious effects on the health and well-being of racialized subjects (Paradies, Harris, & Anderson, 2008).

Social stratification, **ethnicity**, and racism are key elements of health outcomes (Ingleby, 2012). Immigrants and refugees continue to experience intersectional disadvantage in many areas of life. The Access and Equity Inquiry identified significant barriers and challenges in the "lived experience" of immigrants (FECCA, 2012). Collins (1991, p. ii) points to the paradoxical developments in the integration of immigrants in Australia when he states, "the Australian and Canadian experience suggests that prejudice coexists with tolerance, as does racism with social harmony and multiculturalism with ethnic inequality." Pointing to the impacts of the environmental factors on health, Friel (2009, p. 15) states, "any serious effort to promote well-being, prevent ill-health and reduce health inequities must address the social determinants that shape the way people grow, live, work and age." These structural and relations of power and social status are fundamental in determining health outcomes and empowerment for health equity in material, political, and psychosocial aspects of individuals and communities.

Health Outcomes for Immigrants in Australia

In the history of many nations there has been an association of disease and ill health with immigrants or foreigners, with immigrants being seen as a threat to the nation's health, and an attempt to exclude, quarantine, or keep out particular groups based on grounds of communicable disease (Gee & Ford, 2011; Markel & Stern, 2002). These ideas linger on and affect the development of immigration policies. All immigrants to Australia are required to undergo health checks and be in good health prior to admission into the country. This means that all potential immigrants who are not in good health are not granted visas for migration (VandenHeuvel & Wooden, 1999). It is well established that immigrants to a new country have a health advantage over native populations on most indicators of health, including mortality, morbidity, disability, and mental disorder (Fozdar & Torezani, 2008), often referred to as the "healthy immigrant effect." Over time, however, the immigrant health advantage dissipates and their health declines below or to the level of their native-born counterparts (Gushalak, 2007; Markides & Eschbach, 2005).

Gill and Babacan (2012, p. 1) assert that the impact of settlement and acculturation varies widely depending on individual experiences and situations. Determinants of health and well-being such as housing, employment, education, language barriers, family and community networks and supports, changes in lifestyle and diet, and access to essential services play a key role in the settlement time frame. As a result, the health and well-being of **culturally and linguistically diverse (CALD)** communities depend on a complex balance of social, economic, and environmental factors. Health problems are often compounded by a lack of knowledge of health systems and, consequently, many migrants experience difficulties in accessing appropriate health services (Henderson & Kendall, 2011).

The knowledge and skills required to understand and use information relating to health is quite low for many immigrants to Australia, and the health literacy of people born in a non-English-speaking country is far lower at 26 percent as compared to the 40 percent in the Australian-born (ABS, 2008). Additionally, discrimination and racism that migrants experience are also critical factors that impact on health outcomes (Powles & Gifford, 1990). The Access and Equity inquiry concluded that CALD communities face a particular set of challenges when it comes to accessing appropriate health care, including limited English language skills, unfamiliarity with the Western appointment-based system of health care, and a lack of cultural competency among health care professionals (FECCA, 2012, p. 41).

Evidence Concerning Health Outcomes among Immigrants

The institutional arrangements for the collection of data related to immigrants and health have been dismantled in the wake of the retreat from multiculturalism in government policy. This has made it difficult to determine trends and associations between migration and health-based outcomes, which is in itself complex and involves a range of factors ranging from individual to environmental and structural-level determinants (Irving & Mosca, 2010). While individual health services or agencies or state departments collect ethnicity and language data, this is not uniform across the board, and the evidence is sometimes outdated or focused on a particular ethnic group or particular medical condition (Khoo, 2010; Minas et al., 2013), resulting in little understanding of health challenges by immigrant communities. Given this patchy evidence base, some of the past and current evidence suggests the following:

- The Australian Institute of Health and Welfare (AIHW, 2011) reports that Australians have a life expectancy of 82 years—one of the highest among Organisation for Economic Co-operation and Development (OECD) countries—and the second lowest overall mortality of OECD countries. Mortality rates of all immigrant groups were lower than the Australian-born. It was 36 percent lower for Asian-born (both males and females) and 15 percent lower for resident males born in Northwest, Southern, and Eastern Europe, and 24 percent for females. Overseas-born Australian residents also had lower rates of potentially avoidable deaths than their Australian-born counterparts (AIHW, 2014, p. 13).
- Coronary heart disease, cerebrovascular diseases, dementia and Alzheimer disease, and lung cancer were the four leading causes of death for all country/region of birth groups. The United Kingdom- and Ireland-born residents had a similar profile to Australian-born residents for the 10 leading causes of death,

but with higher rates of dementia and Alzheimer disease (14 percent higher) and lung cancer (26 percent higher), and lower rates of colorectal cancer (11 percent lower than the rate for Australian-born residents) and heart failure (13 percent lower). Northwest, Southern, and Eastern Europe-born residents had lower rates for most leading causes of death compared to Australian-born residents, and in particular for chronic obstructive pulmonary disease (COPD), with a rate that was half the rate of Australian-born residents. Asian-born residents had lower rates for all 10 leading causes of death except liver cancer, where the rate for Asian-born residents was twice the rate of Australian-born residents. Residents in the "Other" group had similar or lower rates for all leading causes of death compared to Australian-born residents—in particular, the rate for COPD was 28 percent lower (AIHW, 2014, p. 14).

- Immigration is associated with an increased risk of diabetes, and it is known that approximately 35 percent of people residing in Australia who reported having diabetes in 2001 were born overseas, although only 28 percent of the Australian population in 2001 were born overseas (Colagiuri, Thomas, & Buckley, 2007). The regions of birth with the highest diabetes prevalence, incidence of insulin-treated diabetes, and diabetes-related hospitalizations and/or mortality rates were the South Pacific Islands, Southern Europe, Eastern Europe, and Central Asia, the Middle East, North Africa, and South Asia (Thow & Waters, 2005). AIHW (2005, p. 6) has identified that South Asian communities are likely to have a 2.5 times higher rate of diabetes than the Australian-born.
- Migration and the length of time since migration also play a significant role in dietary change among ethnic communities with the adoption of the unhealthy aspects of mainstream diets upon migration (Anderson et al., 2005). The changing patterns are also pointed to by Mellin-Olsen and Wandel (2005), who found that, post-migration, the cultural importance of breakfast and lunch has diminished and dinner has become the most important meal. It was also found that a rich variety of factors influenced dietary change, including health considerations, children's preferences, work schedules, social relations, stress, traditional beliefs, climate, season, and access to foods.
- A number of condition-specific studies have been conducted. For example, Anikeeva et al. (2010) reviewed health studies in Australia conducted between 1980 and 2008. They examined the Australian National Health Priorities Areas (NHPA), which focused on arthritis and musculoskeletal conditions, asthma, cancer control, cardiovascular health, diabetes mellitus, injury prevention and control, and mental health. The seven NHPAs account for approximately 80 percent of the total burden of disease and injury in Australia. They concluded that the majority of migrants enjoy better health than the

Australian-born population, with the exception of diabetes. They also identified that the immigrant health advantage deteriorates with increasing duration of residence, a finding that was also substantiated in the research conducted by Biddle, Kennedy, and McDonald (2007).

- Migrant workers may be overrepresented in occupational injuries (Trajkovski & Loosemore, 2006), an issue related to factors such as low levels of English literacy, long working hours, lack of safety training, precarious work, cultural factors, and the demands of production. It is also argued that that there is considerable underreporting of work-related injuries by immigrant workers (Reid et al., 2014).
- It is estimated that people from **non-English-speaking background (NESB)** with disability comprise one in 20 Australians or approximately 1 million people (NEDA, 2014, p. 8). Further, there is a higher prevalence of impairment for people born in a non-English-speaking country and aged over 45 years of age, especially for first-wave NES migrants, up to three times that of the Australian-born population. While all people with disability face barriers to social participation—access to employment, technology, social activity, and economic well-being—people from non-English-speaking countries are likely to face greater forms of marginalization (NEDA, 2013). NEDA identifies numerous challenges for culturally diverse communities, including access to services, appropriate services, communication, self-advocacy issues, support for carers, and social exclusion and discrimination (NEDA, 2013, 2014).
- The mental health of immigrants deteriorates after one year spent in the country, although prevalence levels vary across different groups (Chou, 2007). Several factors have been found to be associated with increased risk of mental disorder among immigrants, including limited English proficiency, separated cultural identity, loss of close family ties, lack of opportunity to make effective use of occupational skills, trauma exposure prior to migration (especially for refugees), and the many stresses associated with migration and adjustment to a new country (Minas et al., 2013). The National Mental Health Survey conducted in 2007 (the latest substantive study) found that the overseas-born had lower rates of mental disorders than the Australian-born, including anxiety disorders (11.6 percent of overseas-born compared to 15.4 percent of Australian-born); affective disorders (5.1 percent compared to 6.6 percent); and substance-use disorders (2.8 percent compared to 6 percent) (ABS, 2008, p. 5). Additionally, discrimination experienced by migrants and refugees contributes to depression, poor quality of life, psychological distress, and substance misuse (VicHealth, 2008). For refugees two consistent risk factors are linked to mental disorders: past trauma and post-migration stress. Research

studies have found that post-migration issues—such as socio-economic disadvantage, lack of social support, experiences of discrimination, as well as issues such as unemployment, lack of language fluency, housing, loneliness, culture shock, intergenerational and gender role issues—all contribute to anxiety, depression, and feelings of social isolation among resettled refugees (Correa-Velez, Spaaij, & Upham, 2012; Fozdar & Hartley, 2013).

- Access and equity in health care is a major issue. The Access and Equity Inquiry (FECCA, 2012) identified that greater access to preventative health care and mental health services was needed, pointing out that these services are virtually unavailable to those CALD individuals who cannot afford to pay for them. As has been the case in previous years, consultation participants were concerned with the level of cultural sensitivity and competence within the health care system, and called for more bicultural workers, more extensive use of interpreters, and provision of culturally and linguistically appropriate health care information. Temporary work visa and sponsored visa holders were identified as being at a particular disadvantage in relation to accessing health care services in Australia, and geographical location was identified as having a bearing on the availability of services (FECCA, 2012, p. 41). Access to health care for temporary visa holders and asylum-seekers has been one of the major social justice issues that have emerged in Australia in the last decade.

Health outcomes are often higher for those who have entered in skill streams than from those in family reunification or humanitarian (refugee) streams. The Department of Immigration has conducted the Longitudinal Survey of Immigrants to Australia (LSIA) in three cohorts: September 1993 and August 1995, September 1999 and August 2000, and December 2004 and March 2005 (Sevoyan & Hugo, 2013). The distribution of health outcomes by the type of visa shows that overall the humanitarian migrants score worse on all health outcomes. The authors found that the percentage of humanitarian migrants who reported having a medical condition since migration was about 16 percent compared to 10 percent among family visa holders and 7 percent across skilled immigrant groups.

About half of humanitarian visa holders needed to see a doctor during the last four weeks compared to less than 30 percent of those among skilled migrants and less than 40 percent among family visa holders. The status of mental health of migrants reveals comparable outcomes: the average score on the mental health scale (where higher score signifies worse mental health condition) is higher than 12 among humanitarian migrants, whereas family and skilled immigrant visa holders score from 8 to 9 on average (Sevoyan & Hugo, 2013, p. 11).

Multicultural Health Policy and Culturally Dynamic Health Services

The World Health Organization states that "Health services need to embrace an expanded mandate which is sensitive and respects cultural needs. This mandate should support the needs of individuals and communities for a healthier life, and open channels between the health sector and broader social, political, economic and physical environmental components" (WHO, 2014, p. 1).

The World Health Assembly in 2008 passed a Resolution on the Health of Migrants, which stressed the urgency and importance of understanding immigrant health and seeking equal health rights for migrants, and urged governments to promote immigrant health policies, considering, among other things, the multidimensional effect of migration on health and the increased vulnerability of certain immigrant groups to health risks (WHA, 2008). Public health providers have acknowledged that current models for health service delivery to CALD communities are quite limited (Prasad-Ildes & Ramirez, 2006).

Australian health care systems have an obligation to provide health care to all Australians, and the Charter of Healthcare Rights is built upon the principles of human rights and social justice, namely, access, safety, respect, communication, participation, and privacy. Although the Charter is strong on rights, it is silent on issues of culturally appropriate care. It may be argued that these rights can incorporate notions of culture in care, but this is not explicitly stated in the Charter, so in reality this requires strong advocacy on the part of the patient (Gill & Babacan, 2012). The systemic disadvantages that many immigrants continue to face prevent them from advocating for themselves effectively in health systems. The problems are exacerbated in public health systems due to the cutback in funding for health systems across Australia. Therefore, disparities based on ethnicity, culture, "race," and other factors persist at unacceptably high levels (AHRQ, 2011).

Studies also indicate that immigrant patients are not receiving the same level of health care in terms of diagnosis, treatment, and preventative services as the average population (Johnstone & Kanitsaki, 2006). Other research on patient safety points to adverse events affecting patients from minority backgrounds more frequently, often caused by communication problems, misdiagnosis, and inadvertent errors (Babacan & Gopalkrishnan, 2015). Bischoff (2006) identifies a range of areas of risk for ethnic minorities, including diagnostic testing, medication, pain management, medical follow-up, longer stays in hospital, problems with admission, infection, referral, preparation, complaints, and reporting and participation. More recent studies have identified the impact of racial discrimination on health outcomes and the ways in which these are institutionalized in health care systems (Barraclough & Gardner, 2008; Paradies et al., 2013). More proactive and culturally appropriate services have been advocated. However, the capacity and success of various entities to accomplish real change in achieving a culturally responsive health care service is mixed and patchy. The authors argue that underpinning this response are unacknowledged layers of resistance to the principles and practices of cultural diversity due to new racisms and the invisibility of racism. Also there is the lack of hard data on health disparities demonstrating the experiences that front-line service delivery organizations observe (Johnstone & Kanitsaki, 2007a, b).

The policy responses to improve the responsiveness and effectiveness of health services to Australia's multicultural population have mainly come from state and federal governments. The federal government in Australia has not had a multicultural health policy since the 1990s, although there are multicultural strategies in specific health areas such as mental health and aging. The various state jurisdictions, on the other hand, have been active in policy articulation with policy statements about multicultural health that espouse cultural diversity, access and equity, justice and pluralism. It has been pointed out that no matter how progressive these policies are, they still remain tokenistic as they preserve institutional inequality. Key areas of deficiency focus on under-resourcing of cultural diversity services in health care, cultural skills of health professionals, inadequacy of credentialed language services, and inflexible systems unable to respond to different patient needs (Barraclough & Gardner, 2008; Gill & Babacan, 2012; Johnstone & Kanitsaki, 2007a, b).

Cultural competence has been widely promoted as a way for health care providers and organizations to respond effectively to the cultural and linguistic needs that patients bring to the health care encounter (USDHHS, 2001). One definition of cultural competence is offered by Tong and Cross (1991, p. 12) as "a set of congruent behaviours, attitudes and policies that come together in a system, agency or among professionals and enable that system, agency or those professionals to work effectively in cross-cultural situations." Cultural competence has been criticized for vagueness and inappropriateness of the term, objectification and static views of culture and ethnicity, lack of attention to the intersection of cultural factors with structural dimensions, and the mutual meaning-making between health practitioner and patient (Gopalkrishnan, 2014; Napier et al., 2014; Wight, 2012). To address this critique, alternatives are emerging, such as cultural safety and culturally dynamic partnerships. Policy initiatives clearly need to incorporate notions of establishing culturally safe spaces for cross-cultural interactions, the dynamic and changing nature of cultures, and collaboration and partnership as the basis of working across cultures in health care (Gopalkrishnan, 2014; NACCHO, 2011; Skellet, 2012; Williams, 1999).

Discussion

Immigration programs continue to gain support from governments in Australia, although the processes of immigrant settlement have undergone considerable curtailment. Some analysts view the election of the Howard government in 1996 as the end of Australian multiculturalism and the beginning of a post-multiculturalism period in Australia (Jupp, 2011, p. 47). However, multiculturalism has never been formally abandoned in Australia and it has survived, albeit with less resourcing and less enthusiasm than in its heyday and is undermined by the growing influence of economic rationalism and neo-liberalism in Australian government policy and institutional dynamics (Collins, 2013). The retreat from multiculturalism and lesser resourcing has resulted in the loss of multicultural infrastructure and staff in institutions. There has been a deliberate but silent thrust toward mainstreaming. Mainstreaming is the process of assessing the implications for minorities of any planned action, including legislation, policies, or programs, in any area and at all levels, but embedding it in the core business of an institution. The ultimate goal of mainstreaming is essentially the achievement of equality (UN, 2002) and appears aspirational. However, in adopting a mainstreaming approach, ethno-specific units, cultural brokers, and specific initiatives have been abandoned in the policy and program development processes, and the checks and balances to implement multiculturalism in the core business of the institution have been mostly ignored. Babacan and Gopalkrishnan (2015) have argued that mainstreaming has resulted in the marginalization of ethnic minorities in key areas, including lack of integration in service delivery, lack of resources for diversity initiatives, lack of consumer participation, lack of systemic change, and lack of cultural competencies of professionals. The key reason for these failures is the lack of whole-of-agency approaches and the failure to embed cultural responsiveness into governance and management processes.

Although Australia's multiculturalism record is heralded as a success story, Herscovitch and Bal (2011, p. 6) remind us that "despite much progress having been made, Australia is by no means an unqualified multicultural success story." The authors argue that there is persistent racism experienced by migrants in daily life. They also argue that minorities of non-Anglo Saxon/Celtic backgrounds feel they are not accepted as Australians, and the sense of alienation is particularly acute because the connection between the culture, ethnicity, religion, and language of Australia's Anglo-Celtic, Christian, English-speaking majority and Australian national identity is often made in the public arena. This is borne out in the social cohesion surveys conducted where in 2013 there was a marked shift: the proportion indicating that they have a sense of belonging dropped to 65 percent from 75 percent (Markus, 2013, p. 2).

Negative discourses on multiculturalism, immigration, asylum-seekers, and the war on terror has led to the "*old racism*" (where ethnic communities were viewed as inferior) being largely replaced by the "*new racism*" (also termed "cultural racism," where ethnic communities are differentiated as being a "threat to the cultural integrity" of the Anglo-Celtic host society) (Dunn et al., 2004). Essentially the key element of "old racism"—the so-called "incompatibility" of different ethnic groups and their "inability" to co-exist—remains as an integral aspect of "new racism" (Corlett, 2002). Fear has been used to conduct racialized discourse that casts particular groups as threats (Gopalkrishnan, 2013a). All along discourses have been couched in liberal and egalitarian tropes that position the speaker as rational, fair-minded, and non-prejudiced (Mitchell, Every, & Ranzin, 2011). Such constructions legitimize current inequalities by "blaming the victims" while evading any responsibility and can convey racist views without seemingly being racist. In this way racism and its denial are reproduced in everyday contexts by ordinary members of the majority group (Babacan & Gopalkrishnan, 2011; Mitchell et al., 2011).

Australia arguably has one of the best health systems in the world, but it continues to contribute to health inequities (Friel, 2009). Friel posits that health care systems have been principally concerned with delivery of clinical care and focused on quick wins on medical targets (e.g., waiting times). Poor health care outcomes for ethnic communities are attributed to factors that are beyond the control of care providers—such as individual factors or largely inaccessible cultural systems of value. Others have advocated for culturally sensitive systems and believe multiculturalism has failed to deliver outcomes (Napier et al., 2014). They strongly argue that the failure to recognize the intersection of culture with other structural and societal factors creates and compounds poor health. While cost cutting and targeting has been a focus of neo-liberal governments, the business case for cultural diversity is well established. Not taking into account culturally responsiveness systems will continue to perpetuate health inequities and also multiply financial costs of health care in the long run.

Implications for Immigration and Other Public Policy

Diversity policies are often used as evidence in institutional settings to show that institutions do not have a problem with inclusion. Ahmed (2012) offers accounts from diversity practitioners' experiences of institutions resistant to their work, as captured through their use of the metaphor of the "brick wall." She identifies that there is a gap between symbolic commitments to diversity and the experience of those who embody diversity. In the process racism can be obscured by the institutionalization of diversity. The tendency to use a deficit model of diversity devalues people and reinforces the view of the mainstream population that culturally diverse people are a liability. There is an urgent need to shift away from this model to one that focuses on empowerment and the harnessing and fostering of social networks (Fozdar & Hartley, 2013, p. 49).

Special attention must be paid to the mechanisms of mainstreaming, which render CALD communities invisible in the policy and program delivery processes. The debates about universality versus particularity need to be revisited, as treating everyone the same does not produce equal outcomes, while appearing to be uniform and fair. On the other hand, particular targeting with a narrow focus withers away institutional mechanisms for social inclusion and social justice along the social gradient. Arguments for differentiated universalism recognize a heterogeneous public, and differences such as gender and ethnicity are publicly considered in policy (Kane & Hudson, 2000). Additionally, non-citizens, non-residents, or asylum-seekers are deliberately excluded from nation-state membership, resulting in discrimination against the "other" (McMaster, 2001, p. 161). Friel (2009) argues that a social gradient approach is required so that it can capture the needs of people at different levels. Only by taking such an approach can there be recognition in policies and procedures of the complex needs of participants from CALD backgrounds (NEDA, 2013).

Policy development is not a neutral process and is based on a set of values and principles. Australia is a signatory to many international human rights covenants and declarations. The Attorney General's Department inquiry into human rights identified numerous legislation, policies, and practices that do not adequately reflect human rights considerations or do not fully implement Australia's international human rights obligations, including a federal anti-discrimination framework that does not protect a right of equality or take account of all possible areas of discrimination; national security legislation that reflects an improper balance between the need to protect the community from harm and the need to safeguard individual liberties; and an immigration framework that permits the indefinite detention of people (AHRC, 2012). The gap in Australian policy-making needs to be bridged, creating mechanisms to ensure that human rights are taken into account in reviewing or making policies and legislation. There is public support for this approach, as in a national survey in 2009, overwhelming responses were received with 90 percent of respondents believing parliament should pay attention to human rights when making laws and 85 percent believing governments should pay attention to human rights when they enact laws and policies (CBSR, 2009). Strengthening rights-based approaches is critical in realizing equitable outcomes for immigrants in Australia.

There are major barriers for culturally diverse communities in achieving equitable health outcomes. In relation to health policy, it has been argued by the peak ethnic communities body, FECCA, that the Ottawa Charter for Health Promotion—building healthy public policy, creating supportive environments, strengthening community actions, developing personal skills, reorienting health services, and moving into the future—are of fundamental importance, and should be considered during the formulation of any health policy (FECCA, 2009). However, the constraints on being able to respond in a culturally sensitive manner was identified by the Department of Health and included: varying levels of diversity knowledge and understanding of cultural competence in health service settings; absence of a whole-of-organization approach to delivering culturally responsive services; insufficient alignment between risk management, patient safety, quality-improvement initiatives, and cultural responsiveness; a lack of integration of cultural diversity knowledge with practical strategies for patient-centred care; challenges in managing the multiple planning and reporting requirements for cultural diversity; and absence of clearly specified cultural diversity standards, indicators and benchmarks, and effective assessment tools to measure performance (DOH, 2009).

While expressions of racism, on the main, have changed from overt to covert forms, they nevertheless prevail (Babacan, Babacan, & Gopalkrishnan, 2009; Hollinsworth, 2006). This is further exacerbated by the state positioning itself as "raceless" when in fact it reflects the dominant society norms (Babacan, 1996). Although racism appears contrary to democratic societal values, racism can still be articulated without denouncing democratic principles and, through transformation into more palatable concerns, becomes legitimate concern (Henry, Tator, Mattis, & Rees, 2000). For example, in the context of Australia, Johnson (2000, pp. 64–65) argues that the discourse of nationalism can cover a hidden racist discourse through establishing who and what is Australian and un-Australian, and that "ordinary Australians are not Aboriginal, Asian, homosexual, lesbian, feminist or migrant."

Any policy-making process needs to come to terms with racism and discrimination and needs to recognize that ethnicity/culture-based discrimination is a common challenge with far-reaching health, mental health, social, and economic consequences for individuals and communities (Gridley, 2011). The ramifications of racism for health include reduced and unequal access to societal and health resources, increased exposure to risk factors associated with ill health, stress, and negative emotions contributing to ill mental health, which adversely affects immune, endocrine, and cardiovascular systems; and negative behaviours such as alcohol or substance use (Paradies, Harris, & Anderson, 2008).

Policy frameworks need to be pluralistic and socially inclusive. They need to accommodate different conceptualizations of the individual. Policies need to be less focused on the individual and better able to accommodate the value of the collective and community because for many individuals, well-being outcomes are closely linked with family, kinship, and community (Friel, 2009).

Finally, policy formulation and implementation are not separate but intrinsically linked to implementation. There needs to be appropriate resourcing of implementation, monitoring, accountability, and management systems. This can be achieved through a "stewardship model of government," particularly system stewardship. This implies that although the nature and outcomes of a policy are often adapted by many different actors working together in a system, stewardship involves policy-makers overseeing the ways in which the policy is being adapted, and attempting to steer the system toward certain outcomes across the whole of government (Hallsworth, 2011). The improvements in policy-making will need to be across four areas: processes, qualities, structures, and politics (Kidson, 2013). The Joint Standing Committee on Migration recommended (Recommendation 11) that the Charter of Public Service in a Culturally Diverse Society (a charter adopted by the federal government for the public service) be reviewed and brought up to date and set benchmarks against which access and equity provision is measured (APH, 2013). In health, this will require systematic consideration of the health effects of all government policies on CALD communities.

Conclusion

Australia is recognized as a "successful" settler society with a culturally diverse population base. Multiculturalism in contemporary Australia is focusing on social cohesion and individual forms of diversity with emphasis on individual lifestyle rather than group rights or human rights. It is continuing to evolve in paradoxical ways. On the one hand, there is bipartisan support for a multicultural Australia. On the other hand, there are wavering government and opposition responses to key issues relating to multiculturalism that confront the nation, such as the rights of asylum-seekers, the policy of mandatory detention, and the targeting of particular communities in the war on terror. A climate of concern over safety and security has been created that has impacted very negatively on particular groups of people. The adoption of a "protective framework" has been accompanied by an erosion of civil liberties, freedoms, and human rights, which were traditionally associated with Western democracies. Groups or individuals (e.g., youth, asylum-seekers, refugees, immigrants) who were once considered as being *at risk* and considered as requiring the support of the state are now portrayed as groups/individuals who are *a risk* to society (McCulloch, 2006).

A nation's identity is defined through ethnicity and civic culture and the nation-state plays a critical role in creating a collective consciousness for those who live within its borders (Anderson, 1983). The nation-state is a multi-layered system of governance, characterized by structures, processes, and policies, and the "imagined political community" is given shape by societal institutions (Carter, 2006). The Australian nation-state, in the post–September 11 era, has focused on "social cohesion" and this has become an important element of public debate and policy discourses (Cheong, Edwards, Goulbourne, & Solomos, 2007). This discourse relies heavily on threats posed by cultural, religious, and ethnic diversity. Cultural diversity is increasingly interpreted as a security problem and the practices of prejudice, punishment, control, and suspicion in relation to immigrants characterize public policies (Sales, 2005).

This is highly problematic from a policy perspective as it fails to provide appropriate frameworks for immigrant integration. A key part of integration relates to health outcomes for immigrants, who enter with good health, which deteriorates over time, exacerbated by the challenges of settlement and integration.

The nation-state is and will continue to be a key reference point for citizenship rights and delivery of entitlements. Addressing health disparities will require strong multicultural policies that work across government portfolios. Given the social determinants of health and culturally diverse population demographics, there is now, more than ever, a need for strong policy leadership on multiculturalism. This requires engagement with the politics of recognition and respect for difference. As Jakubowicz and Monani (2010, p. 22) note, "respect for difference does not require endorsement of different values; core values that speak of democracy, freedom, tolerance and opportunity are transcultural, and are the necessary framework for ensuring harmonious social relations."

The nation-state is a contradictory set of relations, institutions, regulations, and apparatuses. It is an arena of struggle and a site of contestation between many conflicting forces in society (Kenny, 2011). Various power relationships within the Australian state can influence the directions and policies of the state, conferring advantage to some and disadvantage to others. The policy domain for multiculturalism will continue to be one of struggle and negotiation in which the paradoxes of reconciling expressions of difference with those of needing to defend unity of the nation-state will play out (Jayasuriya, 2007). Vasta (2007) suggests four prerequisites for expanded multiculturalism:

- mutual accommodation—mutual recognition of core values, differences, and repositioning of social cohesion;
- multiculturalism that embraces the whole society—it should not refer only to minorities;
- equality and full participation; and
- racism—engaging with racism/racial discrimination as a fundamental social phenomenon deeply rooted in the histories, cultures, traditions, and institutions of Western democracies (2007, pp. 25–26).

Multiculturalism not only entails rights for minorities but also deeply concerns societal values and the nature of the society that Australia needs to build. If Australia is to make progress, the current emphasis on policies based on economic rationalist and neo-liberal agendas need to be replaced with a more inclusive multiculturalism that is based on human rights, citizenship, and social justice. To conclude, "We have a responsibility to negotiate and to form practices which are able to deal with difference, since there will always be difference, while trying to remedy the gross inequalities experienced by different groups" (Hall, 1996, p. 17).

Critical Thinking Questions

1. What are the factors that contribute to the healthy immigrant effect in Australia?
2. How can policies of multiculturalism contribute to the improvement of immigrant health in Australia?
3. How can health policies change to reflect the cultural diversity of the population of Australia?
4. What strategies can be adopted to improve cultural responsiveness of health systems and professionals?
5. What role does the nation-state play in immigrant health?

Glossary

Culturally and linguistically diverse (CALD) is commonly used to describe people with a cultural heritage different from that of the majority of people from the dominant Anglo-Australian culture.

Ethnicity is a social construct of group affiliation and identity. An ethnic group is a social group whose members share a sense of common origins; claim a common and distinctive history and destiny; possess one or more dimensions of collective cultural individuality; and feel a sense of unique collective solidarity.

Multiculturalism is (1) a term to describe the cultural and ethnic diversity of a population; (2) a policy of government measures to respond to cultural and ethnic diversity of a population; and (3) an approach in which society values cultural diversity.

Non-English-speaking background (NESB) has been replaced by the term "culturally and linguistically diverse" (CALD).

Racism is a belief that a particular "race," ethnicity, or culture is inferior or superior to others. It represents a pattern of unfair treatment, justified by belief in inferiority of "race," culture, or ethnicity. It is expressed in interactions between individuals and institutions and intends to maintain privileges for members of dominant groups.

Recommended Readings

Babacan, H., & Gopalkrishnan, N. (2015). Integration of ethnic minority groups in healthcare governance. In E. Kuhlmann, R. H. Blank, I. L. Bourgeault, & C. Wendt (Eds.),

International handbook of healthcare policy and governance (pp. 615–630). Basingstoke, UK: Palgrave Macmillan.

This chapter places a cultural diversity lens on health and provides critical analysis of health care policy and governance in Australia.

Collins, J. (2013). Multiculturalism and immigrant integration in Australia. *Canadian Ethnic Studies Journal, 45*(3), 133–49.

This article provides a theoretical and factual analysis of the extent to which immigrants are integrated into economic, social, cultural, and political life in Australia and how successful Australian multiculturalism has been in achieving the objective of immigrant integration.

Hollinsworth, D. (2006). *Race and racism in Australia* (3rd ed.). South Melbourne: Social Science Press.

This book provides an overview of theoretical, historical, and contemporary issues relating to racism in Australia. It is used as a standard text in many university courses and offers a comprehensive exploration of the issues relating to old and new forms of racism.

Jakubowicz, A., & Ho, C. (2013). *"For those who've come across the seas..." Australian multicultural theory, policy, and practice.* North Melbourne: Australian Scholarly Publishing.

This book provides a comprehensive examination of Australian immigration and multiculturalism in the context of a range of policy and practice issues.

Johnstone, M., & Kanitsaki, O. (2008). The problem of failing to provide culturally and linguistically appropriate healthcare. In S. Barraclough and H. Gardner (Eds.), *Analysing health policy: A problem oriented approach* (pp. 176–87). Marrickville: Elsevier.

This chapter provides a detailed examination of health policy-making in Australia and provides an appraisal of the policy process and policy actors.

Related Websites

Australian Human Rights Commission—https://www.humanrights.gov.au

This website for the main human rights body in Australia has numerous resources on racism, other forms of discrimination, and multiculturalism.

Australian Institute of Health and Welfare—http://www.aihw.gov.au

The Institute was established to report on the state of health and welfare in Australia. It provides important health and welfare statistics and research.

Centre for Culture, Ethnicity and Health—http://www.ceh.org.au/
A non-governmental agency providing expertise in cross-cultural health to assist agencies to meet the health needs of migrants and refugees, the Centre has a good resource base with tools, publications, and other useful materials.

Department of Immigration and Border Protection—www.immi.gov.au
The Department is the main federal government agency for immigration and multiculturalism. The website has numerous useful research publications, fact sheets, and statistics.

Immigrant Health Service, Royal Children's Hospital, Melbourne—http://www.rch.org.au/immigranthealth/research/Research_resources/
This is a clearing house for refugee health research in Australia that provides numerous articles on refugee health, classified by subject headings and linked to PubMed or ERIC abstract.

References

ABS. (2008). *Health literacy.* Canberra: Australian Bureau of Statistics.

ABS. (2012). *Cultural diversity in Australia: Reflecting nation-stories from the 2011 census.* Canberra: Australian Bureau of Statistics. Retrieved from http://www.abs.gov.au/ausstats/abs@.nsf/lookup/2071.0main+features902012–2013

ABS. (2013). *2011 census of population and housing.* Canberra: Australian Bureau of Statistics. Retrieved from http://www.abs.gov.au/ausstats/abs@.nsf/lookup/2071.0main+features902012–2013

ABS. (2014). *Characteristics of recent migrants.* Retrieved from http://www.abs.gov.au/ausstats/abs@.nsf/Latestproducts/6250.0Main%20Features2Nov%202013?opendocument&tabname=Summary&prodno=6250.0&issue=Nov%202013&num=&view=

ACOSS. (2012). *Poverty in Australia.* ACOSS Paper 194. Strawberry Hills: Australian Council of Social Service.

ACOSS. (2013). *Australian community sector survey, 2013.* Strawberry Hills: Australian Council of Social Service. Retrieved from http://www.acoss.org.au/images/uploads/Australian_Community_Sector_Survey_2013_ACOSS.pdf

Adelman, H., Borowski, A., Burstein, M., & Foster, L. (1994). *Immigration and refugee policy: Australia and Canada compared.* Melbourne: Melbourne University Press.

Ahmed, S. (2012). *On being included: Racism and diversity in institutional life.* Durham, NC: Duke University Press.

AHRC. (2012). *Gender equality blueprint 2010.* Retrieved from http://www.hreoc.gov.au/sex_discrimination/publication/blueprint/index.html

AHRQ. (2011). *National healthcare disparities report, 2011.* Rockville: Agency for Healthcare Research and Quality, U.S. Department of Health and Human Services. Retrieved from http://www.ahrq.gov/research/findings/nhqrdr/nhdr11/nhdr11.pdf

AIHW. (2005). *Diabetes in culturally and linguistically diverse Australians: Identification of communities at high risk.* Canberra: Australian Institute of Health and Welfare.

AIHW. (2011). *Australia's welfare 2011.* Cat. no. AUS 142. Canberra: Australian Institute of Health and Welfare. Retrieved from http://www.aihw.gov.au/publication-detail/?id=10737420537

AIHW. (2013). *Specialist homelessness services: 2012–2013.* Cat. no. HOU 2. Canberra: Australian Institute of Health and Welfare.

AIHW. (2014). *Mortality inequalities in Australia 2009–2011.* Bulletin no. 124. Canberra: Australian Institute of Health and Welfare.

Anderson, A. S., Bush, H., Lean, M., Bradby, H., Williams, R., & Lea, E. (2005). Evolution of atherogenic diets in South Asian and Italian women after migration to a higher risk region. *Journal of Human Nutrition Dietetics, 18*(1), 33–43.

Anderson, B. (1983). *Imagined communities: Reflections on the origins and spread of nationalism.* London: Verso.

Anikeeva, O., Bi, P., Hiller, J. E., Ryan, P., Roder, D., & Han, G. S. (2010). Review paper: The health status of migrants in Australia: A review. *Asia-Pacific Journal of Public Health, 22*(2), 159–93.

APH. (2013). *Inquiry into migration and multiculturalism in Australia.* Canberra: Joint Standing Committee on Migration, The Parliament of the Commonwealth of Australia.

Babacan, A., & Babacan, H. (2009). *Seeking asylum in a global world: A comparative analysis of refugee and asylum seeker citizenship rights, laws, and policies in Australia, Canada, and New Zealand.* Saarbrücken, Germany: VDM Verlag Dr Muller Publications.

Babacan, H. (1996). The Kurds—who are they? Establishing Kurdish identity in Victoria. In T. Dalton, M. Draper, W. Weeks, & J. Wiseman (Eds.), *Making social policy in Australia* (pp. 154–66). Sydney: Allen and Unwin.

Babacan, H. (2006). Locating identity: Sense of space, place, and belonging. *International Journal of Diversity in Organisations, Communities and Nations, 5*(5), 113–24.

Babacan, H., & Babacan, A. (2007). Sustaining human security. *The International Journal of Environmental, Cultural, Economic and Social Sustainability, 3*(1), 115–22.

Babacan, H., Babacan, A., & Gopalkrishnan, N. (2009). *Situating racism: The local, national, and the global.* Cambridge: Cambridge Scholars' Publishing.

Babacan, H., & Ben-Moshe, D. (2009). *Victorian multicultural policy, valuing diversity.* Discussion Paper. Melbourne: Victorian Multicultural Commission and Institute for Community, Policy and Community Engagement (ICEPA), Victoria University.

Babacan, H., & Gopalkrishnan, N. (2008). Racism and asylum seeker policies. In L. Briskman & A. Babacan (Eds.), *Asylum seekers: International perspectives on interdiction and deterrence* (pp. 143–57). Cambridge: Cambridge Scholars' Publishing.

Babacan, H., & Gopalkrishnan, N. (2011). Creating belonging: Safety, racism, and social cohesion. In A. Babacan & H. Tahiri (Eds.), *Community safety in multicultural Australia: Counter terrorism, social cohesion, and belonging* (pp. 99–116). Cambridge: Cambridge Scholars' Publishing.

Babacan, H., & Gopalkrishnan, N. (2015). Integration of ethnic minority groups in healthcare governance. In E. Kuhlmann, R. H. Blank, I. L. Bourgeault, & C. Wendt (Eds.), *International handbook of healthcare policy and governance.* London: Palgrave Publishers.

Babacan, H., & Herrmann, P. (2013). Nation state, social cohesion, and cultural diversity. In H. Babacan & P. Herrmann (Eds.), *Diversity and the state* (pp. 19–37). New York: Nova Science Publishers.

Babacan, H., & Hollinsworth, D. (2009). *Confronting racism in communities project: A final report on the nature and extent of racism in Queensland.* Brisbane: Centre for Multicultural Pastoral Care.

Barraclough, S., & Gardner, H. (2008). *Analysing health policy: A problem-oriented approach.* Marrickville: Elsevier Science.

Beer, A., & Foley, P. (2003). *Housing need and provision for recently arrived refugees in Australia.* Melbourne: Australian Housing and Urban Research Institute, Southern Research Centre.

Biddle, N., Kennedy, S., & McDonald, J. D. (2007). Health assimilation patterns amongst Australian immigrants. *The Economic Record, 83*(260), 16–30.

Bischoff, A. (2006). *Caring for migrant and minority patients in European hospitals: A review of effective interventions* (vol. 43). Neuchâtel and Basel: Swiss Forum for Migration and Population Studies.

Borooah, V., & Mangan, J. (2007). Love thy neighbour: How much bigotry is there in Western countries? *Kyklos, 60*(3), 295–317.

Briskman, L. (2011). *Australia's wake up call from the UN: Yes, we're a racist country.* Swinburne University Research Bank. Retrieved from http://researchbank.swinburne.edu.au/vital/access/manager/Repository/swin:28174

Carter, D. (2006). *Dispossession, dreams, and diversity: Issues in Australian studies.* Frenchs Forest: Pearson Education Australia.

Castles, S., Vasta, E., & Ozkul, D. (2012). *The internal dynamics of migration processes and their consequences for Australian government migration policies.* Working Paper for the Department of Immigration and Citizenship. Sydney: University of Sydney.

CBSR. (2009). *National human rights consultation—community research phase.* Canberra: Colmar Brunton Social Research—Attorney General's Department.

Cheong, P. H., Edwards, R., Goulbourne, H., & Solomos, J. (2007). Immigration, social capital, and social cohesion: A critical review. *Critical Social Policy, 27*(1), 24–49.

Chou, K. L. (2007). Psychological distress in migrants in Australia over 50 years old: A longitudinal investigation. *Journal of Affective Disorders, 98*(1–2), 99–108.

Colagiuri, R., Thomas, M., & Buckley, A. (2007). *Preventing type 2 diabetes in culturally and linguistically diverse communities in NSW.* Sydney: NSW Department of Health.

Colic-Peisker, V., & Tilbury, F. (2005). *Refugees and employment: The effects of visible difference on discrimination.* Perth: Centre for Social and Community Research, Murdoch University.

Collins, J. (1991). *Migrant hands in a distant land* (2nd ed.). Leichhardt: Pluto Press.

Collins, J. (2013). Rethinking Australian immigration and immigrant settlement policy. *Journal of Intercultural Studies, 34*(2), 160–77.

Corlett, D. (2002). Asylum seekers and the new racism. *Dissent, 8*(Autumn–Winter), 46–47.

Correa-Velez, I., Spaaij, R., & Upham, S. (2012). "We are not here to claim better services than any other": Social exclusion among men from refugee backgrounds in urban and regional Australia. *Journal of Refugee Studies, 26*(2), 163–86.

Dawes, G., & Gopalkrishnan, N. (2014). *Far North Queensland culturally and linguistically diverse communities (CALD) homelessness project.* Cairns: James Cook University.

DIAC. (2006). *Fact sheet 2—Key facts in immigration*. Canberra: Department of Immigration and Citizenship.

DIAC. (2010). *How new migrants fare: Analysis of the continuous survey of Australia's migrants*. Canberra: Department of Immigration and Citizenship. Retrieved from http://www.immi.gov.au/media/publications/research/_pdf/csam-results-2010.pdf

DIAC. (2011). *Migrant economic outcomes and contributions*. Canberra: Department of Immigration and Citizenship. Retrieved from http://www.immi.gov.au/media/publications/research/_pdf/outcomes-contributions-apr11.pdf

DIAC. (2013). *Overseas students in Australia*. DIAC Fact Sheet 50. Canberra: Department of Immigration and Citizenship. Retrieved from http://www.immi.gov.au/media/fact-sheets/50students.htm

DIBP. (2014a). *The place of migrants in contemporary Australia: A summary report*. Canberra: Department of Immigration and Border Protection. Retrieved from http://www.immi.gov.au/pub-res/Documents/research/migrants-contemporary-australia.pdf

DIBP. (2014b). *Setting the migration program for 2015–2016*. Discussion Paper. Canberra: Department of Immigration and Border Protection. Retrieved from https://www.immi.gov.au/pub-res/Documents/discussion-papers/Migration-Programme-2015–16-Discussion-Paper.pdf

DIMA. (2001). *Immigration: Federation to century's end*. Canberra: Department of Immigration & Multicultural Affairs. Retrieved from http://www.immi.gov.au/media/publications/statistics/federation/

DOH. (2009). *Cultural responsiveness framework: Guidelines for Victorian health services*. Melbourne: Department of Health, Victoria Government. Retrieved from http://www.health.vic.gov.au/cald/cultural-responsiveness-framework

Dunn, K., Forrest, J., Burnley, I., & McDonald, A. (2004). Constructing racism in Australia. *Australian Journal of Social Issues, 39*(4), 409–30.

Dunn, K. M., & Nelson, J. K. (2011). Challenging the public denial of racism for a deeper multiculturalism. *Journal of Intercultural Studies, 32*(6), 587–602.

Essed, P. (2002). Everyday racism. In D. Goldberg & J. Solomos (Eds.), *A companion to racial and ethnic studies* (pp. 202–16). Oxford: Blackwell Publishers.

FECCA. (2009). Submission to the National Women's Health Policy. Curtin: Federation of Ethnic Communities Council of Australia.

FECCA. (2012). *Opening the door to access and equity: FECCA access and equity report 2011–2012*. Curtin: Federation of Ethnic Communities Council of Australia.

Ferguson & Associates. (1994). *Mission possible: An overview of literature on issues for young people from non-English speaking backgrounds in Queensland*. Brisbane, Australia: Working Party.

Forrest, J., Hermes, K., Johnston, R., & Poulsen, M. (2012). The housing resettlement experience of refugee immigrants to Australia. *Journal of Refugee Studies, 26*(2), 187–206.

Fozdar, F., & Hartley, L. (2013). Refugee resettlement in Australia: What we know and need to know. *Refugee Survey Quarterly, 32*(3), 23–51.

Fozdar, F., & Torezani, S. (2008). Discrimination and well-being: Perceptions of refugees in Western Australia. *International Migration Review, 42*(1), 30–63.

Friel, S. (2009). *Health equity in Australia: A policy framework based on action on the social determinants of obesity, alcohol, and tobacco.* Canberra: The Australian National Preventative Health Taskforce.

Galbally, F. (1978). *Review of post arrival programs and services for migrants, migrant services, and programs.* Canberra: Australian Government Publishing Service.

Gee, G. C., & Ford, C. L. (2011). Structural racism and health inequalities. *Du Bois Review: Social Science Research on Race, 8*(1), 115–32.

Gill, G., & Babacan, H. (2012). Developing a cultural responsiveness framework in healthcare systems: An Australian example. *Journal of Diversity and Equality in Health and Care, 9*(1), 45–56.

Gopalkrishnan, N. (2006). Globalization, migration, and fear of the "other." *Proceedings of the International Conference on Racisms in the New World Order* (pp. 136–42). Maroochydore: University of the Sunshine Coast.

Gopalkrishnan, N. (2013a). CALD communities and racism in times of crisis. *Mosaic, 31,* 1–4.

Gopalkrishnan, N. (2013b). From covert to overt: The role of crisis in transforming racism. In N. Gopalkrishnan & H. Babacan (Eds.), *Proceedings of the third International Conference on Racisms in the New World Order: Realities of culture, colour, and identity* (pp. 95–105). Cairns: James Cook University.

Gopalkrishnan, N. (2014). Building resilient communities through culturally dynamic partnerships. *International Journal of Social Work and Human Services Practice, 2*(6), 220–27.

Gridley, H. (2011). *The Australian Psychological Society submission to the Joint Standing Committee on Migration, inquiry into the economic, social, and cultural impacts of migration to Australia.* Melbourne: The Australian Psychological Society.

Gushalak, B. (2007). Healthier on arrival? Further into the "healthy immigrant effect." *Canadian Medical Association Journal, 176*(10), 1439–40.

Gutmann, A. (2003). *Identity in democracy.* Princeton, NJ: Princeton University Press.

Hall, S. (1996). Introduction: Who needs "identity"? In S. Hall & P. D. Gay (Eds.), *Questions of cultural identity* (pp. 1–17). London: Sage Publications.

Hallsworth, M. (2011). *System stewardship? The future of policy making?* Working Paper. London: Institute for Government.

Harrison, D. (2007, October 3). African refugees face integration issues. *The Age.* Retrieved from http://www.theage.com.au/news/national/refugee-cut-notracist/2007/10/03/1191091178266.html

Henderson, S., & Kendall, E. (2011). Culturally and linguistically diverse peoples' knowledge of accessibility and utilisation of health services: Exploring the need for improvement in health service delivery. *Australian Journal of Primary Health, 17*(2), 195–201.

Henry, F., Tator, C., Mattis, W., & Rees, T. (2000). *The colour of democracy: Racism in Canadian society.* Toronto: Harcourt Brace and Company.

Herscovitch, B., & Bal, D. (2011). National identity and civics classes: The limitations of "The people of Australia—Australia's multicultural policy." In L. Harbon & L. Woodrow (Eds.),

Multiculturalism: Perspectives from Australia, Canada ,and China (pp. 6–12). Sydney: The University of Sydney.

Ho, C. (2013). From social justice to social cohesion: A history of Australian multicultural policy. In A. Jakubowicz & C. Ho (Eds.), *"For those who've come across the seas ...": Australian multicultural theory, policy, and practice* (pp. 31–44). North Melbourne: Australian Scholarly Publishing.

Hollinsworth, D. (2006). *Race and racism in Australia.* South Melbourne: Thomson.

Hugo, G. (2014). *Migration update report.* Paper presented at the 2014 Migration Update Conference, September 11, Adelaide.

Ingleby, D. (2012). Ethnicity, migration, and the "social determinants of health" agenda. *Psychosocial Intervention, 21*(3), 331–41.

Irving, G., & Mosca, D. (2010). *Future capacity needs in managing the health aspects of migration.* Background Paper for World Migration Report 2010. Geneva: International Organization for Migration.

Jakubowicz, A., & Ho, C. (2013). *"For those who've come across the seas ...": Australian multicultural theory, policy, and practice.* North Melbourne: Australian Scholarly Publishing.

Jakubowicz, A., & Monani, D. (2010). *International student futures in Australia: A human rights perspective on moving forward to real action.* Canberra: Australian Human Rights Commission, Academy of the Social Sciences in Australia, and Universities Australia. Retrieved from http://www.assa.edu.au/publications/occasional/107

Jayasuriya, D. L. (2007). Integration in a diverse plural society. *Dialogue, 26*(2), 48–53.

Jayasuriya, L. (1997). *Immigration and multiculturalism in Australia: Selected essays by Laksiri Jayasuriya.* Perth: School of Social Work and Social Administration, The University of Western Australia.

Johnson, C. (2000). *Governing change: Keating to Howard.* St. Lucia: University of Queensland Press.

Johnstone, M., & Kanitsaki, O. (2006). Culture, language, and patient safety: Making the link. *International Journal for Quality in Health Care, 18*(5), 383–88. doi: 10.1093/intqhc/mzl039

Johnstone, M., & Kanitsaki, O. (2007a). Healthcare provider and consumer understandings of cultural safety and cultural competency in health care: An Australian study. *Journal of Cultural Diversity, 14*(2), 96–105.

Johnstone, M., & Kanitsaki, O. (2007b). The problem of failing to provide culturally and linguistically appropriate healthcare. In S. Barraclough & H. Gardner (Eds.), *Analysing health policy—a problem-oriented approach* (pp. 176–86). Australia: Churchill Livingstone Elsener.

Jordan, K., Krivokapic-Skoko, B., & Collins, J. (2011). Immigration and multicultural place-making in rural and regional Australia. In G. Luck, D. Race, & R. Black (Eds), *Demographic change in Australia's rural landscapes: Implications for society and the environment* (pp. 259–81). Collingwood, Australia: Springer.

Jupp, J. (2007). *From White Australia to Woomera* (2nd ed.). Cambridge: Cambridge University Press.

Jupp, J. (2011). Politics, public policy, and multiculturalism. In J. Jupp & M. Clyne (Eds.), *Multiculturalism and integration: A harmonious relationship* (pp. 41–52). Canberra: ANU E-Press.

Jupp, J., McRobbie, A., & York, B. (1991). *Settlement needs of small, newly arrived ethnic groups.* Canberra: AGPS.

Kane, J., & Hudson, W. (2000). *Rethinking Australian citizenship.* Cambridge: Cambridge University Press.

Kenny, S. (2011). *Developing communities for the future.* South Melbourne: Cengage Learning.

Khoo, S. (2010). Health and humanitarian migrants' economic participation. *Journal of Immigrant and Minority Health, 12*(3), 327–39.

Kidson, M. (2013). *Organising policy making.* London: Institute for Government.

Levey, G. B. (2012). *Political theory and Australian multiculturalism.* Oxford: Berghahn Books.

Marginson, S., Nyland, C., Sawir, E., & Forbes-Mewett, H. (2010). *International student security.* Port Melbourne: Cambridge University Press.

Markel, H., & Stern, A. M. (2002). The foreignness of germs: The persistent association of immigrants and disease in American society. *The Milbank Quarterly, 80*(4), 757–88.

Markides, K. S., & Eschbach, K. (2005). Aging, migration, and mortality: Current status of research on the Hispanic paradox. *Journals of Gerontology, Series B: Social Sciences and Psychological Sciences, 60B*(II), 68–75.

Markus, A. (2013). *Mapping social cohesion: The Scanlon Foundation surveys 2013.* Melbourne: Scanlon Foundation and Monash University.

Markus, A., Jupp, J., & McDonald, P. (2009). *Australia's immigration revolution.* Sydney: Allen & Unwin.

McCulloch, J. (2006). State of emergency: The militarisation of civil society and the decline of politics post 9/11. *Australian Marxist Review,* (44), April, 1–3.

McMaster, D. (2001). *Asylum seekers: Australia's response to refugees.* Carlton South: Melbourne University Press.

Mellin-Olsen, T., & Wandel, M. (2005). Changes in food habits among Pakistani immigrant women in Oslo, Norway. *Ethnicity and Health, 10*(4), 311–39.

Minas, H., Kakuma, R., Too, L. S., Vayani, H., Orapeleng, S., Prasad-Ildes, R., ... Oehm, D. (2013). Mental health research and evaluation in multicultural Australia: Developing a culture of inclusion. *International Journal of Mental Health Systems, 7*(23), 3–25.

Missingham, B., Dibden, J., & Cocklin, C. (2006). A multicultural countryside? Ethnic minorities in rural Australia. *Rural Society, 16*(2), 131–49.

Mitchell, M., Every, D., & Ranzin, R. (2011). Everyday antiracism in interpersonal contexts: Constraining and facilitating factors for "speaking up" against racism. *Journal of Community & Applied Social Psychology, 21*(4), 329–41.

NACCHO. (2011). *NACCHO cultural safety training standards: A background paper.* Canberra: National Aboriginal Community Controlled Health Organisation.

Napier, A. D., Ancarno, C., Butler, B., Calabrese, J., Chater, A., Chatterjee, H., ... Woolf, K. (2014). Culture and health. *The Lancet, 384*(9954), 1607–39.

NEDA. (2013). *What does the data say: People from NESB background with a disability in Australia.* Harris Park: National Disability Ethnic Alliance. Retrieved from http://www.neda.org.au/index.php/reports/item/what-does-the-data-say

NEDA. (2014). *National disability strategy 2014 progress report to COAG.* Harris Park: National Disability Ethnic Alliance. Retrieved from www.neda.org.au

Nelson, J. K. (2013). Denial of racism and its implications for local action. *Discourse and Society,* 24(1), 89–109.

NPC. (1988). *A proposed settlement strategy.* Canberra: National Population Council.

OECD. (2011). *International migration outlook 2011.* Paris: Organisation for Economic Co-operation and Development.

OMA. (1989). *National agenda for a multicultural Australia.* Canberra: Office of Multicultural Affairs, Department of Prime Minister and Cabinet.

Paradies, Y., Harris, R., & Anderson, I. (2008). *The impact of racism on Indigenous health in Australia and Aotearoa: Towards a research agenda.* Casuarina: Cooperative Research Centre for Aboriginal Health.

Paradies, Y., Priest, N., Ben, J., Truong, M., Gupta, A., Pieterse, A., ... Gee, G. (2013). Racism as a determinant of health: A protocol for conducting a systematic review and meta-analysis. *Systematic Reviews, 2*(85), 1–7.

Powles, J., & Gifford, S. (1990). How healthy are Australia's immigrants? In J. Reid & P. Trompf (Eds.), *The health of immigrant Australia: A social perspective* (pp. 77–107). Marrickville: Harcourt Brace Jovanovich.

Poynting, S., & Noble, G. (2004). Living with racism: The experience and reporting by Arab and Muslim Australians of discrimination, abuse, and violence since 11 September 2001. *Report to the Human Rights and Equal Opportunity Commission.* Sydney: Centre for Cultural Research, University of Western Sydney.

Poynting, S., Noble, G., Tabar, P., & Collins, J. (2004). *Bin Laden in the suburbs: Criminalising the Arab other.* Sydney: The Federation Press.

Prasad-Ildes, R., & Ramirez, E. (2006). What CALD consumers say about mental illness prevention. *Australian e-Journal on the Advancement of Mental Health, 5*(2), 126–31.

Pyke, J., Bertone, S. H. B., Gill, G., & Grossman, M. (2011). *The community safety of international students in Melbourne: A scoping study.* Melbourne: Victoria University.

RCOA. (2013). *Housing issues for refugees and asylum seekers in Australia.* Sydney: Refugee Council of Australia. Retrieved from https://www.refugeecouncil.org.au/r/rpt/1309_HousingLitRev.pdf

Reid, A., Lenguerrand, E., Santos, I., Read, U., La Montagne, A. D., Fritschi, L., & Harding, S. (2014). Taking risks and survival jobs: Foreign-born workers and work related injuries in Australia. *Safety Science, 70,* 378–86.

Sales, R. (2005). Secure borders, safe haven: A contradiction of terms? *Ethnic and Racial Studies, 28*(3), 445–62.

Sevoyan, A., & Hugo, G. (2013). *Exploring migrant health in Australia.* Paper presented at the 28th USSP International Population Conference, Busan, Korea.

Skellet, L. (2012). Cultural awareness and cultural safety. *Australian Pharmacist, 31*(5), 382–84.

Soroka, S. N., Johnston, R., & Banting, K. (2007). Ties that bind? Social cohesion and diversity in Canada. In K. Banting, T. J. Courchene, & F. L. Seidle (Eds.), *Belonging? Diversity, recognition, and shared citizenship in Canada* (pp. 561–600). Montreal: IRPP.

Thow, A., & Waters, A. M. (2005). *Diabetes in culturally and linguistically diverse Australians—Identification of communities at high risk.* Canberra: Australian Institute of Health and Welfare.

Tong, C., & Cross, T. (1991). Cross cultural partnerships for child abuse prevention with Native American communities. Portland, OR: Northwest Indian Child Welfare Institute.

Trajkovski, S., & Loosemore, M. (2006). Safety implications of low-English proficiency among migrant construction site operative. *International Journal of Project Management, 24*(5), 446–52.

UN. (2002). *Gender mainstreaming: An overview.* New York: United Nations Publications.

USDHHS. (2001). National standards for culturally & linguistically appropriate services in health care: Final report. Rockville, MD: OPHS Office of Minority Health, U.S Department of Health & Human Services.

Van den Berg, R. (2002). *Nyoongar people of Australia: Perspectives on racism and multiculturalism.* International Studies in Sociology and Social Anthropology series, vol.

VandenHeuvel, A., & Wooden, M. (1999). *New settlers have their say—How immigrants fare over the early years of settlement.* Canberra: Department of Immigration and Multicultural Affairs.

Vasta, E. (2007). *Accommodating diversity: Why current critiques of multiculturalism miss the point.* Working Paper no. 53. Oxford: Centre on Migration, Policy, and Society, University of Oxford.

VicHealth. (2008). *Ethnic and race-based discrimination: As a determinant of mental health and wellbeing.* Research Summary 3. Carlton: Victorian Health Promotion Foundation.

WHA. (2008). *Resolution on the "health of migrants."* Document EB122.R5. Geneva: World Health Assembly, WHO.

WHO. (2014). *The Ottawa Charter for health promotion.* Geneva: World Health Organization. Retrieved from http://www.who.int/healthpromotion/conferences/previous/ottawa/en/index1.html

Wight, J. (2012). The varied expressions of "cultural competence": Findings from an exploratory study with health and human services practitioners. *Australian Mosaic, 32*, 41–43.

Williams, R. (1999). Cultural safety—What does it mean for our work practice? *Australian and New Zealand Journal of Public Health, 23*(2), 213–14.

CHAPTER 4

Public Policy, Immigrant Experiences, and Health Outcomes in Canada

Ilene Hyman and Agnes Meinhard

Chapter Objectives

This chapter focuses on Canadian immigration and multiculturalism as a case study. The specific objectives of this chapter are:

- to identify patterns of immigration and integration in Canada and their impact on immigrant health;
- to discern the impact of Canada's official multiculturalism policy on immigrant integration and health; and
- to discuss the role of public policy in addressing barriers to immigrant integration in Canada.

Introduction

Many frameworks have been proposed to understand the determinants of health outcomes. For example, the social determinants of health (SDOH) identified by Raphael (2016) reflect the fact that health is largely influenced by social and economic factors and thus requires health promotion and policy that move beyond biomedical and behavioural risk factor approaches. The World Health Organization Commission on the Social Determinants of Health distinguishes between structural and intermediary determinants (World Health Organization, 2007); the former includes government policies (macroeconomic, social, and public) that give rise to a set of unequal socio-economic positions, which leads to differences in social cohesion and social capital. These affect equity in health and well-being by means of a series of intermediary social factors (e.g., living conditions, health behaviours, psychosocial factors). Therefore, in order to understand the factors that affect immigrant health in Canada, it is critical to consider the role of government policy. For example, policies of **social inclusion** can have a major effect on various structural determinants such as social exclusion, social cohesion, and social capital, which in turn have an impact on immigrant integration and health.

In Canada, the federal government has been, and in most cases continues to be, the leading force behind immigration policy and practice, setting admission levels, defining admission procedures, and managing the admission system (Hiebert & Sherrell, 2009). Regarding integration, Canada is well known for its official policy of **multiculturalism**, which is considered a strategy for immigrant integration, rather than isolation or assimilation (Reitz, 2012). The 1971 Multiculturalism Policy of Canada forms the basis of Canada's approach to citizenship and immigration:

> In 1971, Canada was the first country in the world to adopt multiculturalism as an official policy. By so doing, Canada affirmed the value and dignity of all Canadian citizens regardless of their racial or ethnic origins, their language, or their religious affiliation. The 1971 Multiculturalism Policy of Canada also confirmed the rights of Aboriginal peoples and the status of Canada's two official languages. (Government of Canada, 2012)

While the Act also confirmed the rights of Indigenous peoples in Canada, colonization and government policies toward its Indigenous peoples have cut across the social determinants of health, impacting on access to education, housing, food security, and employment, and permeating societal systems and institutions, including the health care, child welfare, and criminal justice systems to adversely affect the health and well-being of Indigenous peoples (Allan & Smylie, 2015).

Integration is a broad term that encompasses many different dimensions: economic integration into the labour market; political (or civic) integration into the electoral process and other forms of political participation; and social integration into the networks and spaces of civil society, from informal networks of friends and neighbours to membership in more formal organizations (Kymlicka, 2010). The literature also describes integration as a two-way interactional process between a host society and "immigrants" (regardless of generation) that is influenced both by institutional structures and societal attitudes on the one hand, and migration factors such as human capital and collective social capital on the other (Frideres, 2008).

Therefore, immigrants may be well integrated in one domain of life (e.g., employment) but poorly integrated in other domains (e.g., social and political) during different stages of the settlement process. The lack of integration, often associated with social exclusion and absences in the availability of social networks and support, is linked with adverse changes to immigrant health and well-being (Hyman, 2009; Galabuzi & Teelucksingh, 2010).

In this chapter we focus on the role that multiculturalism policy can play in creating an inclusionary and healthy society. We maintain that broader social inclusionary policies aimed at eliminating systemic barriers to economic, political, and social integration are necessary and a prerequisite for immigrant health and well-being. We demonstrate this by looking at the health outcomes of Canadian immigrants and how they are influenced by Canada's multiculturalism policy, both historically and currently. Has this policy successfully prevented racism and discrimination that leads to social exclusion and its impact on health? Has it contributed to creating social capital, which helps in integration? How can government policies and programs address social exclusion and build social capital? We conclude by considering the leadership role multiculturalism policy can take in developing and implementing national social inclusion policies that ensure the full and valued participation of all Canadians, thus helping to improve immigrant health.

Recent Immigration Patterns in Canada

Canada's commitment to humanitarian values, and the need to sustain social and economic bases in light of declining rates of natural population growth, will ensure that immigration will continue to play a major role in its evolution. Since 2006, Canada has accepted approximately 250,000 immigrants per year, or about 0.7 percent of the Canadian population (Keung, 2012). Newcomers to Canada fall into two broad classifications: permanent residents and temporary residents, the former group coming to Canada with the objective of resettling, while the latter come to visit, study, or work.

Permanent residents in Canada fall into different categories, depending on their reasons for immigrating: economic class, family class, and refugees. In 2008, Canada received over 247,000 permanent residents, 192,000 temporary foreign workers, and 79,000 international students (Citizenship and Immigration Canada, 2010a). Since 2012, Canada's immigration system has been undergoing a significant and rapid transformation that will increase the proportion of economic class immigrants and reduce the proportion of immigrants entering through family and humanitarian classes (Ali, 2014). It is also estimated that at least 20,000 immigrants are without status in Canada (Ontario Council of Agencies Serving Immigrants, n.d.), most of whom entered through a legal pathway such as a visitor permit, temporary work permit, or as refugee claimants who stayed in Canada beyond the expiration of their permit.

Immigration has historically played an important role in shaping Canada's population into the culturally diverse nation it is today. According to the 2006 Census of Canada, one in five Canadians—6.2 million or 19.8 percent—is foreign-born (Statistics Canada, 2006). Statistics Canada projections suggest that by the year 2031, as much as 25–28 percent of the population could be foreign-born (Statistics Canada, 2010).

Throughout much of the 20th century, the majority of immigrants to Canada were from the United Kingdom, the United States, and Europe. By the 1980s, the majority of immigrants to Canada were not from Europe or the United States. In 2001, of all immigrants to Canada, 53 percent were from Asian and Pacific countries, 19.2 percent were from Africa and the Middle East, 17.3 percent were from the United Kingdom and Europe, 8.0 percent were from South and Central America, and 2.4 percent were from the United States (Citizenship and Immigration Canada, 2010b). Canada is part of the same trend as other high-income Western nations that will increasingly be relying on racialized immigrants to sustain their economic, cultural, and social vitality.

The 2011 National Household Survey (NHS) estimated that over 6 million Canadians identified themselves as members of the visible minority population, representing 19.1 percent of the population. By comparison, this proportion was 16.2 percent in the 2006 Census. The increase is due largely to the number of immigrants who arrived in Canada in recent decades from non-European countries as well as increases in the Canadian-born population who are the children and grandchildren of visible-minority immigrants. In 2011, 13.7 percent of newcomers were born in Europe, while another 3.9 percent were born in the United States. The remaining 82.4 percent came from Asia (including the Middle East), the Caribbean and Central and South America, Africa and Oceania, and other regions (Statistics Canada, 2011). Due to the changing mix of immigration since the 1970s, almost one-quarter of young people aged 20 to 24 now belong to a visible-minority group, and this proportion is much higher in big cities (Jackson, 2013). Projections by Statistics Canada indicate that the proportion of Canadians who belong to a visible minority could double by 2031 (Statistics Canada, 2010).

Immigrants to Canada tend to be highly educated, in part reflecting the fact that the majority of immigrants who come to Canada do so through the economic class. In fact, the proportion of men and women holding a university degree is significantly higher among recent immigrants (58 percent and 49 percent, respectively) than among the Canadian-born population (19 percent and 23 percent, respectively) (Galarneau & Moricette, 2008) (Figure 4.1).

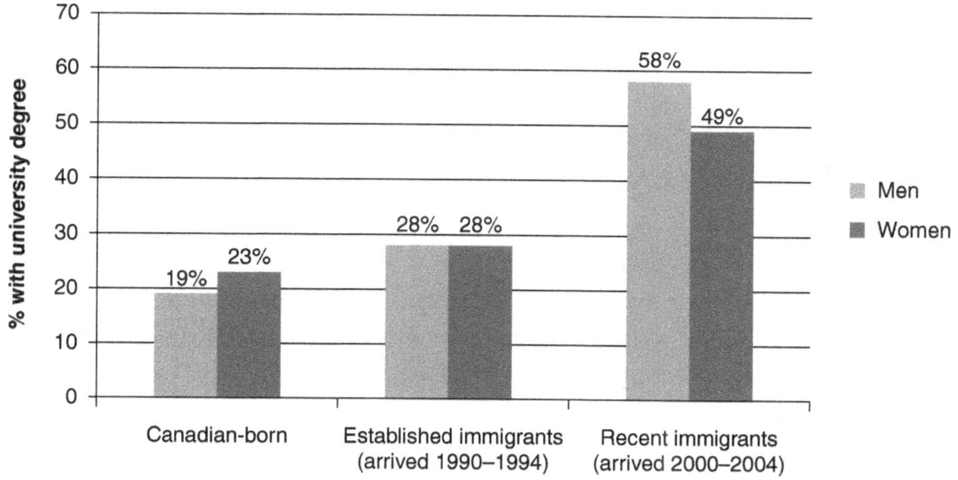

Figure 4.1: Percentage of Recent and Long-Term Immigrant and Canadian-Born Populations with a University Degree, by Sex, 2006

Source: Statistics Canada. (2008). *Canada's ethnocultural mosaic, 2006.* Census. Ottawa: Author. Catalogue no. 97-562-X. Retrieved from http://www12.statcan.gc.ca/english/census06/analysis/ethnicorigin/pdf/97-562-XIE2006001.pdf

Overview of Canadian Integration Policies

In 1971, the federal government of Canada recognized multiculturalism as a fundamental characteristic of Canadian society through the adoption of a formal multiculturalism policy. The policy recognized the contribution to the nation of many ethnocultural groups, in addition to the original French and British pioneers who had made Canada their home. It encouraged a vision of Canada based on the values of equality and mutual respect with regard to race, national or ethnic origin, and religion. The 1971 Multiculturalism Policy of Canada also confirmed the rights of Indigenous peoples and the status of Canada's two official languages (Kymlicka, 2010).

By 1981, as Canada's racial diversity was beginning to grow, more attention was being devoted to racial discrimination, and a special unit for race relations was formed. In 1982, with the patriation of the Canadian Constitution, multicultural policies were firmly entrenched in the Charter of Rights and Freedoms, guaranteeing among others, equal protection and benefit of the law, and freedom from discrimination on the basis of gender, religion, and racial or ethnic origin. When the multiculturalism policy was first announced in 1971, the Canadian social mosaic was still dominated by people of European Christian heritage. Its original emphasis was on cultural retention and cultural sharing, and it was supported by funding initiatives aimed at the preservation of language and culture (Fleras & Kunz, 2001). As the racial and religious makeup of new immigrants was shifting from mostly European Christian to mostly Asian non-Christian, a growing number of Canada's newcomers found themselves facing the consequences of social exclusion in many spheres of life (Omidvar & Richmond, 2005).

In 1988, Parliament passed the Canadian Multiculturalism Act, which provided a legal framework to guide federal responsibilities and activities with respect to multiculturalism in Canada. The Act went beyond simply guaranteeing equal opportunity for all Canadians, regardless of origin. It emphasized the right of Canada's ethnic, racial, and religious minorities to preserve and share their unique cultural heritage and it underlined the need to address race relations and eliminate systemic inequalities. It required all federal institutions to carry out their activities in a manner that is sensitive and responsive to the multicultural reality of Canada and report annually on how their institution met these requirements. It also included a provision for funding to mainstream institutions such as police forces, hospitals, and schools to implement multiculturalism policies and programs aimed at reducing barriers to access (Mock, 2002; Kunz & Sykes, 2007; Policy Research Initiative, 2009a, b).

From the start, supporters and critics of multiculturalism have debated its role and impact on the integration of immigrants, racial and ethnic groups, and religious minorities in Canada. It is difficult to weigh these arguments because they are often based on different conceptions of multiculturalism. We summarize some of the arguments both in favour of and against multiculturalism, bearing in mind that not only are the arguments based on different conceptions of multiculturalism, but some are also influenced by what is happening outside of Canada. Nevertheless, we present these arguments because they are an indication of some of the concerns regarding multiculturalism as a policy.

According to an Angus Reid poll, 55 percent of Canadians thought that our multiculturalism policy has been very good or good, and 30 percent thought it has been bad or very bad. More than half of respondents (54 percent) believed Canada should be a melting pot, while one-third of Canadians (33 percent) endorsed the concept of the mosaic (Angus Reid, 2010). This is an intriguing contradiction that seems to indicate both an acceptance of the diversity that is characteristic of Canada today, and a desire for all these diverse people to become "Canadian," however that is defined in the mind of the respondent. Indeed, in the minds of the majority of several hundreds of university undergraduates surveyed over the course of a decade, the defining feature of Canadian culture is multiculturalism.[1]

Supporters of multiculturalism policy argue that it promotes integration by removing barriers to participation in Canadian life. There is strong evidence that multiculturalism policy has played a positive role in the successful integration of immigrants and ethnic and religious minorities in Canada as compared to many other countries that lack an official multiculturalism policy (Kymlicka, 1998, 2010; Banting et al., 2007; Bloemraad, 2006). Among the examples of success provided by Kymlicka (2010) were the high level of mutual identification and acceptance among immigrants and native-born Canadians, the high likelihood of immigrants in Canada becoming citizens, high rates of intermarriage, high levels of official language proficiency, and the fact that Canadian immigrants are more likely to participate in the political process as voters, party members, or even candidates for political office than in the United States, Australia, or any European country, none of which has an official multiculturalism policy (Howe, 2007). Findings from the OECD (2006) suggest that the children of immigrants have better educational outcomes in Canada than in any other Western democracy. According to a survey conducted by Focus Canada in 2006, 83 percent of Canadians agree that Muslims make a positive contribution to Canada (Adams, 2009), suggesting that Canada has been less affected by the global surge in anti-Muslim sentiments and by the resulting polarization of ethnic relations experienced in many European countries (Kymlicka, 2010).

Shared identity and sense of belonging are considered important indicators of the effectiveness of multiculturalism policy in Western democratic nation-states, such as Canada, where there is no common ethnicity or culture (Bush, 2008; Edwards, 2010). According to data from the 2003 Canadian General Social Survey (GSS), 84 percent of recent immigrants and an even higher proportion of non-recent immigrants reported a strong sense of belonging to Canada, compared to 85 percent of the Canadian-born population (Statistics Canada, 2003). Data from the 2002 Ethnic Diversity Survey (EDS) suggest that Canadians identifying as "visible minorities" express a stronger sense of belonging than other Canadians (Reitz & Banerjee, 2007). There is evidence that immigrants in Canada, regardless of their religious affiliation, increasingly share Canada's liberal-democratic norms, or what the authors called "Charter values," including the rights of gays and women (Soroka, Johnston, & Banting 2007).

Critics, on the other hand, maintain that multiculturalism threatens national cohesion and contributes to ghettoization (Bissoondath, 2002; Wong, 2010). In a recent poll, Canadians widely agreed that "Canada should not promote cultural differences at the expense of shared Canadian values" (Policy Research Initiative, 2009a, b). This, of course, has never been the objective of Canadian multiculturalism. Other scholars critique multiculturalism policy by suggesting that it is used as a means by which certain social groups are kept in a dependent position through the accentuation of differences, thus entrenching their second-class status and reducing the challenge they pose to the so-called "dominant" group (Li, 2003; Bannerji, 2000; Henry & Tator, 2006; Kallen, 1982).

Others maintain that multiculturalism policy can act as a barrier to immigrant integration and social inclusion. Richmond and Shields (2005) observe that the recognition of differences that is the core of multiculturalism policy is not the same as valued recognition. Inclusive citizenship is emerging as a 21st-century goal not only for multiculturalism policy but also for Canadian social policy as a whole (Richmond & Shields, 2005; Roeher Institute, 2003). Inclusive citizenship is about valued participation, valued recognition, and belonging, wherein citizens are nurtured to their fullest capacities. The concept of inclusive citizenship goes beyond the idea of integrating new immigrants into the host society. It implies that while newcomers are being integrated, the rest of Canadian society is also changing to reflect the diversity of the whole—redefining what it means to be Canadian.

In summary, the focus of and challenges to multiculturalism policy have evolved over time from celebrating difference in the 1970s, to managing diversity in the 1980s, and to constructive engagement in the 1990s (Fleras & Kunz, 2001). The 2009 policy objectives for the Multiculturalism Program focus on building an integrated, socially cohesive society and making institutions more responsive to the needs of Canada's diverse population (Citizenship and Immigration Canada, 2010a, b). These aims are consistent with addressing broader social inclusionary processes that influence inequities and impact on nation building as a whole.

The Economic Backdrop against Which Immigration Is Occurring

Canadian society, economy, and labour markets have been reshaped by demographic shifts, new economic realities, globalization, emerging technologies, and changing culture and attitudes. These changes have the potential to affect the economically and socially vulnerable the most and this appears to be the case for immigrants of colour to Canada.

Income inequality has been a major problem in Canada and other advanced economies for many years now. The bottom two quintiles of the income scale have seen their market incomes decline in real terms since the early 1980s (though transfers have resulted in some degree of after-tax and transfer growth). At the same time, the top 1 percent of economic families has accumulated an ever-increasing share of Canada's wealth. Income inequality, a feature of all market economies, is now giving way to income polarization. While this phenomenon is still more acute in the United States than in Canada, some recent studies suggest the gap between rich and poor—and between the super-rich and the middle class—is now growing faster in Canada than in the United States (Torjman & Battle, 2011). Income polarization can have serious effects on the economy and society. At an extreme, it can undermine social cohesion, unravelling the fabric of a country. The government of Canada, in partnership with the provinces, has an array of social programs that includes the Canada Pension Plan, medicare, and Employment Insurance. Reforms to federal income security programs and the tax-transfer system have also taken place over the past 20 years. While social spending as a percentage of GDP spiked the early 1990s due to economic recession and rising Employment Insurance and social assistance costs, there have been drastic cuts to government programs as a results of neo-liberal and neo-conservative ideology, and the redistributive impact of Canada's tax and transfer policies has fluctuated over time.

By the late 1990s, after-tax income inequality rose partly as a result of cuts to Employment Insurance and other federal cuts to social spending in response to rising deficits. Many of the core social programs and policies designed in the middle of the last century have not kept pace with these broader changes. Income polarization has not, until now, been a big issue on the federal agenda. Immigrants bear the brunt of this polarization since they make up a large part of the impoverished. Scholars in the area argue that it is time for the federal government to analyze and consider the longer term effects of income and to consider strategic policy reforms to head off a looming problem (Corak, 2008; Frenette & Morissette, 2003). Many of the main pillars of Canada's social architecture have not evolved to appropriately address current economic and demographic realities.

Evidence of Social Exclusion among Canadian Immigrants

One of the most insidious processes undermining the achievement of immigrant integration and inclusion is **racism** and the multi-dimensional forms of **social exclusion** that result from it. Racism is the belief that race is the primary determinant of human traits and capacities, and that racial differences produce an inherent superiority of a particular race (*Merriam-Webster Dictionary*, 2008). However, the Canadian Race Relations Foundation defines "racism" not only as an attitude, but also as the specific actions resulting from this attitude that marginalize and oppress certain people. Racism is usually understood in the interpersonal sense—that is, discriminatory interactions, both conscious and unconscious, between individuals (Karlsen & Nazroo, 2002). A less visible form of racism is systemic or institutional racism. This refers to "the collective failure of an organization or social structure to provide an appropriate and professional service to people because of their colour, culture, or ethnic origin ... [it]... can be seen or detected in processes, attitudes, and behaviour that amount to discrimination through unwitting prejudice, ignorance, thoughtlessness, and racist stereotyping which disadvantages people in ethnic minority groups" (Macpherson, 1999, article 6.34).

The concept of **racialization** refers to the social *process* whereby certain groups come to be designated as different and consequently subjected to differential and unequal treatment (Galabuzi, 2004, 2006). Lack of equal access to opportunities, marginalization, and exclusion among ethno-racial groups suggest that their perceived racial membership plays a significant role in shaping their collective experience—that is, they are *racialized*, rather than "merely" *racial*, groups. Unlike the term "visible minorities," which Canada's Employment Equity Act defines as "non-Caucasian in race or non-white in colour," the term "racialized groups" makes clear that race is not an objective biological fact, but rather a social and cultural construct that exposes individuals to racism.

The right to equal treatment is a fundamental human right, as outlined in the Canadian Human Rights Act (Department of Justice, 1985). Despite this, there has been a failure, both presently and historically, to fully recognize that racial and religious discrimination persists across all dimensions of Canadian society (Canadian Race Relations Foundation, n.d.). Historical examples of discrimination and racism in Canada include the establishment of the residential school system for Indigenous children, the internment of the Japanese Canadians during the Second World War, the denial of entry to Canada to Jews during the Nazi persecution, the establishment of the head tax for the Chinese, the establishment of the Oriental Exclusion Act, the exclusion of African Canadians to services and employment, discriminatory immigration provisions against African Americans, and denial of the vote to Asians and Indigenous peoples (Gogia & Slade, 2011).

Despite the proliferation of methods to measure racism, including surveys and interviews, analysis of secondary data, and social psychological experimentation, there are no sources that regularly collect information on this construct in Canada. Recent research attests to the existence of perceived racism in Canada despite the fact that equal treatment is a fundamental human right.

- According to data from the 2003 Canadian Ethnic Diversity Survey, 20 percent of visible minorities, compared with 5 percent of non–visible minorities, reported having experienced discrimination or unfair treatment in the five years preceding the survey (Canadian Ethnic Diversity Survey, 2003). Significant differences in experiences and perceptions of racism were noted between dominant groups with European heritage and racialized groups (Reitz & Banerjee, 2007; Nakhaie et al., 2007).
- Immigrants were twice as likely as non-immigrants to experience discrimination (in jobs or promotions, in a store, on the street), and racialized groups were twice as likely as non-racialized groups to experience discrimination (Perreault, 2008, quoting data from the 2004 GSS Survey on Victimization).
- Police reports on hate crimes in 2006 showed that the majority of hate crimes were motivated by race/ethnicity (61 percent), followed by religion (27 percent) and sexual orientation (10 percent). Half of all the racially motivated crimes targeted people who were in black racialized groups. Nearly two-thirds of religiously motivated hate crimes were directed at the Jewish faith (Dauvergne et al., 2008).
- According to the International Youth Survey, immigrant and second-generation youth were significantly more likely than Canadian-born (third or more generation) youth to report that they had been discriminated against at least once in their lifetime because of race, religion, or spoken language (Zeman & Bressan, 2006).

- The Ontario Roots of Youth Violence report identified racism and poverty as a form of violence that disproportionately affects black and Indigenous communities and, to a lesser extent, other visible minorities (McMurtry & Curling, 2008).
- Public opinion polls, student surveys, and other research indicate that people of the Islamic faith and those with Muslim or Arab-sounding names experienced significant discrimination beyond the immediate backlash after the events of September 11, 2001 (Rousseau et al., 2010; Kymlicka, 2010; Policy Research Initiative, 2009a, b; Patychuk & Hyman, 2009).

While most people refrain from direct expressions of racism, they may condone, overlook, or be patently unaware of the fundamental ways in which society's political, economic, and social institutions contribute to social exclusion. These include, for example, the lack of recognition of international credentials; lack of policies to ensure the accessibility (financial, linguistic, cultural, geographic) of public services for all; and lack of policies to ensure greater representation in decision making. Systemic institutional racism is evident if we consider the following facts about the experiences of racialized groups in Canada:

- Data from the 2011 National Household Survey (NHS) (which replaced the long-form Census[2]) indicate that racial status remains a significant factor in shaping advantage and disadvantage in the Canadian job market and in influencing the overall level of poverty and income inequality (Jackson, 2013).
- Recent Canadian immigrants earn substantially less than the average Canadian, with the gap growing since 1980 despite immigrants gaining on the general population in average level of educational attainment (CICS Immigration Consulting, 2014; Picot & Hou, 2003).
- The incidence of low income for non-whites in 2010 was 21.5 percent using the Low-Income Measure (LIM), which was much higher than the 13.3 percent rate for whites (Statistics Canada, 2014; Jackson, 2013). The median total income of non-whites in 2010 was just $20,153, or one-third (32 percent) less than $29,649 for whites (Statistics Canada, 2014; Jackson, 2013).
- The unemployment rate in 2011 was 9.9 percent for visible-minority workers compared to 7.3 percent for white workers, a difference of 2.6 percentage points. The difference in unemployment rates between visible minorities and white workers was significantly greater for women (10.6 percent vs. 6.7 percent) than for men (9.3 percent vs. 7.8 percent) and also varied by ethno-racial group.

- Despite their higher levels of education, racialized groups in Canada are more likely to be unemployed or employed in precarious work (defined as atypical employment contracts, limited social benefits, poor statutory entitlements, job insecurity, short tenure, and low wages) than non-racialized Canadians (Martin Prosperity Institute, 2013; Lightman et al., 2008; Galabuzi, 2006).
- Muslim Canadians face major obstacles to integration, and experience high unemployment despite high levels of education (Adams, 2009).
- Recent studies on the diversity of decision-making bodies in three sectors indicate a massive under-representation of Canada's visible minorities (Cukier & Yap, 2009; Bradshaw et al., 2009; Yap, 2004).
- Many consider the exclusion of Roma refugee claimants in Canadian refugee policy to be a form of institutional racism (Levine-Rasky et al., 2014).

Demographic changes, occurring as they did during two economic downturns, resulted in a slowing down of the economic integration of newcomers, with an accompanying racialization of poverty (Picot et al., 2008; Saloojee, 2005). The 2008 recession widened the gap between the labour market experience of both established and recent immigrants and the Canadian-born (Kelly, Park, & Lepper, 2011). According to Jackson (2013) of the Broadbent Institute, racial differences in unemployment rates for non-immigrants cannot be explained by the undervaluation of international educational credentials and work experience or by levels of education, since visible-minority Canadian-born young people are more highly educated than their white counterparts. He suggests that racialized Canadians are disadvantaged in the job market because of overt racial discrimination in layoffs and in hiring and the lack of social capital to facilitate employment. Previous studies based on Census data, notably by Grace-Edward Galabuzi of Ryerson University, have carefully shown that race is a significant independent factor influencing success in the Canadian job market. Increasing religious diversity in Canada and escalations of racial tension and violence in the wake of 9/11 and other international incidents also contributed to the marginalization and social exclusion of certain immigrant groups (Kymlicka, 2007; Policy Research Initiative, 2009a, b; Mock, 2002; Kunz & Sykes, 2007).

The 2004 United Nations Mission on contemporary racism concluded that racial discrimination in Canada was tangible as reflected in the high incidence of poverty, overrepresentation in the prison population, racial profiling, and under-representation of ethnic and racial minorities in the upper and middle layers of political, administrative, economic, cultural, and media institutions and mechanisms (Diene, 2004, p. 21, cited in Cassin et al., 2007).

Evidence Concerning Health Outcomes among Immigrants

It would be surprising if these developments did not affect the health of immigrants, especially those who are members of racialized groups. It is well documented that recent immigrants to Canada enjoy a health advantage over long-term immigrants and the Canadian-born population (Hyman, 2001, 2007). This "healthy immigrant effect" is believed to result from, in part, a self-selection process in which people who are able and motivated to move do so, while those who are sick or disabled, or who reside in institutions, do not. It is also the result of immigration procedures that exclude immigrants with serious medical conditions and select immigrants with higher education, language ability, and job skills. The latter characteristics facilitate social and economic integration and are associated with good health. The healthy immigrant effect has also been observed in other high-income countries, including Australia, the United States, and the United Kingdom (Biddle et al., 2007; Frisbie et al., 2001; Muenning & Fahs, 2002).

However, the relative good health of immigrants upon arrival in Canada is not a guarantee of good health in the long term. On the contrary, studies show that deteriorating health status becomes a reality for many immigrants. For example, the Longitudinal Survey of Immigrants to Canada (LSIC) asked newcomers to answer whether they perceived their health to be excellent, good, fair, or poor one year and four years after their arrival in Canada. The data showed a substantial deterioration in immigrant self-reported health status over the four years following arrival (De Maio & Kemp, 2010). The evidence for declining health, especially when it comes to chronic diseases (e.g., heart disease, arthritis, and diabetes), is well demonstrated (Creatore et al., 2010; Newbold, 2006).

Several major reviews suggest that the health of Canadian immigrants is either better than or similar to that of their native-born counterparts, particularly in the areas of mental health, chronic conditions, disability/functional limitations, and risk behaviours (Vang et al., 2015; Gushulak et al., 2011; Kirmayer et al., 2011; De Maio, 2010). A number of these studies found that Canadian immigrants initially reported fewer mental health problems than their Canadian-born counterparts, once again demonstrating the healthy immigrant effect. In fact, Malenfant (2004) found that suicide rates (often used as an indicator of mental health) among immigrants were approximately half those of the Canadian-born population. However, caution must be exercised when drawing conclusions on the mental health status of Canadian immigrants as all positive (Hansson et al., 2010). For example, when Kliewer and Ward (1988) investigated suicide rates among 25 immigrant groups, they found evidence of convergence such that immigrants from low-risk countries (i.e., countries with lower suicide rates than Canada) who came to Canada had increased suicide rates, and among immigrants from high-risk countries, suicide rates decreased. There is strong evidence that the frequency of mental health problems increases with length of stay in Canada and with generational status (Hansson et al., 2010; Smith et al., 2007; Bergeron et al., 2009; Ali, 2002). Second-generation youth also engage in high-risk behaviours such as harmful drinking and illicit drug use more so than first-generation youth (Georgiades et al., 2006).

There is also strong evidence that Canadian immigrants experience lower rates of chronic diseases (e.g., cancer, diabetes, heart disease) and conditions (e.g., obesity, asthma) than their Canadian-born counterparts (Vang et al., 2015; Gushulak et al., 2011; De Maio, 2010). But again there is evidence of heterogeneity and changes over time. For example, Creatore et al. (2010) found that recent immigrants and refugees from South Asia, Latin America, the Caribbean, and sub-Saharan Africa to Ontario had a two to three times greater risk of developing type 2 diabetes than immigrants and refugees from Western Europe or North America. Moreover, this elevated risk began earlier in life (i.e., from 20 to 40 years of age), compared with European and North American immigrant populations, who tend to develop the disease at a somewhat older age (i.e., between 35 to 49 years of age). Immigration from low- to high-income Western countries is associated with an increased risk of heart disease, which, over time, surpasses that of the host population (Tremblay et al., 2006). On average, immigrants are substantially less likely to be obese or overweight upon arrival in Canada, but weight converges to native-born levels over time spent in Canada (McDonald & Kennedy, 2005).

The lack of clear findings on immigrant health at a national level may reflect the need for finer intersectional analysis of health problems among Canada's heterogeneous immigrant groups and particularly the impact of social determinants such as racism and social exclusion.

There is strong evidence from Canadian and international studies that compared to other groups, refugees generally have poorer health due to their experience of displacement and the difficult resettlement process (Kirmayer et al., 2011). Refugees may have experienced traumatic events such as war, family separation, physical and psychological torture, refugee camp internment, acute deprivation, periods of prolonged desertion, and poor access to health care prior to arrival (Marwah, 2014). The compounding effects of these experiences can lead to severely compromised physical, mental, and social health. There is qualitative evidence that immigration policies denying rights and privileges to refugees, such as health insurance and barriers to government services such as welfare and housing, intersect with socio-cultural variables to increase the vulnerability of refugees (Simich et al., 2005; Canadian Council for Refugees, 2004; Caulford & Vali, 2006).

On June 30, 2012, the Government of Canada introduced major amendments to the Interim Federal Health (IFH) program that provides health care coverage for refugees, particularly those who are not covered by provincial or territorial health insurance programs. These amendments limited access to health coverage (except in cases of public health or public safety risk) to refugee claimants from Designated Countries of Origin (i.e., countries considered to be safe/non-refugee-producing countries) and rejected refugee claimants who had exhausted the appeal and judicial review process. As a result, Canada now has a conditional and differential model of health coverage, where the type and level of IFH coverage depends on the refugee category (Marwah, 2014).[3]

Clearly not all immigrant groups experience the same risk of transitioning to poor health post-migration. Immigrant subgroups observed to be at the highest risk of transitioning to poor health includes seniors, women, low-income immigrants, and recent immigrants who are members of a racialized group (Figure 4.2). This highlights the need to examine critical intersections of health with age, gender, ethnicity, racialization, socio-economic status, and geography (Ng et al., 2005; Newbold, 2005; De Maio & Kemp, 2010).

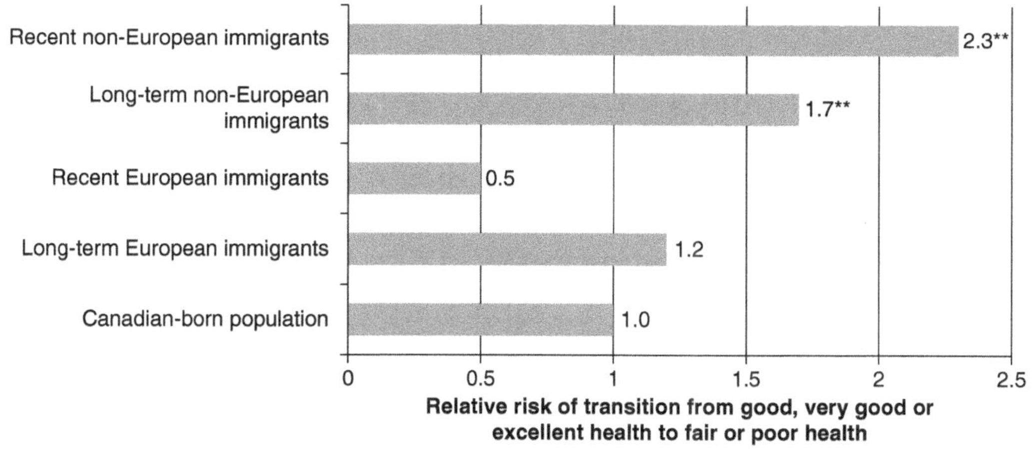

Figure 4.2: Relative Risk of Transition from Good to Poor Health by Immigrant Type

Note: Analysis based on individuals reporting good, very good, or excellent health and controls for age, sex, income adequacy, education, smoking, inactive leisure, social support, and body mass image.

** Statistically significant difference from estimate for Canadian-born ($p < 0.01$)

Source: Ng, E., Wilkins, R., Gendron, F., & Berthelot, J. M. (2005). Dynamics of immigrants' health in Canada: Evidence from the National Population Health Survey. *Healthy today, healthy tomorrow? Findings from the National Population Health Survey, 2.* Catalogue no. 82-618-MWE2005002. Ottawa: Statistics Canada. Retrieved from http://www.statcan.gc.ca/pub/82-618-m/2005002/pdf/4193621-eng.pdf

Interrelationships between Multiculturalism Policy, Social Exclusion, and Health

Despite the many successes of multiculturalism policy, racism remains a major obstacle to full integration and inclusive citizenship (Wood & Wortley, 2010; Reitz & Banerjee, 2007; Mock, 2002; Reitz et al., 2009; Weinfeld, 1981). This poses challenges for multiculturalism policy in Canada in terms of how it can be used to address racism and hierachies of oppression (Shields et al., 2006; Saloojee, 2005; Shields, 2004).

Racism influences health indirectly through differential exposures related to other determinants of health, for example, education and employment. In fact, the WHO considers racism to be a root cause of poverty. In Canada, recent data from the Longitudinal Survey of Immigrants to Canada (LSIC) show that perceived discrimination has a negative impact on immigrants' life satisfaction (Houle & Schellenberg, 2010) and health (De Maio & Kemp, 2010). De Maio and Kemp (2010) explored relationships between perceived racial discrimination, self-reported health, and mental health among new immigrants in Canada. Using data from the LSIC (approximately 12,000 immigrants arriving between October 2000 and September 2001 surveyed six months, two years, and four years after arriving in Canada), the study observed a decline in physical health status (self-reported health) and the deterioration of mental well-being. Similar findings were reported by Fuller-Thompson et al. (2011).

The consequences of social exclusion for racialized groups include a lack of recognition and acceptance, feelings of powerlessness, economic vulnerability, diminished life experiences, and limited life prospects (Omidvar & Richmond, 2005; Saloojee, 2005). Of particular concern for racialized immigrants are recent studies suggesting that perceptions and experiences of racial discrimination increase over length of stay (Gee et al., 2006).

Evidence for Social Capital, Immigrant Integration, and Health in Canada

Social capital refers to the "the norms and networks facilitating collective action for mutual benefit" (Woolcock, 1998, p. 155). It is predicated on reciprocity, trust, and the active and willing engagement of citizens within a participative community (Portes, 1998; Coleman, 1988). One of the hypothesized outcomes of social capital is a vibrant civic life (Stone & Hughes, 2002). Two types of social capital commonly referred to are bonding social capital, characterized by strong ties within groups populated by like-minded individuals who share a collective orientation (Wuthnow, 2002; Putnam, 1993), and bridging social capital, characterized by weaker, intergroup ties that cross religious, class, age, ethno-racial, and economic groups (Putnam, 1993).

Much attention, both in the form of research and discourse, has been paid to the concept of social capital since the publication of *Bowling Alone*, Putnam's (2000) treatise linking social capital to a country's social and economic development. The concept of social capital has implications for economic and social development, immigrant integration, health, poverty, social exclusion, and neighbourhood revitalization (Galabuzi & Teelucksingh, 2010; Long & Perkins, 2007; Putnam, 1993, 2007; Shookner, 2002). Social capital can enhance positive outcomes or, on the negative side, impede access to opportunity either through social closure or by virtue of its absence (Putnam, 1993, 2000).

There is a vast literature on the mechanisms linking social capital to health (Carpiano, 2007; Kawachi et al., 2008; Browning & Cagney, 2003; Browning & Cagney, 2002; Kim et al., 2008; Macintyre & Ellaway, 2003). Neighbourhood social cohesion may influence health-related behaviours by the adoption of health-promoting activity and healthy norms, and exerting social control over deviant behaviour (Altschuler et al., 2004). Higher levels of community cohesion may result in higher degrees of social organization that enhances access to services that influence health. For example, Kawachi (1999) suggested that the ability to arrange child care at short notice depends on the level of trust between neighbours and the expectation that a good deed will be reciprocated in the future. Social cohesion might influence health through psychosocial processes such as through the provision of affective support and enhancing self-esteem and mutual respect (Kawachi & Berkman, 2000). Being able to depend on neighbours for help may attenuate the adverse effects on mental well-being of living in socio-economically deprived neighbourhoods. However, some studies suggested that in stressful/disadvantaged neighbourhoods, isolation from neighbours might exert a protective effect on mental health (Dupéré & Perkins, 2007; Caughy et al., 2003).

Both bridging and bonding social capital are important for the new immigrant (Kunz, 2003). Bridging social capital ultimately provides links with others and paves the way for a shared understanding of the new society. Bonding provides a sense of support and identity to the newcomer. However, without bridging social capital, the newcomer may be insufficiently integrated in the Canadian mosaic (Berger et al., 2008). Having access to close networks of people of the same cultural origin—as well as to programs that support these networks—is associated with the social and economic integration of immigrants (Esses et al., 2009). According to the Canadian Ethnic Diversity Survey (2003), immigrants are more likely than the Canadian-born population to report a strong sense of belonging to their ethnic or cultural group and are more likely to participate in ethnic or immigrant associations (6 percent vs. 1 percent). Family and friendship networks for new immigrants in Canada provide an extremely important support system, particularly during early stages of settlement. This is associated with better perceived health (Van Kemenade et al., 2006; Kunz,

2003). Reciprocity in social relationships was associated with good health in both immigrant and non-immigrant women, but the relationship was stronger among immigrant women (Van Kemenade et al., 2006).

In addition to bridging and bonding social capital, one can differentiate between *individual social capital* (i.e., the social networks through which an individual finds the resources he or she needs), and *collective social capital* (i.e., the networks formed by social groups within a neighbourhood or community to achieve the resources needed to attain their goals). Collective social capital plays an additional role in providing voice to the various ethnic groups that make up Canada's mosaic. As indicated above, evidence suggests that very few of Canada's "visible minorities" sit in decision-making positions in any of the sectors. Groups that have strong collective social capital are more likely to have their voices heard in community and public policy debates (De Leon et al., 2009).

Collective social capital can occur in geographic or community networks. Geographic networks refer to proximal social ties within a confined physical space, such as a building, or several city blocks, or a whole neighbourhood. Immigrants in Canada are likely to reside in "ethnic enclaves" (i.e., organized on the basis of cultural and national origins rather than race) within racially diverse neighbourhoods as opposed to urban ghettos, which are residentially segregated on a racial, ethnic, and/or religious basis, although there are some examples of concentrations of racialized people of colour at the scale of city blocks or apartment buildings (Qadeer & Kumar, 2003). Ethnic enclaves can facilitate access to entry-level employment, financial capital, information about business opportunities and access to markets; provide an informal infrastructure for social service delivery; and contribute to a sense of belonging (Qadeer & Kumar, 2003; Li, 2003; Portes, 1998). Neighbourhood ethnic enclaves in Canada generally represent opportunities for social inclusionary pathways, but there are risks of social exclusion if segregation coincides with structural factors such as low income, underemployment, and poor housing (Omidvar & Richmond, 2005; Portes, 1998).

Community networks refer to organizational social ties based on interests and shared values, not necessarily on geographic proximity. These networks are critical for early and long-term immigrant integration and inclusion. Studies of social support among recent immigrants show that many newcomers prefer to stay within their own social/ethnic groups for support and experience discomfort and other barriers in seeking formal mainstream support (Simich et al., 2004). The more institutionally complete a community is in terms of businesses, churches, banks, and social services, the more it can offer newcomers and established members in terms of resources that increase ethnic attachment and bonding (Kunz, 2005, p. 55). Over the long term, community organizations are important drivers of social capital through direct-service provision and their ability to respond to the social needs arising in their communities (Jedwab,

2008). Some ethnic and/or religious communities (e.g., Ismaili Muslim community, Jewish community) provide linguistically and culturally accessible support in health promotion and chronic disease management that can complement mainstream services, including information sessions and support groups for community members. However, many communities do not have the resources or infrastructures to provide such services without government support. The collective social capital of these groups is weaker and the sustainability of their organizations is precarious.

Research from Western countries shows that building mutual support and solidarity within communities (however defined) can be a basis for effective integration into mainstream society (Banting, Courchene, & Seidle, 2006; Berry et al, 2006; Banting & Kymlicka, 2006; Harty & Murphy, 2005). Bloemraad (2006) compared the integration experiences of Vietnamese immigrants in Boston and Toronto and found that civic integration was much stronger among the latter. After considering alternative explanations, she concluded that Canadian multiculturalism policy may enable newcomer communities to integrate by facilitating community self-organization, leadership, and partnerships. These features also help to enhance the participation of communities in other realms, and the benefits are reciprocal. For example, the advantages of diverse leadership are well documented and include increased productivity, effectiveness, responsiveness, and innovation (Conference Board of Canada, 2008; Maytree Foundation, n.d.).

The Role of Multiculturalism Policy in Addressing Social Exclusion

Broad national policies and programs are more effective than smaller piecemeal measures at reducing social exclusion and improving health and quality of life (National Council of Welfare, 2007; Beckfield & Krieger, 2009; Fang et al., 2009; Tugwell et al., 2006). For example, government policies have played an important role in promoting health equity (Bryant et al., 2010), education, crime reduction, and social welfare (Cottingham et al., 2004), and in reducing unemployment (Benach et al., 2010). Laws and policies aimed at eliminating institutional racism in all sectors may be more effective than piecemeal anti-racism initiatives or programs that attempt to foster relationships across various ethnic, religious, and racialized communities or act to change public attitudes.

One of the most promising ways to promote an anti-racist perspective is through the adoption and support of racial impact analyses at all levels of government. This analysis involves a careful examination of the actual or likely impact of a proposed policy, legislation, program, or practice in order to minimize resulting disparities or to foster racial equity, racial justice, and inclusion. As such it is considered a vital tool for identifying, reducing, and eliminating long-standing institutional and structural access barriers that contribute to inequities. Color of Change (2008) has called for racial impact analyses on all legislation, policies, program, and practices previously passed (and yet to be considered) to determine their impact, either positive or negative, on racial equity and justice.

Multiculturalism policy needs to be better integrated with social inclusion policies targeting multiple levels and government sectors (Hyman et al., 2014). Multiculturalism policy may not be specific enough nor sufficiently coordinated to address racial inequities in Canada that result from institutional barriers, including existing immigration and settlement, human rights, and employment policies (Reitz & Banerjee, 2007). Institutional racism contributes to the immigrant's sense of alienation and may be more harmful than interpersonal discrimination (Wood & Wortley, 2010). The identification and elimination of institutional and structural barriers that impede integration and equality of opportunity for all Canadians is consistent with the aims of social inclusion policy. Saloojee (2005) suggests that government policy should take a leadership role in adopting an inclusion framework that incorporates an anti-racist perspective. In this way multiculturalism policy could be integrated with social inclusion policy aimed at ensuring equitable outcomes and the full and valued participation of all Canadians regardless of their race, ethnicity, religion, socio-economic status, dis/ability, gender, sexual orientation, and language proficiency. It is established that government social policy aimed at reducing population inequalities leads to better health outcomes (Wilkinson & Pickett, 2010; Raphael, 2012).

The Role of Multiculturalism Policy in Building Collective Social Capital

Many examples were provided to show that supporting and building collective neighbourhood and community capacity yields positive results for healthy integration. Bonding social capital facilitates immigrant integration and intra-community cohesion by enhancing social and economic networks within a community. Bridging social capital has been associated with individual integration and represents a promising collective pathway to partnerships across communities and to national cohesion as a whole. This poses a challenge for multiculturalism policy in terms of how it can promote and support the development of social capital within and across communities.

Wong (2010) proposed the idea of *interactive multiculturalism* that has a civic component where there are common spaces for people to meet and interact (e.g., formal institutions, voluntary organizations):

> Common spaces are defined as locations in time and space where diverse groups of Canadians can meet and interact. Examples include workplaces, political parties, schools, neighbourhood facilities, and public transport systems, which

> have been described as the vehicles through which a multicultural, multi-racial, multi-religious population develops synergies that are strong enough to lead to a collective national identity. (Dib et al., 2008, p. 162)

With the support of multiculturalism policy, public institutions can play an important role in the creation of common spaces and in ensuring that all public spaces are more sensitive and responsive to diversity (Wood & Wortley, 2010).

Programs that foster intercommunity partnerships and social, civic and political engagement are essential to building social capital across and between communities. For example, initiatives such as DiverseCity (Maytree Foundation, 2010) in Toronto are promoting ethnic and racial leadership and participation in all sectors as a key to increased productivity and responsiveness. Similarly, umbrella organizations that act as a collective voice for immigrant-serving organizations contribute to the development of bonding and bridging social capital but have no regular source of funding (Laidlaw Foundation, 2004). Multiculturalism policy may consider the provision of sufficient support to organizations that have a broad mandate of building social capital to increase the participation of newcomer and racialized communities and their members in different areas of the public, private, and non-profit sectors.

Finally, multiculturalism policy needs to explicitly recognize the importance of social capital in its support of community building and in broader social inclusion policies at multiple levels. Governments can strengthen social inclusion, build social cohesion, and empower communities by identifying key factors that demonstrate the value of social capital and supporting successful models of social, cultural, economic, and political participation in local communities.

Conclusions

Canada is the only country in the world where multiculturalism policy is enshrined in the country's constitution. We have presented evidence of its successes in helping immigrants to integrate; however, it has not been able to address some of the systemic determinants, such as discrimination, that create social and health inequities. Today's new waves of immigrants, mostly from non-European countries, are facing economic and social challenges that may not have been encountered by earlier waves of immigrants to the same extent; this has consequences for their health and well-being.

This chapter suggests that multiculturalism policy can help to tackle some of these issues by addressing racism and social exclusion and strengthening collective social capital. In addition to providing specific programs aimed at immigrant groups to help them integrate successfully, multiculturalism policy should also focus on broader social inclusionary processes at all levels of government and in all sectors of society as these have been shown to be critical determinants of health and well-being.

But it is unclear to what extent multiculturalism can deal with many of the economic and social realities that many immigrants face in unemployment, under-employment, and insecure employment with low wages. Growing inequality and welfare state retrenchment have affected the health and well-being of all Canadians, and especially of recent immigrants to Canada, many of whom are people of colour. The healthy immigrant effect and the deterioration of health of recent immigrants over time highlight the depth of these challenges.

Critical Thinking Questions

1. What are the factors that contribute to the healthy immigrant effect in Canada?
2. What are the key social determinants of immigrant health in Canada?
3. How can multiculturalism policy contribute to maintaining and/or improving immigrant health in Canada?
4. What other types of policies are needed to support immigrant health in Canada and social cohesion overall?
5. Is there sufficient evidence that social capital can be facilitated through governmental policies and injections of funding?

Glossary

Integration is a broad term that is typically used to describe the settlement experiences and participation of immigrants in the country of adoption. Integration may encompass many different dimensions: economic integration into the labour market; political (or civic) integration into the electoral process and other forms of political participation; and social integration into the networks and spaces of civil society, from informal networks of friends and neighbours to membership in more formal organizations (Kymlicka, 2010).

Multiculturalism refers to "a system of beliefs and behaviors that recognizes and respects the presence of all diverse groups in an organization or society, acknowledges and values their socio-cultural differences, and encourages and enables their continued contribution within an inclusive cultural context which empowers all within the organization or society" (Rosaldo, 1996, p. 2). In Canada, multiculturalism most often refers to a set of ideas and ideals celebrating the nation's cultural diversity. At the policy level it refers to the "management of diversity through formal initiatives in the federal provincial and municipal domains" (Dewing & Leman, 2006, p. 1).

Racialization refers to the social process whereby certain groups come to be designated as different and unequal based on socially constructed perceptions of external features (such as skin colour, physical features, accents, etc.) in ways that lead to negative social, economic, health, and political impacts (Galabuzi, 2006).

Racism is the belief that race is the primary determinant of human traits and capacities and those racial differences produce an inherent superiority of a particular race (*Merriam-Webster Dictionary*, 2008). The Canadian Race Relations Foundation (CRRF) defines racism not only as an attitude, but also as the specific actions resulting from this attitude that impact upon, marginalize, and oppress some people. Beliefs of race are reflected in institutional and individual practices to create and reinforce oppressive systems of race relations and social position (Krieger, 2003).

Social capital can be defined as the "the norms and networks facilitating collective action for mutual benefit" (Woolcock, 1998, p. 155). Social capital exists within and through structures of relationships occurring among both individuals and groups. It is based on the social norms and shared values that direct behaviour, reciprocity, trust, and the active and willing engagement of citizens within a participative community (Portes, 1998; Coleman, 1988). Two types of social capital commonly referred to are (1) bonding social capital, characterized by strong ties within groups populated by like-minded individuals who share a collective orientation (Wuthnow, 2002; Putnam, 1993); and (2) bridging social capital, characterized by weaker, intergroup ties that cross religious, class, age, ethno-racial, and economic groups (Putnam, 1993). Frank (2003) also includes linking social capital that builds links not just horizontally but vertically among groups occupying different layers in the economic or political system.

Social exclusion originated as a formal concept in France in the 1970s when it emerged in response to the erosion of the welfare state, downward economic shifts, and increasing population diversity (Ebersold, 1998). The notion of social exclusion gained prominence when large segments of the population were excluded from the labour market. This contributed to homelessness, alarming increases in child poverty, and elevated rates of family breakdown (Shields et al., 2006). Social exclusion, or the "unequal access to critical resources that determine the quality of membership in society, ultimately produces and reproduces a complex of unequal outcomes" (Galabuzi, 2008, p. 236).

Social inclusion is considered by many to be a normative, values-based concept identifying the type of society we want to live in and the changes needed to build that society (O'Hara et al., 2006). Sen (1999, p. 124) defines an inclusive society as "characterized by a widely shared social experience and active participation, by a broad equality of opportunities and life chances for individuals and by the achievement of a basic level of well-being for all citizens." The removal of barriers is critical for full participation.

Recommended Readings

De Maio, F. G., & Kemp, E. (2010). The deterioration of health status among immigrants to Canada. *Global Public Health*, 5(5), 462–78.

This article examines health transitions among new immigrants to Canada and determines which are largely driven by discrimination and inequality.

Hyman, I., & Jackson, B. (2010). The healthy immigrant effect: A temporary phenomenon? *Health Policy Research Bulletin*, 17, 17–21.

This article reviews key Canadian findings on the healthy immigrant effect.

Hyman, I., Meinhard, A., & Shields, J. (2011). *The role of multiculturalism policy in addressing social inclusion processes in Canada*. Prepared for the Canadian Multicultural Education Foundation. Edmonton: CMEF.

This report reviews the successes and failures of Canada's Multiculturalism Policy and recommends future directions.

Hyman, I., & Wray, R. (2013). *Health inequalities and racialized groups—A review of the evidence*. Toronto: Toronto Public Health.

This review examines Canadian and U.S. data on racialization and health outcomes and makes the case for initiating data collection on discrimination and health in Canada.

Ng, E., Wilkins, R., Gendron, F., & Berthelot, J. M. (2005). Dynamics of immigrants' health in Canada: Evidence from the National Population Health Survey. *Healthy today, healthy tomorrow? Findings from the National Population Health Survey*, 2. Catalogue no. 82–618-MWE2005002. Ottawa: Statistics Canada. Retrieved from http://www.statcan.gc.ca/pub/82–618–m/2005002/pdf/4193621–eng.pdf

This was one of the first research papers to draw attention to the differences in health outcomes among immigrants originating from different regions of origin.

Related Websites

CERIS—http://ceris.ca/who-we-are/

CERIS is Ontario's leading network of researchers, policy-makers, and practitioners working in the field of migration and settlement. It serves as the knowledge-exchange hub for all three communities and works in the interest of all migrants and the general public. It recently added synthesis reports on five main areas of Canadian immigration on the domestic front: (1) settlement and integration, (2) foreign credential recognition, (3) citizenship, (4) multiculturalism, and (5) refugees. It also provides a searchable online library.

Citizenship and Immigration Canada. Multiculturalism—www.cic.gc.ca/english/multiculturalism/citizenship.asp

This is the official Canadian government website on multiculturalism policy that reviews current and past initiatives in this area.

Health Canada. Health Policy Bulletin—www.hc-sc.gc.ca/sr-sr/pubs/hpr-rpms/bull/2010–health-sante-migr/index-eng.php

This issue of the *Health Policy Bulletin* is devoted entirely to migration and health in Canada, including definitions, historical perspectives, social determinants of immigrant health, health of temporary migrants, mental health and other specific health outcomes, and health care utilization.

Metropolis Canada—www.metropolis.net/index_e.html

Metropolis is an international network for comparative research and public policy development on migration, diversity, and immigrant integration in cities in Canada and around the world. The Metropolis Canada website has publications on many aspects of immigration in Canada.

Notes

1. This finding comes from an informal survey done yearly by the second author in her undergraduate classes in Toronto. Without priming, students are asked to list three defining features of Canada. Among 75 percent of the students, multiculturalism ranks first or second.
2. The NHS data likely understate pay and income differences between whites and non-whites due to under-sampling of lower income groups, and are not directly comparable to Census data from previous years. This is unfortunate since other Statistics Canada surveys of earnings and income such as the Labour Force Survey do not gather data based on racial status.
3. With the new Liberal government, all refugee health care benefits were fully restored to pre-2012 levels by April 1, 2016.

References

Adams, M. (2009). Muslims in Canada 2007. *PRI Horizons, 10*(2), 19–26.

Ali, J. (2002). *Mental health of Canada's immigrants, supplement to Health Reports.* Catalogue no. 82–003. Ottawa: Statistics Canada.

Ali, J. (2014). *Welcome to Canada? A critical review and assessment of Canada's fast-changing immigration policies.* RCIS Working Paper no. 2014/6.

Allan, B., & Smylie, J. (2015). *First peoples, second class treatment: The role of racism in the health and well-being of Indigenous peoples in Canada.* Toronto: The Wellesley Institute.

Altschuler, A., Somkin, C. P., & Adler, N. E. (2004). Local services and amenities, neighborhood social capital, and health. *Social Science & Medicine, 59*(6), 1219–29.

Angus Reid. (2010). *Canadians endorse multiculturalism, but pick melting pot over mosaic.* Retrieved from http://www.angus-reid.com/polls/43492/canadians-endorse-multiculturalism-but-pick-melting-pot-over-mosaic

Bannerji, H. (2000). *The dark side of the nation.* Toronto: Canadian Scholars' Press Inc.

Banting, K. T., Courchene, T., & Seidie, L. (Eds.) (2006). *Belonging? Diversity, recognition, and shared citizenship in Canada.* Ottawa: Institute for Research on Public Policy.

Banting, K., & Kymlicka, W. (2006). Introduction: Multiculturalism and the welfare state: Setting the context. In K. Banting & W. Kymlicka (Eds.), *Multiculturalism and the welfare state: Recognition and redistribution in contemporary democracies* (pp. 1–48). Oxford: Oxford University Press.

Banting, K., Thomas, J., Courchene, T., & Seidle, L. (2007). *Belonging? Diversity, recognition, and shared citizenship in Canada.* Montreal: Institute for Research in Public Policy.

Beckfield, J., & Krieger, N. (2009). Epi + demos + cracy: Linking political systems and priorities to the magnitude of health inequities—Evidence, gaps, and a research agenda. *Epidemiology Reviews, 31*(1), 152–77.

Benach, J., Muntaner, C., Chung, H., Solar, O., Santana, V., Friel, S., ... & Marmot, M., (2010). The importance of government policies in reducing employment related health inequalities. *British Medical Journal, 340*(2154).

Berger, I., Foster, M. K., & Meinhard, A. (2008). *Civic engagement, social cohesion, and integration in Canada.* 12th Biennial Jerusalem Conference in Canadian Studies.

Bergeron, P., Auger, N., & Hamel, D. (2009). Weight, general health, and mental health: The status of various subgroups of immigrants in Canada. *Canadian Journal of Public Health, 100*(3), 215–20.

Berry, J., Phinney, J., Sam, D., & Vedder, P. (2006). Immigrant youth: Acculturation, identity, and adaptation. *Applied Psychology: An International Review, 55*(3), 303–32.

Biddle, N., Kennedy, S., MacDonald, J. T. (2007). Health assimilation patterns amongst Australian immigrants. *Economic Record, 83*(260), 16–30.

Bissoondath, N. (2002). *Selling illusions: The cult of multi-culturalism in Canada* (2nd ed.). Toronto: Penguin Canada.

Bloemraad, I. (2006). *Becoming a citizen: Incorporating immigrants and refugees in the United States and Canada.* Berkeley: University of California Press.

Bradshaw, P., et al. (2009). *Results of a national survey of diversity on Canadian nonprofit boards.* Presented at the Association for Nonprofit and Social Economy Research, ANSER, Carlton University, Ottawa.

Browning, C. R., & Cagney, K. A. (2002). Neighborhood structural disadvantage, collective efficacy, and self-rated physical health in an urban setting. *Journal of Health and Social Behavior, 43*(4), 383–99.

Browning, C. R., & Cagney, K. A. (2003). Moving beyond poverty: Neighborhood structure, social processes, and health. *Journal of Health and Social Behavior, 44*(4), 552–71.

Bryant, T., Raphael, D., & Rioux, M. (2010). *Staying alive: Critical perspectives on health, illness, and health care* (2nd ed.). Toronto: Canadian Scholars' Press Inc.

Bush, N. (2008). Multicultural nations: Issues of race and national identity in Britain and Canada. Theses and dissertations, Paper 113. Retrieved from http://digitalcommons.ryerson.ca/dissertations/113

Canadian Council for Refugees. (2004). *Impacts on children of the Immigration and Refugee Protection Act.* Montreal: Author.

Canadian Ethnic Diversity Survey. (2003). Ethnic Diversity Survey 2002. Statistics Canada, *The Daily.* Retrieved from www.statcan.ca/Daily/English/030929/d030929.pdf

Canadian Race Relations Foundation. (n.d.). Racism fact sheet. Retrieved from http.//www.crrf-fcrr. ca/images/stories/pdf/ePubFaShAckRac.pdf

Carpiano, R. M. (2007). Neighborhood social capital and adult health: An empirical test of a Bourdieu-based model. *Health & Place, 13*(3), 639–55.

Cassin, A. M., Krawchenko, T., & VanderPlaat, M. (2007). *Racism and discrimination in Canada: Laws, policies, and practices.* Multiculturalism and Human Rights Research Reports no. 3. Atlantic Metropolis Centre/Centre Metropolis Atlantique. Retrieved from: http://atlantic.metropolis.net/ResearchPolicy/Racism%20and%20Descrimination%20in%20Canada%20–%20%20Report%20May%202007.pdf

Caughy, M. O. B., O'Campo, P. J., & Muntaner, C. (2003). When being alone might be better: Neighborhood poverty, social capital, and child mental health. *Social Science & Medicine, 57*(2), 227_37.

Caulford, P., & Vali, Y. (2006). Providing health care to medically uninsured immigrants and refugees. *CMAJ: Canadian Medical Association Journal, 174*(9), 1253(2).

CICS Immigration Consulting. (2014). *New Statistics Canada report shows high education levels among immigrants.* Retrieved from http://www.cicsimmigration.com/statistics/

Citizenship and Immigration Canada. (2010a). *Facts and figures 2009: Summary tables—permanent and temporary residents.* Retrieved from http://www.cic.gc.ca/English/resources/statistics/facts2009/index.asp

Citizenship and Immigration Canada. (2010b). *The current state of multiculturalism in Canada and research themes on Canadian multiculturalism 2008–2010.* Working Paper. Retrieved from http://www.cic.gc.ca/english/resources/publications/multi-state/index.asp

Coleman, J. (1988). Social capital in the creation of human capital. *American Journal of Sociology, 94,* 95–120.

Color of Change. (2008). *Ontario's racial equity justice review with respect to recent federal policies, programs, and initiatives.* Retrieved from http://www.ocasi.org/downloads/Federal_Government_Racial_Equity.Racial_Justice_Review_October6_2008.pdf

Conference Board of Canada. (2008). *The value of diverse leadership.* Retrieved from http://www.diversecitytoronto.ca/wpcontent/themes/openair/download/The_Value_of_Diverse_Leadership_CBC_final.pdf

Corak, M. (2008). Immigration in the long run: The education and earnings mobility of second generation Canadians. *IRPP Choices, 13*(3), 1–32.

Cottingham, P., Maynard, R., & Stagner, M. (2004). Synthesizing evidence on the impacts of programmes and policies in education, crime and justice, and social welfare: Practical recommendations. *Evaluation and Research in Education, 18*(1), 28–53.

Creatore, M., Moineddin, R., Booth, G., Manual, D., & Glazier, R. (2010). Age and sex patterns of diabetes among immigrants to Canada. *Canadian Medical Association, 182*(8), 781–89.

Cukier, W., & Yap, M. (2009). *Diversity counts: A snapshot of diversity in the Greater Toronto Area.* Toronto: The Diversity Institute in Management and Technology, Ted Rogers School of Management, Ryerson University.

Dauvergne, M., Scrim, K., & Brennan, S. (2008). *Hate crime in Canada.* Statistics Canada. Catalogue no. 85F0033M. Canadian Centre for Justice Statistics (17). Retrieved from www.statcan.gc.ca/pub/85f0033m/85f0033m2008017-eng.htm

De Leon, E., Maronick, M., De Vita, C., & Boris, E. T. (2009). *Community-based organizations and immigrant integration in the Washington, D.C. metropolitan area.* Washington, D.C.: The Urban Institute.

De Maio, F. G. (2010). Immigration as pathogenic: A systematic review of the health of immigrants to Canada. *International Journal for Equity in Health, 9*(27), 1–20.

De Maio, F. G., & Kemp, E. (2010). The deterioration of health status among immigrants to Canada. *Global Public Health, 5*(5), 462–78.

Department of Justice. (1985). *Canadian Multiculturalism Act. Section 3. Canadian Multiculturalism Policy.* Retrieved from http://laws-lois.justice.gc.ca/eng/acts/C–18.7/

Dewing, M., & Leman, M. (2006). *Canadian multiculturalism.* Library of Parliament, Canada. Retrieved from http://www2.parl.gc.ca/content/lop/researchpublications/936–e.htm

Dib, K., Donaldson, I., & Turcotte, B. (2008). Integration and identity in Canada: The importance of multicultural common spaces. *Canadian Ethnic Studies, 40*(1), 161–87.

Dupéré, V., & Perkins, D. D. (2007). Community types and mental health: A multilevel study of local environmental stress and coping. *American Journal of Community Psychology, 39*(1–2), 107–19.

Ebersold, S. (1998). *Exclusion and disability.* Organisation for Economic Co-operation and Development, Centre for Educational Research and Innovation. Retrieved from http://www.oecd.org/dataoecd/20/17/1856907.pdf

Edwards, B. F. R. (2010). Who do we think we are: Writings on citizenship and identity in the twenty-first century. *Journal of Canadian Studies, 44*(1), 221–28.

Esses, V., Hamilton, L. K., Bennet-AbuAyyash, C., & Burnstein, M. (2009). *Characteristics of a welcoming community.* Report to CIC. Retrieved from http://ceris.metropolis.net/research-policy/Characteristics%20of%20a%20Welcoming%20Community-%20Symposium.pdf

Fang, R., Kmetic, A., Millar, J., & Drasic, L. (2009). Disparities in chronic disease among Canada's low-income populations. *Previous Chronic Disorder, 6*(4). Retrieved from http://www.cdc.gov/pcd/issues/2009/oct/08_0254.htm

Fleras, A., & Kunz, J. L. (2001). *Media and minorities: Representing diversity in a multicultural Canada.* Toronto: Thompson Educational Publishing.

Frank, J. (2003). Making social capital work for public policy. *Horizons, 6*(3), 3–6. Ottawa: Policy Research Initiative.

Frenette, M. & Morissette, R. (2003). *Will they ever converge? Earnings of immigrant and Canadian-born workers over the past two decades.* Ottawa: Statistics Canada.

Frideres, J. (2008). Creating an inclusive society. In J. Biles, M. Burstein, & J. Frideres (Eds.), *Immigration and integration in Canada* (pp. 77–102). Kingston: McGill-Queen's University Press.

Frisbie, W. P., Youngtae, C., & Hummer, R. A. (2001). Immigration and the health of Asian and Pacific Islander adults in the United States. *American Journal Epidemiology, 153*(4), 372–80.

Fuller-Thomson, E., Noack, A. M., & George, U. (2011). Health decline among recent immigrants to Canada: Findings from a nationally-representative longitudinal survey. *Canadian Journal of Public Health/Revue Canadienne de Santé Publique, 102*(4), 273–80.

Galabuzi, G. E. (2004). Social exclusion. In D. Raphael (Ed.), *Social determinants of health: Canadian perspectives* (pp. 235–51). Toronto: Canadian Scholars' Press Inc.

Galabuzi, G. E. (2006). *Canada's economic apartheid: The social exclusion of racialized groups in the new century*. Toronto: Canadian Scholars' Press Inc.

Galabuzi, G. E. (2008). Social exclusion. In D. Raphael (Ed.), *Social determinants of health: Canadian perspectives* (2nd ed., pp. 252–268). Toronto: Canadian Scholars' Press Inc.

Galabuzi, G. E., & Teelucksingh, C. (2010). *Social cohesion, social exclusion, social capital.* Regional Municipality of Peel. Retrieved from http://www.peelregion.ca/social-services/pdfs/discussion-paper-1.pdf

Galarneau, D., & Morissette, R. (2008). Immigrants' education and required job skills. Statistics Canada, Perspectives. Catalogue no. 75–001–X, p. 6. Ottawa: Statistics Canada.

Gee, G. C., Ryan, A., Laflamme, D. J., & Holt, J. (2006). Self-reported discrimination and mental health status among African descendants, Mexican Americans, and other Latinos in the New Hampshire REACH 2010 Initiative: The added dimension of immigration. *American Journal of Public Health, 96*(10), 1821–28.

Georgiades, K., Boyle, M. H., Duku, E., & Racine, Y. (2006). Tobacco use among immigrant and nonimmigrant adolescents: Individual and family level influences. *Journal of Adolescent Health, 38*(4), 1–7.

Gogia, N., & Slade, B. (2011). *About Canada: Immigration.* Halifax: Fernwood Publishers.

Government of Canada. (2012). *Canadian multiculturalism: An inclusive citizenship.* Retreived from www.cic.gc.ca/english/multiculturalism/citizenship.asp

Gushulak, B. D., Pottie, K., Roberts, J. H., Torres, S., & DesMeules, M. (2011). Migration and health in Canada: Health in the global village. *Canadian Medical Association Journal, 183*(12), E952–58.

Hansson, E., Tuck, A., Lurie, S., & McKenzie, K., for Task Group of the Services Systems Advisory Committee, Mental Health Commission of Canada. (2010). *Improving mental health services for immigrant, refugee, ethno-cultural and racialized groups: Issues and options for service improvement.* Ottawa: Mental Health Commission of Canada.

Harty, S., & Murphy, M. (2005). *In defence of multicultural citizenship.* Cardiff: University of Wales Press.

Henry, F., & Tator, C. (2006). *Racial profiling in Canada: Challenging the myth of "a few bad apples."* Toronto: University of Toronto Press.

Hiebert, D., & Sherrell, K. (2009). *The integration and inclusion of newcomers in British Columbia.* Metropolis British Columbia, Centre of Excellence for Research on Immigration and Diversity (CERID). Vancouver: CERID.

Houle, R., & Schellenberg, G. (2010). *New immigrants' assessments of their life in Canada.* Statistics Canada. Catalogue no. 11F0019M–No. 322. Retrieved from http://www.statcan.gc.ca/pub/11f0019m/11f0019m2010322–eng.pdf

Howe, P. (2007). The political engagement of new Canadians: A comparative perspective. In K. G. Banting, T. J. Courchene, & F. L. Seidle (Eds.), *Belonging? Diversity, recognition, and shared citizenship in Canada* (pp. 611–646). Montreal: Institute for Research on Public Policy.

Hyman, I. (2001). *Immigration and health.* Health Policy Working Paper Series. Working Paper no. 01–05. Ottawa: Health Canada.

Hyman, I. (2007). *Immigration and health: Reviewing evidence of the healthy immigrant effect in Canada.* CERIS Working Paper no. 55. Toronto: Joint Centre of Excellence for Research in Immigration and Settlement.

Hyman, I. (2009). *Racism as a determinant of immigrant health.* Ottawa: Public Health Agency of Canada and Metropolis Canada. Retrieved from http://canada.metropolis.net/pdfs/racism_policy_brief_e.pdf

Hyman, I., Mercado, R., Galabuzi, G. E., & Patychuk, D. (2014). A critical review of social exclusion and inclusion indicators: Implications for the development of a Canadian framework. In K. Murphy Kilbride (Ed.), *Immigrant integration: Research implications for future policy* (pp. 85–102).

Jackson, A. (2013). *Racial discrimination and the economic downturn.* Toronto: Broadbent Institute. Retrieved from https://www.broadbentinstitute.ca/en/blog/racial-discrimination-and-economic-downturn

Jedwab, J. (2008). The rise of the unmeltable Canadians? Ethnic and national belonging in Canada's second generation. *Canadian Diversity, 6*(2), 25–34.

Kallen, E. (1982). Multiculturalism: Ideology, policy, and reality. *Journal of Canadian Studies,17*(1), 51–63.

Karlsen, S., & Nazroo, J. Y. (2002). Relation between racial discrimination, social class, and health among ethnic minority groups. *American Journal of Public Health, 92*(4), 624–31.

Kawachi, I. (1999). Social capital and community effects on population and individual health. *Annals of the New York Academy of Sciences, 896*(1), 120–30.

Kawachi, I., & Berkman, L. (2000). Social cohesion, social capital, and health. In L.F. Berkman & I. Kawachi (Eds.), *Social epidemiology* (pp. 174–190). New York: Oxford University Press.

Kawachi, I., Subramanian, S. V., & Kim, D. (2008). Social capital and health. In I. Kawachi, S.V, Subramanian, & D. Kim (Eds.), *Social capital and health* (pp. 1–26). New York: Springer.

Kelly, P., Park, S., & Lepper, L. (2011). *Economic recession and immigrant labour market outcomes in Canada, 2006–2011.* TIEDI Analytical Report 22. Toronto: Immigrant Employment Data Initiative (TIEDI).

Keung, N. (2012). Canada to keep same immigration levels for 2013. *Toronto Star,* December 26.

Kim, D., Subramanian, S. V., & Kawachi, I. (2008). Social capital and physical health. In I. Kawachi, V. Subramanian, & D. Kim (Eds.). *Social capital and Health* (pp. 139–190). New York: Springer.

Kirmayer, L. J., Narasiah, L., Munoz, M., Rashid, M., Ryder, A. G., Guzder, J., ... & Pottie, K. (2011). Common mental health problems in immigrants and refugees: General approach in primary care. *Canadian Medical Association Journal, 183*(12), E959–67.

Kliewer, E. V., & Ward, D. (1988). Convergence of immigrant suicide rates to those in the destination country. *American Journal of Epidemiology, 127*(3), 640–53.

Krieger, N. (2003). Does racism harm health? Did child abuse exist before 1962? On explicit questions, critical science, and current controversies: An eco-social perspective. *American Journal of Public Health, 93*(2), 194–99.

Kunz, J. L. (2003). Social capital: A key dimension of immigrant integration. *Canadian Issues,* April, 33–34. Concord, ON: Canadian Studies Association.

Kunz, J. L. (2005). Orienting newcomers to Canadian society: Social capital and settlement. In *Social Capital in Action: Thematic Policy Studies* (pp. 52–64). Ottawa: Policy Research Initiative.

Kunz, J. L., & Sykes, S. (2007). *From mosaic to harmony: Multicultural Canada in the 21st century: Results of regional roundtables.* Report to Government of Canada. Ottawa: Policy Research Institute.

Kymlicka, W. (2007). Ethnocultural diversity in a liberal state: Making sense of the Canadian model(s). In K. Banting, T. J. Courchene, & F. L. Seidle (Eds.), *Belonging? Diversity, recognition, and shared citizenship in Canada* (pp. 39–86). Montreal: Institute for Research in Public Policy.

Kymlicka, W. (1998). *Finding our way: Rethinking ethnocultural relations in Canada.* Toronto: Oxford University Press.

Kymlicka, W. (2010). *The current state of multiculturalism in Canada and research themes on Canadian multiculturalism 2008–2010.* Paper prepared for CIC. Retrieved from http://www.cic.gc.ca/english/resources/publications/multi–state/index.asp

Laidlaw Foundation. (2004). *What role do ethnoracial umbrella organizations play in developing social capital and promoting social inclusion?* Retrieved from http://www.laidlawfdn.org/what-role-do-ethnoracial-umbrella-organizations-play-developing-social-capital-and-promoting-social

Levine-Rasky, C., Beaudoin, J., & St. Clair, P. (2014). The exclusion of Roma claimants in Canadian refugee policy. *Patterns of Prejudice, 48*(1), 67–93. doi:10.1080/0031322X.2013.857477

Li, P. (2003). *Destination Canada: Immigration debates and issues.* Toronto: Oxford University Press.

Lightman, E., Mitchell, A., & Wilson, B. (2008). *Poverty is making us sick: A comprehensive survey of income and health in Canada.* Toronto: Community Social Planning Council of Toronto and Wellesley Institute. Retrieved from http://socialplanningtoronto.org/healthequitylightman2008.pdf

Long, D. A., & Perkins, D. D. (2007). Community social and place predictors of sense of community: A multilevel and longitudinal analysis. *Journal of Community Psychology, 35*(5), 563–81.

Macintyre, S., & Ellaway, A. (2003). Neighborhoods and health: An overview. In I. Kawachi & L. F. Berkman (Eds.), *Neighborhoods and health* (pp. 20–42). Oxford: Oxford University Press.

Macpherson, W. (1999). *The Stephen Lawrence inquiry. Report of an inquiry by Sir William Macpherson of Cluny* (Chapter 6). London: Stationery Office.

Malenfant, E. C. (2004). Suicide in Canada's immigrant population. *Health Reports, 15*(2), 9–17.

Martin Prosperity Institute. (2013). *Untapped potential: Creating a better future for service workers.* Institute for Competitiveness & Prosperity. Working Paper 17, p. 10. Toronto: Author.

Marwah, S. (2014). Refugee health care cuts in Canada—System level costs, risks, and responses. Wellesley Institute Advance Urban Health. Toronto: Wellesley Institute.

Maytree Foundation. (2010). DiverseCity: The greater Toronto leadership project 2010. Retrieved from http://maytree.com/integration/diversecity-leadership-project

McDonald, J. T., & Kennedy, S. (2005). Is migration to Canada associated with unhealthy weight gain? Overweight and obesity among Canada's immigrants. *Social Science & Medicine, 61*(12), 2469–81.

McMurtry, R., & Curling, A. (2008). *The review of the roots of youth violence: Literature reviews.* Toronto: Government of Ontario.

Merriam-Webster Dictionary. (2008). Racism. Retrieved from http://www.merriam-webster.com/dictionary/racism

Mock, K. (2002). *Redefining multiculturalism*. Adapted from a presentation at the University of Victoria Conference Changing Multicultural Identities, University of Victoria. Victoria: University of Victoria.

Muenning, P., & Fahs, M. C. (2002). Health status and hospital utilization of recent immigrants to New York City. *Preventative Medicine* 35(3), 225–231.

Nakhaie, R. M., Smylie, L. K., & Arnold, R. (2007). Social inequalities, social capital, and health of Canadians. *Review of Radical Political Economics, 39*(4), 562–85.

National Council of Welfare. (2007). Welfare Incomes. Retrieved from http://www.ncwcnbes.net/en/home.html

Newbold, K. B. (2005). Health status and health care of immigrants in Canada: A longitudinal analysis. *Journal of Health Services Research and Policy*, 10(2), 77–83a.

Newbold, K. B. (2006). Chronic conditions and the healthy immigrant effect: Evidence from Canadian immigrants. *Journal of Ethnic and Migration Studies, 32*(5), 765–84.

Ng, E., Wilkins, R., Gendron, F., & Berthelot, J. M. (2005). Dynamics of immigrants' health in Canada: Evidence from the National Population Health Survey. *Healthy today, healthy tomorrow? Findings from the National Population Health Survey, 2*. Catalogue no. 82–618-MWE2005002. Ottawa: Statistics Canada. Retrieved from http://www.statcan.gc.ca/pub/82–618–m/2005002/pdf/4193621–eng.pdf

OECD (Organisation for Economic Co-operation and Development). (2006). *Where immigrant students succeed: A comparative review of performance and engagement in PISA 2003*. OECD, Program for International Student Assessment. Paris: OECD.

O'Hara, P. (2006). *Social inclusion health indicators: A framework for addressing the social determinants of health*. Edmonton: Edmonton Social Planning Council and Inclusive Cities Canada.

Omidvar, R., & Richmond, T. (2005). Immigrant settlement and social inclusion in Canada. In T. Richmond & A. Saloojee (Eds.), *Social inclusion: Canadian perspectives* (pp.155–179). Halifax: Fernwood Publishing.

Ontario Council of Agencies Serving Immigrants (OCASI). (n.d.). Questions and answers about non-status Canadians. Retrieved from w.ocasi.org/downloads/Status_Questions.pdf

Patychuk, D., & Hyman, I. (2009). *Income adequacy and processes of marginalization and social exclusion*. Public Health Agency of Canada (PHAC), Strategic Initiatives and Innovations Directorate. Ottawa: PHAC.

Perreault, S. (2008). *Visible minorities and victimization—2004*. Catalogue no. 85F0033MIE—no. 015. Ottawa: Statistics Canada.

Picot, G., & Hou, F. (2003). *The rise in low-income rates among immigrants in Canada*. Analytic Studies Research Paper Series 11F0019MIE2003198. Analytic Studies Branch. Ottawa: Statistics Canada.

Picot, G., Hou, F., & Coulombe, S. (2008). Poverty dynamics among recent immigrants to Canada. *International Migration Review, 42*(2), 393–424.

Policy Research Initiative. (2009a). Religious diversity in a multicultural Canada. *Horizons, 10*(2), 6–13.

Policy Research Initiative. (2009b). *Understanding Canada's "3M" (multicultural, multi-linguistic, and multi-religious) reality in the 21st century*. Ottawa: Government of Canada.

Portes, A. (1998). Social capital: Its origins and applications in modern sociology. *Annual Review of Sociology, 24*, 1–24.

Putnam, R. (1993). *Making democracy work: Civic traditions in modern Italy*. Princeton, NJ: Princeton University Press.

Putnam, R. (2000). *Bowling alone: The collapse and revival of American community*. New York: Simon & Schuster.

Putnam, R. D. (2007). E pluribus unum: Diversity and community in the twenty-first century. The 2006 Johan Skytte prize lecture. *Scandinavian Political Studies, 30*(2), 137–174.

Qadeer, M., & Kumar, S. (2003). Toronto's residential mosaic. *Ontario Planning Journal, 18*(5), 7–9.

Raphael, D. (Ed.). (2012). *Tackling health inequalities: Lessons from international experiences*. Toronto: Canadian Scholars' Press Inc.

Raphael, D. (Ed.). (2016). *Social determinants of health: Canadian perspectives*, (3rd ed.). Toronto: Canadian Scholars' Press Inc.

Reitz, J. G. (2012). The distinctiveness of Canadian immigration experience. *Patterns of Prejudice, 46*(5), 518–38.

Reitz, J. G., & Banerjee, R. (2007). Ethnocultural communities: Participation and social cohesion. In K. Banting, T. J. Courchene, & F. L. Seidle (Eds.), *Belonging? Diversity, recognition, and shared citizenship* (pp. 489–546). Montreal: Institute for Research on Public Policy.

Reitz, J. G., Breton, R., Dion, K. K., & Dion, K. L. (2009). *Multiculturalism and social cohesion potentials and challenges of diversity VIII*. New York: Springer.

Richmond, T., & Shields, J. (2005). NGO-government relations and immigrant services: Contradictions and challenges. *Journal of International Migration and Integration/Revue de l'integration et de la migration internationale*, 6(3-4), 513–526.

Roeher Institute. (2003). *Policy approaches to framing social inclusion and social exclusion: An overview*. Toronto: The Roeher Institute.

Rosaldo, C. (1996). *Toward a definition of multiculturalism*. Retrieved from http://www.rosado.net/pdf/Def_of_Multiculturalism.pdf

Rousseau, C., Hassan, G., Moreau, N., & Thombs, B. (2010). Perceived discrimination and its association with psychological distress in newly arrived immigrants before and after 9/11. *American Journal of Public Health, 101*(5), 909–15.

Saloojee, A. (2005). Social inclusion, anti-racism, and democratic citizenship. In T. Richmond & A. Saloojee (Eds.), *Social inclusion: Canadian perspectives*. Halifax: Fernwood Publishing.

Sen, A. K. (1999). *Development as freedom*. London: Oxford University Press.

Shields, J. (2004). No safe haven: Markets, welfare, and migrants. In P. Kretsendemas & A. Aparacio (Eds.), *Immigrants, welfare reform, and the poverty of policy* (pp. 35–60). New York: Praeger.

Shields, J., Rah, K., & Scholtz, R. (2006). *Voices from the margins: Visible minority immigrant youth experiences with employment exclusion in Toronto*. Joint Centre of Excellence for Research on Immigration and Settlement. Working Paper Series, (47), 62. Toronto: CERIS.

Shookner, M. (2002). *An inclusion lens: Workbook for looking at social and economic exclusion and inclusion.* Population Health Research Unit, Dalhousie University, for the Population and Public Health Branch. Halifax: Health Canada.

Simich, L., Beiser, M., Stewart, M., & Mwakarimba, E. (2005). Providing social support for immigrants and refugees in Canada: Challenges and directions. *Journal of Immigrant Health, 7*(4), 259–68.

Simich, L., Mawani, F. N., Wu, F., & Noor, A. (2004). *Meanings of social support, coping, and help-seeking strategies among immigrants and refugees in Toronto.* CERIS Working Paper no. 31. Toronto: CERIS.

Smith, K. L. W., Matheson, F. I., Moineddin, R., & Glazier, R. H. (2007). Gender, income, and immigration differences in depression in Canadian urban centres. *Canadian Journal of Public Health, 98*(2), 149–53.

Soroka, S., Johnston, R., & Banting, K. (2007). Ties that bind: Social cohesion and diversity in Canada. In K. Banting, T. J. Courchene, & F. L. Seidle (Eds.), *Belonging? Diversity, recognition, and shared citizenship in Canada.* Montreal: Institute for Research in Public Policy.

Statistics Canada. (2003). *Ethnic Diversity Survey: Portrait of a multicultural society.* Catalogue no. 89–593–XIE. Ottawa: Author.

Statistics Canada. (2006). *Immigration in Canada: A portrait of the foreign-born population, 2006 census.* Catalogue no. 97–557–XIE. Ottawa: Author.

Statistics Canada. (2008). *Canada's ethnocultural mosaic, 2006.* Census. Catalogue no. 97–562–X. Ottawa: Author. Retrieved from http://www12.statcan.gc.ca/english/census06/analysis/ethnicorigin/pdf/97–562–XIE2006001.pdf

Statistics Canada. (2010). Projections of the diversity of the Canadian population study. *The Daily.* Retrieved from http://www.statcan.gc.ca/daily-quotidien/100309/dq100309a–eng.htm

Statistics Canada. (2011). *Immigration and ethnocultural diversity in Canada.* Ottawa: Author.

Statistics Canada. (2014). *2011 National Household Survey.* Catalogue no. 99–010–X2011038. Ottawa: Author.

Stone, W., & Hughes, J. (2002). *Social capital. Empirical meaning and measurement validity.* Research Paper, Australian Institute of Family Studies, 27.

Torjman, S., & Battle, K. (2011). Inequality is not inevitable. In *The Canada we want in 2020: Toward a strategic policy roadmap for the federal government* (pp. 102–111). Ottawa: Caledon Institute.

Tremblay, M. S., Bryan, S. N., Perez, C. E., Ardern, C. I., & Katzmarzyk, P. T. (2006). Physical activity and immigrant status: Evidence from the Canadian Community Health Survey. *Canadian Journal of Public Health, 97*(4), 277–82.

Tugwell, P., O'Connor, A., Andersson, N., Mhatre, S., Kristjansson, E., & Jacobsen, M. (2006). Reduction of inequalities in health: Assessing evidence-based tools. *International Journal for Equity in Health, 5*(1), 11.

Vang, Z., Sigouin, J., Flenon, A., & Gagnon, A. (2015). The healthy immigrant effect in Canada: A systematic review. *Population Change and Lifecourse Strategic Knowledge Cluster Discussion Paper Series/Un Réseau stratégique de connaissances Changements de population et parcours de vie Document de travail, 3*(1), 4.

Van Kemenade, S., Roy, J., & Bouchard, L. (2006). *Social networks and vulnerable populations. Findings from the GSS. Social capital and health: Maximizing the benefits.* Health Policy Research, Health Canada. Retrieved from http://hc-sc.gc.ca/sr-sr/pubs/hpr-rpms/bull/2006–capital-social-capital/2006–capital-social-capital-4_e.html

Weinfeld, M. (1981). Canada. In R. G. Wirsing (Ed.), *Protection of ethnic minorities* (pp. 41–78). New York: Pergamon Press.

Wilkinson, R., & Pickett, K. (2010). *The spirit level: Why equality is better for everyone.* London: Penguin.

Wong, L. L. (2010). Debunking the fragmentation critique of MC. *Diverse,* Summer 2010. Retreived from http://diversemagazine.ca/culture-questioning%201.htm

Wood, P. B., & Wortley, S. (2010). *AlieNation: Racism, injustice, and other obstacles to full citizenship.* CERIS Working Paper no. 78. Toronto: CERIS Retrieved from http://ceris.metropolis.net/Virtual%20Library/other/CWP78.pdf

Woolcock, M. (1998). Social capital and economic development: Toward a theoretical synthesis and policy framework. *Theory and Society, 27*(2), 151–208.

World Health Organization (WHO). (2007, April). *A conceptual framework for action on the social determinants of health.* Discussion paper for the Commission on Social Determinants of Health. Geneva: Author.

Wuthnow, R. (2002). Religious involvement and status-bridging social capital. *Journal for the Scientific Study of Religion, 41*(4), 669–84.

Yap, M. (2004). *Gender and racial differentials in compensation, promotions, and separations* (Doctoral dissertation, University of Toronto).

Zeman, K., & Bressan, A. (2006). *Factors associated with youth delinquency and victimization in Toronto.* Retrieved from http://dsp-psd.pwgsc.gc.ca/collection_2008/statcan/85–561–M/85–561–MIE2008014.pdf

CHAPTER 5

Public Policy, Immigrant Experiences, and Health Outcomes in the United Kingdom

Jenny Phillimore and Hannah Bradby

Chapter Objectives

This chapter focuses on UK immigration as a case study. The objectives of this chapter are:

- to provide knowledge about the development of diversity in the United Kingdom and the difference between old and new migration;
- to promote understanding of the problems associated with measuring health outcomes by ethnicity;
- to consider the challenges associated with health provision in an era of super-diversity; and
- to promote appreciation of the ways in which welfarism diversifies and restricts access to health services for vulnerable migrants.

Introduction

The British Isles have long received immigrants from across the globe. Arrivals settled and formed diverse populations in urban and maritime centres, but mass migration did not occur until after the Second World War. The devastation of war, and the consequent rationing and austerity, prompted significant emigration to Australia, Canada, and South Africa, leaving skilled and unskilled labour shortages. Britain's enormous 19th-century global power had transmitted cultural values, religion, educational systems, and language skills such that people in the colonial protectorates and colonies were familiar with aspects of British society. Appeals for immigrants to work in the "mother country" resulted in arrivals from the Caribbean and Indian subcontinent from the late 1940s onward.

The resultant mass immigration of semi-skilled and unskilled men and women, followed by their families, changed the nature of British cities. Public policy responses to immigration, the emergent realization of its permanent rather than temporary nature, and the establishment of populations with distinct ethnic and/or religious affiliations through the second half of the 20th century have come to be known as the British version of multiculturalism and are explored in this chapter. With the 21st century came changes to European legislation and shifting global migration patterns that have been referred to as the mobility turn (Urry, 2007). Policy that had developed in response to **post-colonial migration**, whereby a large number of people came to the United Kingdom from a limited number of colonially linked settings, has been shown to be inadequate in the face of new patterns of migration. In particular, the arrival of smaller numbers of people from a greater range of settings has created "superdiverse" populations with a dizzying range of health care needs that the multicultural model cannot accommodate. This chapter describes the changes from "old" post–Second World War migration to the new migration patterns and looks at some of the ways in which policy has responded, the resultant experiences of migrants in accessing services, and how these play out in terms of health outcomes.

"Old" Migration

Until the 1990s, migration to Britain, now frequently described as "old migration," generally consisted of the arrival of economic migrants from former colonies. The start of this mass migration is epitomized by images of the ocean liner *Empire Windrush* docking in Tilbury, Essex, in 1946, carrying some 500 men and women migrants from the Caribbean. Through the 1960s Caribbeans settled in large numbers in London and were employed in public transport and in hospitals, with settlement patterns in specific enclaves associated with specific island identities. Indians also arrived in large numbers in the 1960s, showing more scattered patterns in terms of residential location and the industries in which they gained employment.

These waves of migrant arrivals were greeted with overt racism and discrimination, as epitomized by the "No dogs, no Irish, no blacks" notices displayed in boarding houses. Economic expansion during the late 1950s and 1960s meant that despite routine and institutional discrimination, migrants could get jobs relatively easily and migration continued through informal networks of patronage rather than statutory recruitment. Initially there was almost no specific action taken to meet the health or other welfare needs of these migrants since they were seen as a reserve army of labour who would return to their original homes in a few years.

However, within two decades it became clear that rather than returning, these immigrants were being joined by their families and establishing communities in British cities. Hostile responses to the development of a critical mass of immigrants are well documented with Enoch Powell most famously warning of the "rivers of blood" that would flow as a result of tensions between new communities and the white working classes in his infamous 1968 address to the General Meeting of the West Midlands Area Conservative Political Centre. Powell was sacked from his post as a government minister, but his warning was heeded and immigration restrictions were rapidly imposed, which massively reduced the rights of people from the former colonies to migrate to the United Kingdom. At the same time, the government recognized the need to address the racism and discrimination that was apparent in almost every area of life by introducing race equality legislation.

"East African Asians" arrived in the 1970s following expulsions from Uganda, Kenya, and Tanzania. Predominantly a business community, who were also British passport holders with experience of urban life in East Africa, they were well equipped to establish themselves in self-employment in Britain. Pakistanis, a more homogeneous group, were predominantly small-scale landowning farmers and were recruited as semi-skilled labour in the Midlands steel industry and the textile industry in Manchester and the Pennine towns, including Bradford and Leeds. Chinese, from Hong Kong rather than the mainland, arrived in various phases, predominantly settling in family-run restaurants and take-away businesses highly dispersed across the United Kingdom, with "Chinatowns" in London and Manchester acting as cultural and community hubs. Bangladeshis arrived after the other major groups in the late 1970s at a time when employment opportunities were increasingly restricted due to legislative change and economic recession. This limited their ability to accumulate capital and restricted the possibilities of family unification (Ahmad & Bradby, 2007).

Throughout the 1970s and 1980s these migrant communities consolidated by settling permanently, marrying and raising children, and bringing other family members to Britain to join them. Local authorities, recognizing the power of the minority vote, especially where ethnic-specific enclaves emerged, established a range of ethnic-specific services for communities, recognizing them as a permanent feature. These included consultation networks based around ethnic identity, culturally specific services, and interpretation. The approach was criticized by the national government as divisive, but it was continued—for example, there are Asian women's centres (in Birmingham and Bradford) that still exist, although they survive on much lower levels of funding.

The concentration of migrants in particular neighbourhoods enabled the establishment of voluntary sector provision of welfare services within and for these minority communities. This tendency has been criticized on the grounds that it was a low-cost option for the British state (Rex, 1991), which mitigated the need to reconfigure services for a diversifying population by passing on responsibility for making accommodations to those very groups. For self-employed migrants, family and community networks were crucial in establishing successful small businesses (Werbner, 1990). Furthermore, supportive family networks potentially acted as a buffer against prejudice and racism, providing role models, according status to individuals for skills or knowledge not acknowledged outside the community, offering social and moral support, and providing resources for recreation and relaxation (Ahmad & Bradby, 2007). In exploring the health deficits of minorities below, it is worth asking whether the injuries to health might have been worse without such strong networks.

Although we have described "old" post-colonial migration as being relatively simple compared to more recent "new migration," the economic downturn of the 1980s showed the diversity of opportunity across "migrant" and "ethnic minority" populations. While certain ethnic groups were faring poorly across a whole raft of social policy areas, others were thriving. Those migrants who had arrived to work in once-flourishing manufacturing industries were hugely affected by the decline of manufacturing in the 1980s: factories that shifted their production overseas withdrew jobs on which whole communities depended. The concentration of migrants from Pakistan in the textile industry of the northeast and the relative homogeneity of their skills meant that large numbers suffered from its rapid regional decline. The education outcomes of Bengali, Pakistani, and African-Caribbean children were far lower than the national average, with average health outcomes poor and communities located in some of the most deprived areas of Britain. Outcomes were variable given that the Chinese and Indians were faring better than the general population on both educational and health outcomes.

The differential outcomes of different migrant groups contributed to the growing dissatisfaction with terminology that inappropriately referred to the British-born descendants of immigrants as "immigrants" and that homogenized "minorities," regardless of their place of origin. With the development of a range of local authority and voluntary sector initiatives alongside national policy, the politics of what was then called "race relations" was politically contested and studied academically. Over the subsequent decades, anti-racism, multiculturalism, and the relative virtues of acculturation, assimilation, and integration would continue to be debated.

Until 1991, the only indication of a person's non-indigenous status in statutory data was his or her country of birth. Among various disadvantages of this proxy measure was its inability to indicate British-born people of minority background and to distinguish people who were born in colonial settings because of their British parents' employment. In the national census of 1991, for the first time, people were asked to select a category that best described their ethnic identity. The question varied very slightly across the countries of the United Kingdom, and was updated for the 2001 census. The following categories were used in England and Wales:

- White—British or Irish or Any Other White background (write in)
- Mixed—White and Black Caribbean or White and Black African or White and Asian or Any Other Mixed background (write in)
- Asian or Asian British—Indian or Pakistani or Bangladeshi or Any Other Asian background (write in)
- Black or Black British—Caribbean or African or Any Other Black background (write in)
- Chinese or other ethnic group—Chinese or Any Other (write in)

In filling out the census, respondents were expected to select a single main category, which was the first descriptor for each bullet point, shown above, and then to choose a subcategory from the options that followed. Since there was historically no legal definition of population diversity in the United Kingdom, this census definition of ethnicity comfounds aspects of nationality, country of birth, geographical origin, and skin colour. The inadequacies of this approach were highlighted by the emergence of "Mixed" and "White Irish" categories between the 1991 and 2001 censuses in response to both popular and policy concerns that these groups were not represented. Other obvious compromises in this classification are that everyone tracing their origins from sub-Saharan Africa are covered by a single category, as is everyone with an Indian identity. Such compromises reflected the dimensions of ethnic identity that were perceived to be of policy importance, with a question on religious identity included in the 2001 England and Wales census for the first time, as minority religious affiliation became a preoccupation of the public policy agenda. The lack of institutionalized or legal "racial" categories in the United Kingdom means that classifications inevitably reflect powerfully felt **racialized** folk typologies that both constrain and inform people's identities (Bradby & Nazroo, 2010). Conceiving a classification that usefully captures the experience of identity and the effect of structural factors without **essentializing** difference has proved to be an ongoing challenge. Critique of the homogenizing assumptions of ethnic classifications echo earlier objections to race classifications and have provided impetus for identifying alternative conceptualizations, to which we will return.

Health Effects

The postwar generation of pioneer migrants from the Commonwealth to Britain are likely to have been protected by the "healthy migrant effect" as young seekers of employment. However, as the century wore on, there were clearly significant problems in the accessibility and appropriateness of health services for newly arrived migrants. Strikingly, the 1970s saw the reappearance of rickets in inner city populations—a disease of urban poverty that had been largely eradicated in the majority population; it was recast as an exotic disease (Donovan, 1984).

Termed "Asian rickets," its cause was attributed to deficient South Asian diets, codes of gender, and dress. South Asian skins were assumed to be too pigmented to convert Northern hemisphere sunlight into vitamin D, with modest clothing seen as further hampering the process. In the long term, the solution to the problem was declared as lying in "health education and a change towards the Western diet and lifestyle" (Goel et al., 1981, p. 405) without consideration of the chronic health problems associated with the Western diet and lifestyle. The fortification of a staple food with vitamin D that worked for the general population was deemed inappropriate for South Asian minorities on the pretext that such fortification of ghee or chapatti flour could lead to vitamin D toxicity (Bradby & Nazroo, 2010).

In addition to special initiatives to address minority group's educational deficits, cultural guidebooks appeared (e.g., Henley, 1979) to inform service providers about the peculiarities of minority ethnic cultures. Presenting minorities as static, homogeneous cultural entities, such cultural guides confirmed a view that all members of a "culture" shared common features of diet, worship, and family life. This static and essentialist view of ethnicity and culture as properties of minorities (but not the general population) implied that professionals could accommodate minority patients' "special needs" within an otherwise unchanged health service (Bradby, 2012). Racism and discrimination did not fit well with this formulation of ethnic minority "special" needs beyond an implicit sense that with adequate information, racism would somehow disappear.

Research into the health of minority ethnic groups grew through the 1980s in the wake of the *Black Report* (Black and Smith, 1992), which had shown health outcomes to be structured by social class and gender, and suggested that ethnic group could also be significant, although this suggestion was based on the limitations of country of birth data. It was clear from these data that babies born to women who were themselves born in the Indian subcontinent had elevated risk of poor birth outcomes (Peel & Clarke, 1990). A high-profile government initiative addressing birth outcomes of these migrants was named "The Asian Mother and Baby Campaign" (Bahl, 1987). Seeking to assert a connection between a minority culture and its relationship with specific health outcomes had a damaging culture-blaming effect, despite progressive intentions (Rocheron, 1988). Furthermore, rather than reconfiguring mainstream services to cater for the universal needs of all birthing mothers, health education and community group bridging and advocacy projects were relied upon to teach new minorities to use the health services in a "proper" way.

Epidemiological studies of population and environmental characteristics sought to compare the health of minority ethnic communities with the majority community "norm" in terms of **morbidity**, mortality, or health-related behaviour, including use of services. This approach tended to focus on instances where excess morbidity, mortality, or damaging health behaviour among the minority in question were found. During the 1980s, minority ethnic health was explored as a comparative problem, rather than as a significant or interesting phenomenon in its own right, with a particular focus on those conditions where minority ethnic groups had a raised incidence or prevalence of a condition, irrespective of whether the condition was of significance for the minority or the majority population. Thus, tuberculosis rates remained higher among some minority ethnic groups compared with the general population, but, given that overall **prevalence rates** were low, and treatment was effective, no great public health significance pertained. By contrast, cancers, accounting for around one-sixth of all deaths among minority ethnic groups, were neglected as the relative prevalence rates for minorities were lower than in the general population. The emphasis on relative risk has parallels with the culture of "special initiatives" in health and welfare services, which consistently treats minority groups' needs as exceptional rather than universal (Ahmad & Bradby, 2007).

Differences in health across ethnic groups, in terms of both morbidity (the presence of illness and disease) and mortality, have been repeatedly documented in the United Kingdom (Marmot et al., 1984; Harding & Maxwell, 1997) using country of birth as a proxy. Broad trends were as follows (Bradby & Nazroo, 2010):

- Men born in the Caribbean had low mortality rates overall, and particularly low mortality rates for coronary heart disease, but high rates of mortality from stroke, as did women born in the Caribbean.
- This high mortality rate from stroke and low mortality rate from coronary heart disease were also found among those born in West/South Africa, who also had a high overall mortality rate.
- Men and women born in the Indian subcontinent and East Africa (presumed to be South Asian migrants) had high rates of death from coronary heart disease, with the highest rates found among those born in Bangladesh. Those born in the Indian subcontinent also had high mortality rates from stroke.
- Those born in Ireland had high mortality rates for most diseases.
- On the whole, the non-white migrant groups had lower mortality rates from respiratory disease and lung cancer.
- There were very high death rates among non-white migrants for conditions relating to diabetes.

The Policy Studies Institute Fourth National Survey of ethnic minorities (Nazroo, 1997) showed significant differences in health outcomes between ethnic minorities (which overlapped with recent migrants), as well as a sizable gap between variously collated groups of minorities and the general population. Findings from the 1999

Health Survey for England (Erens, Primatesta, & Prior, 2001) using ethnic differences in self-reported general health showed considerable heterogeneity in experience, with the non-white groups having a variably increased risk of poor health compared with the white groups. Most notable, perhaps, was the wide variation for the three South Asian groups identified, with Indians having better health than Pakistanis, who had better health than Bangladeshis (Bradby & Nazroo, 2010).

Such evidence of statistically significant difference in health outcomes pointed to unmet need in the 1990s, but was also been part of a reification of administrative categories around fixed ethnic groups. While the use of routine administrative categories for "ethnic monitoring" has been introduced to the National Health Service (NHS), acknowledging this as a potential dimension of inequality, the quality of the data is very poor. The reasons for this are multiple and include the lack of identification that people have with predetermined categories.

The emergence of evidence of differential health outcomes for minority groups in Britain throughout the 1970s and 1980s informed the creation of statutory ethnic categories in the 1990s. The prevailing assimilationist assumptions of the 1950s and 1960s that immigrants from colonial settings would either return "home" or would assimilate in the general population informed the approach to ethnic minorities in the 1970s and 1980s. Health deficits of minorities were linked to a deviation from the British "norm" through the methods of research and the response to findings, while minorities' health advantages were overlooked. The parcelling out of ethnic groups to minority and majority has meant an inability to appreciate the dynamic, contingent nature of cultural change such that the British population as a whole has been remade. However, without using the crude proxy of country of birth and then the census classification of ethnic group, inequalities would not have been measured. The government had hoped that conceptualizations of ethnicity would encompass the labile complexity of a characteristic that combines elements of transmitted culture with an aspect of self-identification or subjectivity (Bradby, 1995). However, the process of creating administrative categories for census purposes rendered the content-dependent contingencies of ethnicity arising from migration into static, essentialist conceptualizations of ethnic minority groups (Bradby, 2003). These rigid cateogories have left us unprepared to apprehend and respond to the ongoing diversification of diversity as patterns of migration have developed.

Emergence of "New" Migration

While the socio-economic problems and poor health outcomes of old migrants remained largely unresolved, the late 1980s and early 1990s began to see a major shift in the nature of migration. Family reunion and, to a smaller extent, economic migration from the former colonies continued, but it began to be matched by the arrival of migrants from other locations. Individuals began arriving to the United Kingdom from almost every country in the world and they settled not just in the big cities but across a wide range of rural and urban areas. Since new migrants tended to arrive in smaller numbers than previous migrations, to come from a larger number of different places, and to be more dispersed in the United Kingdom, there was much less likelihood of forming the kind of diasporic communities that had emerged with post–Second World War migration. Further, new migrants came for a wider range of reasons. A booming economy and associated labour and skills shortage served as a pull factor in the late 1980s and 1990s, but many migrants arrived spontaneously as forced migrants escaping major conflicts in the Great Lakes region of Africa and in the Middle East. The rise of asylum-seeking to a high point of just over 100,000 applicants per annum in 2003 was one of the factors that contributed to escalating government, media, and public concerns about rising levels of immigration. The period from 1996 to the present was the most intense period of immigration policy-making ever with new legislation emerging on an almost annual basis.

The creation of the National Asylum Seeker Support Service (NASS) in 1999 and an associated dispersal program led to asylum-seekers arriving in southeast England being involuntarily dispersed across the United Kingdom to the cheapest and least popular available housing. This was part of a bid to reduce the overall costs of supporting asylum-seekers, to reduce the "burden" of support on the southeast of England, and to create a deterrent for would-be applicants who were thought to be arriving in the hopes of being housed in London. Dispersal was hugely criticized. Most existing minority and asylum support services, largely offered by civil society, were located in the southeast or London. Asylum-seekers were sent to towns and cities with little experience of diversity and no capacity to support individuals who had often experienced high levels of trauma. Asylum-seekers were allocated housing of poor quality that they had to share with strangers and were given support vouchers, which meant they were unable to use transport or shop for essentials outside of expensive, nominated supermarkets. Much has been written about the experiences of these asylum-seekers, ranging from murder at the hands of racist attackers, to illness associated with poor housing conditions and diet, and high levels of depression and PTSD (Phillimore, 2011; Phillips, 2006). Over time vouchers were replaced with cash, but asylum-seekers' right to work was removed, as was fee remission that enabled them to attend English language classes without payment.

Asylum-seeking was just one of the migration routes through which new migration developed. In 2004 the European Union expanded and Sweden, Great Britain, and Ireland opened their labour markets to eight of the new members from Eastern and Central Europe. The new Labour government of the time saw the so-called A8—the eight Eastern and Central European accession countries that had not had access to the UK labour market previously—as an ideal source of workers to address the demands of its booming economy and predicted that 13,000 migrants would move to the United Kingdom in the first 12 months after accession. Within months it was clear that this figure was an underestimate with some 900,000 migrants estimated to have arrived in the decade following accession. While asylum-seeking had led to the development of pockets of superdiversity in largely urban areas, accession migration saw the emergence of communities of migrants almost everywhere in the United Kingdom.

Rural areas such as Devon, Cornwall, Cambridgeshire, Herefordshire, and Shropshire experienced unprecedented immigration. Such areas had little experience of diversity and lacked basic resources such as interpreters. Most A8 migrants were young and single with larger numbers of men than women arriving. A decade on, there were two more accession countries, Romania and Bulgaria. Many European Union migrants have settled with their partners and children. The largest number of immigrants come from Poland, and figures monitoring their progress are beginning to emerge in outcome measuring. Early indicators suggest there is a healthy migrant effect with low use of health services. Evidence is, however, emerging of high levels of exploitation by employers in some areas wherein migrants are housed in non-standard accommodation such as sheds and greenhouses, and expected to work long hours with poor health and safety provision and low job security. The effects of these poor working conditions, without the support of established minority networks, may emerge in later years as health problems (Pemberton et al., 2014). For the time being, poor socio-economic outcomes are observed in terms of heavy reliance on in-work benefits with some people dependent on multiple jobs to secure sufficient resources. Concerns are growing about high levels of industrial injury and mental health problems among these new migrant populations. In addition, public health officials have expressed worries that allegedly high levels of smoking and alcohol abuse among young male A8 migrants threaten to reverse recent improvements in population smoking-cessation rates.

Policy Responses to New Migration

As migration routes diversified and migrant numbers increased, a key government response that has endured since the election of New Labour in the late 1990s and the formation of the Coalition in 2000 is the use of welfare restrictionism as a tool of immigration control. "Welfare chauvinism" or "welfarism," where resident populations view immigrants as less deserving than themselves of employment opportunities and statutory benefits, has been a feature of the rise of populist anti-immigration political parties across Europe. In the United Kingdom, the main political parties have been promoting a "welfarist" perspective, even in the face of evidence that health care tourism is more myth than reality (Hanefeld, Horsfall, Lunt, & Smith, 2013; Hanefeld, Lunt, & Smith, 2013). Successive administrations have sought to reduce new migrants' access to welfare benefits and health care. The provision of health care free at the point of delivery has been a foundation of the British welfare system. Legislation such as the Borders, Citizenship and Immigration Act (2009) emerged on an almost annual basis seeking to restrict or ration new migrants' access to the welfare state, with different rights and entitlements associated with different migrant statuses.

The argument justifying such restrictionism is twofold; it is intended to both reduce the so-called pull factor of the allegedly generous welfare state and to reduce the costs of migration to the United Kingdom. The impact of restrictionism has received little research attention, largely because data that would enable the effect of service withdrawal on new migrants to be systematically investigated are lacking. Qualitative evidence suggests that some groups of migrants, particularly pregnant women, asylum-seekers, and refugees, are faring badly (Phillimore, 2011, 2015). Restrictionism and the way it is applied differently to different immigration statuses also increased intra-ethnic group diversity with students, accession migrants, economic migrants, refugees, and asylum-seekers all having different rights and entitlements to welfare. This diversification of diversity has been described as a key dimension of the demographic complexity, termed "superdiversity" (Vertovec, 2007). In brief, it is argued that the labelling of immigrants (and their UK-born children) by ethnicity has become even less appropriate than it was in the post-colonial immigration period because of intra-ethnic group diversity whereby people identify and have experiences based upon a wide variety of variables—which include immigration status, rights and entitlements—intersecting with class, education, reason for migration, religion, language, age, gender, sexuality, and embodiment.

The diversification of diversity and resultant superdiverse populations have led to a range of concerns about the ability to meet the health and well-being needs of migrant populations and their integration in economic and social terms. With the right-wing United Kingdom Independence Party (UKIP) gaining support for its populist expression of anti-migrant policy, mainstream politicians have sought to address a backlash against multiculturalism. One approach used has been a clampdown on so-called "health tourism" and a move away from any kind of specialized health provision with the government also threatening to radically reduce the extent to which interpretation services are made available within state institutions, including the National Health Service, in a combined attempt to reduce costs and show the public that they will not provide special services to migrants.

There is evidence that while immigrants as individuals utilize health services at a level similar to the general population, the emergence of superdiversity in already deprived, densely populated, inner city areas has placed some stresses on an already overstretched health service, particularly in relation to increased numbers of non-English speakers (George et al., 2011). Despite the economic contribution of migrants and their under-reliance on benefits and social housing (compared to the general population), there have been scant attempts to invest in service provision in the areas under pressure with the financial benefits of migration enjoyed by employers and the Exchequer. Professionals find themselves with insufficient resources to cover interpretation costs, language classes are underfunded to the extent that they are too expensive for individuals on low incomes, and there is no attempt to help new arrivals understand the institutional culture of the National Health Service. For instance, general practitioners report confusion and frustration with the lack of clarity around new patients' entitlements (Woodhead, 2013). Headlines report migrants "mis-using" accident, emergency, and maternity services. Professionals report lack of flexibility in systems designed after the Second World War for white, middle-class, nuclear families and caseloads that do not account for the newness and naivety of migrants used to radically different approaches to health care (Phillimore, 2015).

Lived Experience: Integration, Disadvantage, and Discrimination

Labour Market Outcomes

The share of overseas-born workers in the United Kingdom has increased from 7.2 percent to 13.2 percent of the working population between 1993 and 2012 (Rienzo, 2013) and grown fastest in low-skilled and low-paid sectors and occupations. For example, foreign-born workers employed as process operatives (e.g., transport drivers, food services) have increased from 8.5 percent to 25.3 percent in the decade up to 2012. There are gender differences in occupations, with men concentrated in elementary work and women in associate professional and elementary work (e.g., cleaners, kitchen and catering assistants). Although traditionally migrant employment has been concentrated in London, since the 2004 accession EU-born migrants have begun to spread more evenly across the United Kingdom. A recent review of migrant poverty for the Joseph Rowntree Foundation argued that many economic migrants were vulnerable to a circle of poverty wherein poor-quality and precarious employment made them vulnerable to homelessness and ill health as well as shaping future opportunities. While migrants could often be found working in jobs similar to the UK-born population, they were likely to be paid less and have fewer rights. Vulnerability to illegal wage deductions, long hours, and health and safety infractions took their toll. Migrants were more likely to be found in low-paid, low-skilled work than the UK-born, and were frequently underemployed with deskilling common, particularly on entry to the labour market (Datta et al., 2006).

Poverty and Income

Eurostat data (2011) suggest that non-European Economic Area (EEA) migrants are more likely to be vulnerable to poverty, with some 35 percent at risk of poverty, compared with EEA-born migrants whose risk is similar to the general population (18 percent). A recent analysis indicated that migrants from outside Europe were more likely to be struggling financially and to be sending remittances overseas (26.5 percent) than EEA-born immigrants (Pemberton et al., 2014). Immigrants from outside Europe were also much less likely to take a holiday, save regularly, possess a car, or be up-to-date with their bills (Pemberton et al., 2014) while food shortages have been identified among those working in seasonal or irregular work (Jayaweera, 2014). Analysis has revealed new migrants typically earn less than their British-born counterparts: over 30 percent less for men and 15 percent less for women (Dickens & McKnight, 2008). This pay gap reduces as their stay in Britain extends: for migrant men, it takes around 20 years to close the gap, and for women up to six years. Further, a survey of new migrants in 2008 showed that one in five earned less than minimum wage (Markova & Black, 2008).

Many immigrants work long and non-standard hours, with few born outside of the United Kingdom having written employment contracts or access to statutory rights such as paid holiday, sick pay, or maternity pay. New migrants have also been found to be subject to high levels of exploitation in the workplace and lack information about their rights. In particular, domestic workers, some 20,000 arriving per annum, must remain in continuous full-time employment with the same employer while in the United Kingdom. This dependence makes them vulnerable to unrealistic demands, such as being permanently on call or not having their own living space (Anderson, 2000).

Housing and Homelessness

Immigrants born outside the United Kingdom were much less likely to live in a house in a decent state of repair or to possess contents insurance than European migrants, who themselves had poorer outcomes in these areas than UK-born residents (Pemberton et al., 2014). Evidence suggests that many immigrants practise income maximization strategies whereby they work long hours and share overcrowded, poor-quality housing in a bid to pay low levels of rent. Imigrants are much more likely to be living in private rented housing than the UK-born (Pemberton et al., 2014). It is clear that there is a "migrant housing market" consisting of landlords who are prepared to rent to individuals unable to pay a deposit or agency fee required to access decent-quality housing. Such landlords often charged inflated rents and do little in the way of housing maintenance while tolerating or even encouraging high levels of overcrowding. Many immigrants do not have tenancy agreements and thus are subject to unlawful eviction if they lose their income or complain about housing conditions. Immigrants have been found to experience a range of physical and mental health problems—including gastro-intestinal complications, respiratory problems, and depression—associated with poor conditions (Jayaweera, 2014).

Racism and Discrimination

The use of aggregated ethnic group categories from 1991 onward may have masked unjust inequities in service access and service uptake by immigrants and their descendants, which may have been attributable to individual or institutional forms of discrimination. For instance, an examination of the use of primary and outpatient services by ethnic group found no gross pattern of inequity, although once disaggregated, certain minorities were shown to underuse services (Smaje & Le Grand, 1997). The extent to which the underuse of services is due to racism or other forms of discrimination is extremely hard to assess, partly because of the politically fraught nature of the debate regarding what constitutes racism. For instance, the use of mental health services varies dramatically by ethnic group, with detention overused and community services underused by certain racialized minorities, especially young men of Caribbean origin and increasingly of Pakistani origin (Rogers & Pilgrim, 2010). The cause of the overuse of detention for certain minorities has been hotly debated, and various racist mechanisms have been proposed, but not proven (Bradby, 2009). The ability to investigate racism and to distinguish it from other forms of discrimination in the production and delivery of health and welfare services has been hampered by the discussion of racism in public services being strongly influenced by debates about the culture and practice of policing. High-profile official investigations of racist police practice resulted in a published definition of institutional racism (Macpherson, 1999), which, while worthless for analysis of other forms of services, has been treated as centrally important (Bradby, 2009).

Health Outcomes

While we have queried the usefulness of a monitoring system based on ethnic group categories, it has enabled identification of some inequalities in health outcome between the groups identified in the 1991 census, as described above. However the NHS and most other institutions have not adapted ethnic categories to take into account the emergence of new migration. Although outcomes for Polish and Somali migrants are recorded in some databases—for example, social housing waiting lists—they are not included in NHS monitoring. Further, despite both identity and outcomes being affected by immigration status, given that this now determines rights of access to welfare, there is no mechanism to examine outcomes by this variable. Emergent superdiversity and the arrival of people from every country in the world are reflected only by an increase in the proportion of respondents falling into the "other" ethnic category.

The lack of evidence regarding outcomes and experiences of new migrants is problematic and will endure without complete rethinking of monitoring systems. Small pockets of scholarship note particular concerns in some different groups. Interviews with accession country migrants suggest that the youthfulness of these predominantly economic migrants is accompanied by low levels of health concerns, but that where health problems do arise, there is a tendency to return to their country of origin to access health services (Migge & Gilmartin, 2011; Phillimore et al., 2010). The complexity of the issues in hand makes for great methodological and practical challenges when seeking to research the full range of issues relevant to newly arrived migrants, even in a single locality (Randhawa, 2014).

In terms of poor health outcomes, concerns have been greatest about asylum-seekers, refugees, and undocumented immigrants, all of whom have been the main target of welfarism. There is some evidence that the health outcomes of asylum-seekers are poor. In particular, maternal mortality rates are extremely high, with 12 percent of maternal mortalities occurring among asylum-seekers even though they comprise just 0.3 percent of the overall population (Phillimore, 2015). Around 25 percent of asylum-seekers are granted refugee status with the process having taken many years, until the introduction of the National Asylum Model in the mid-2000s. New refugees have the same welfare rights and entitlements as the general population. In England and Wales they are evicted from their asylum accommodation after a maximum of 28 days and after having been notified that their asylum claim was successful. Only those who are deemed vulnerable are offered social housing. Cases of malnutrition and extreme levels of deprivation have been recorded where new refugees have had to wait several weeks or months for the national insurance number that would allow them to claim welfare benefits.

Even those who are housed by the state face major problems with obvious implications for their health. They are placed in social housing, which is provided on an unfurnished basis and lacks basic amenities such as beds, washing machines, stoves, and utensils. Those asylum-seekers whose cases are refused can apply for low levels of support vouchers, providing they agree to return to the country from which they have fled as soon as possible. Many asylum-seekers will not make this commitment as they wish to continue to fight their case and so are offered no financial support or housing whatsoever, forcing them to rely heavily on their local asylum-seeker and refugee communities for support. Thus, the poorest and most vulnerable provide support to the destitute, but the lack of quantitative monitoring data about the impact of immigration policies and legislation on different migrant groups means that emergent health problems and stark inequalities in outcomes largely go unnoticed.

Conclusions

British statutory data employ administrative categories that reflect the mass migration of the 1960s, while the apparent hypermobility of humanity is giving rise to populations that are termed "superdiverse" because of the ongoing diversification of diversity. This diversification means an uncoupling of any assumption that knowing a person's ethnicity will offer any insight into his or her migration status and, conversely, migration status no longer offers much clue about ethnicity since the range of groups migrating is so broad. This, in turn, means that generalizations about health status and dimensions of diversity, being made from survey data from the 1990s, are much harder to make given the extent to which the speed, spread, and scale of migration have increased. Matters are further complicated when welfarism further differentiates migrants in terms of access to different kinds of health service.

While the enduring nature of health inequalities of some minority populations is acknowledged, insufficient attention is paid to structural factors that can help explain why some ethnic groups thrive while others do not. The absence of data about emergent categories of diversity, such as migration status and religion, and the impacts of welfarism means that an understanding of post-millennium inequality will be more inadequate than ever. Further, a combination of austerity cuts and claims about the failure of multiculturalism as an integration strategy means that there is neither the finance nor the political will to measure outcomes of new migrants, and levels of interest in meeting the needs, imagined or otherwise, of minority populations is low. How to research, understand, and meet the health needs of migrant and minority populations is perhaps the biggest challenge facing health and welfare providers in this century and one that we have as yet made little progress in resolving.

Critical Thinking Questions

1. How have health outcomes been measured for diverse groups in the United Kingdom?
2. What are the main problems associated with using ethnicity as a lens through which to measure health outcomes?
3. In what ways is a multicultural approach to health service provision problematic?
4. How might welfarism lead to increased diversity in access to health care?
5. What challenges to health care provision might emerge with the diversification of diversity?

Glossary

Essentializing refers to the attribution of "natural" (given or biologically determined) characteristics to a socially constructed group of people. It has the effect of homogenizing heterogeneity and promoting stereotypes and discrimination.

Morbidity is a term used in public health to mean illness or disease. Morbidity and mortality rates are often used to describe the health of specific populations.

Post-colonial migration is a migratory movement between two territories that were formerly linked by a colonial regime, which may have given rise to a common language, legal system, and educational curricular, thus facilitating migration. The term could also imply return migration to a country once a period of colonial rule has ended.

Prevalence rate is the proportion of a population that has a particular disease or condition. It is often used in combination with "incidence," which is the rate of new cases of a disease or condition in a population.

Racialized is the description of social phenomena in terms of a system of distinct races that reinscribes that racial system. For instance, where urban crime rates are attributed to racial characteristics of a group of young people, socio-economic factors are overlooked.

Recommended Readings

Ahmad, W., & Bradby. H. (2007). Locating ethnicity and health: Exploring concepts and contexts. *Sociology of Health & Illness, 29*(6), 795–810.

With the rapid development of ethnicity and health as a field of sociological research, this article seeks to re-evaluate the development of ideas about ethnicity, "race," and culture and considers how they have been applied to the question of health.

Bradby, H., & Nazroo, J. (2010). Health, ethnicity, and race. In W. Cockerham (Ed.), *The new companion to medical sociology* (pp. 113–129). Malden, MA: Blackwell.

This chapter explores the relationship between ethnicity, race, and health, drawing on sociological evidence from the United Kingdom and the United States.

George, A., Meadows, P., Metcalf, H., & Rolfe, H. (2011). *Impact of migration on the consumption of education and children's services and the consumption of health services, social care, and social service.* Report to the Migration Advisory Committee. Retrieved from www.gov.uk/government/uploads/system/uploads/attachment_data/file/257236/impact-of-migration.pdf

The main aims of the study were to estimate migrants' consumption of under-18 education, health and personal social services and the related costs, and to assess the implications for UK immigration policy.

Nazroo, J. Y. (2001). *Ethnicity, class, and health.* London: Policy Studies Institute.

Ethnicity, Class, and Health examines the existing evidence on ethnic differences in health and the explanations for them. It looks at how rates of illness vary across and within ethnic groups and considers how far differences in health might be consistent across subgroups and generations.

Phillimore, J. (2011). Approaches to health provision in the age of super-diversity: Accessing the NHS in Britain's most diverse city. *Critical Social Policy, 31*(1), 5–29.

This article argues that models of health provision need to be rethought to take into account the new reality of superdiversity in a way that is affordable, politically acceptable, and meets the needs of all.

Related Websites

Centre on Dynamics of Ethnicity—www.ethnicity.ac.uk/

This website is concerned with understanding changing ethnic inequalities and identities in the United Kingdom.

Centre on Migration, Policy, and Society (COMPAS)—www.compas.ox.ac.uk/

The mission of COMPAS is to conduct research to develop theory and knowledge through research on migration flows and dynamics, urban changes and settlement, and migrant welfare.

Centre for Research and Analysis of Migration—www.cream-migration.org/

The Centre for Research and Analysis of Migration, located at University College London's Department of Economics, has links to publications, blogs, and other websites.

Institute for Research into Superdiversity (IRiS)—www.birmingham.ac.uk/research/activity/superdiversity-institute/index.aspx

IRiS is an interdisciplinary centre looking at population dynamics, integration, identity, and access to social welfare with a strong emphasis on health.

Migration Watch UK—www.migrationwatchuk.com/

Migration Watch UK is an anti-migration think tank that seeks to counter what is seen as the liberal pro-migration bias.

References

Ahmad, W. I. U., & Bradby, H. (2007). Locating ethnicity and health: Exploring concepts and contexts. *Sociology of Health & Illness, 29*(6), 795–810.

Anderson, B. (2000). *Doing the dirty work?: The global politics of domestic labour.* London: Zed Books.

Bahl, M. V. (1987). *Asian mother and baby campaign—A report by the director Miss Veena Bahl.* London: Department of Health and Social Security.

Black, D. & Smith, C. (1992). The Black Report. In P. Townsend, N. Davidson, & M. Whitehead (Eds.), *Inequalities in health: The Black Report and the health divide.* New York: Penguin.

Bradby, H. (1995). Ethnicity: Not a black and white issue. A research note. *Sociology of Health & Illness, 17*(3), 405–417.

Bradby, H. (2003). Describing ethnicity in health research. *Ethnicity and Health, 8*(1), 5–13.

Bradby, H. (2009). Understanding and apprehending institutional racism in mental health services: Compromised conceptualisation. *Sociological Research Online, 15*(3), 8.

Bradby, H. (2012). Race, ethnicity, and health: The costs and benefits of conceptualising racism and ethnicity. *Social Science & Medicine, 75*(6), 955–958.

Bradby, H., & Nazroo J. Y. (2010). Health, ethnicity, and race. In W. C. Cockerham (Ed.), *The new companion to medical sociology* (pp. 113–129). Malden, MA: Blackwell.

Datta, K., McIlwaine, C., Evans, Y., Herbert, J., May, J., & Wills, J. (2006) *Work and survival strategies among low-paid migrants in London.* London: Department of Geography, Queen Mary, University of London. Retrieved from http:// www.geog.qmul.ac.uk/globalcities/wpaper3.pdf

Dickens, R., & Mcknight, A. (2008). *Assimiliation of migrants into the British labour market, working paper.* Centre for Economic Performance. London: London School of Economics.

Donovan, J. (1984). Ethnicity and health: A research review. *Social Science and Medicine, 19*(7), 663–670.

Erens, B., Primatesta, P., & Prior, G. (2001). *Health survey for England 1999: The health of minority ethnic groups.* London: The Stationery Office.

Eurostat. (2011). Migration and migrant population statistics. Retreived from http://tinyurl.com/ploh-4nf

George, A., Meadows, P., Metcalf, H., & Rolfe, H. (2011). Impact of migration on the consumption of education and children's services and the consumption of health services, social care, and social services. *Report to the Migration Advisory Committee.* Retrieved from https://www.gov.uk/government/uploads/system/uploads/attachment_data/file/257236/impact-of-migration.pdf

Goel, K. M., Campbell, S., Logan, R. W., Sweet, E. M., Attenburrow, A., & Arneil, G. C. (1981). Reduced prevalence of rickets in Asian children in Glasgow. *The Lancet, 318*(8243), 405–407.

Hanefeld, J., Horsfall, D., Lunt, N., & Smith, R. (2013). Medical tourism: A cost or benefit to the NHS? *PloS ONE, 8*(10), e70406. doi:10.1371/journal.pone.0070406.

Hanefeld, J., Lunt, N., & Smith, R. (2013). Health tourism and the NHS: Facts or fiction? *The Lancet, 382*(9890), e2.

Harding, S., & Maxwell, R. (1997). Differences in the mortality of migrants. In F. Drever & M. Whitehead (Eds.), *Health inequalities: Decennial supplement* (pp. 108–121). London: The Stationery Office.

Henley, A. (1979). *Asian patients in hospital and at home.* London: King Edward's Hospital Fund for London.

Jayaweera, H. (2014). Health of migrants in the UK: What do we know? *Migration Observatory Briefing, COMPAS*, Sept 30. Oxford: University of Oxford.

Macpherson, W. (1999). *The Stephen Lawrence Inquiry: Report of an inquiry by Sir William Macpherson of Cluny.* London: Home Office Cm 4262-I. Retrieved from http://www.archive.official-documents.co.uk/document/cm42/4262/4262.htm

Markova, E., & Black, R. (2008). The experiences of "new" East European immigrants in the UK labour market. *Journal of Poverty and Social Justice, 16*(1), 19–31.

Marmot, M., Abraham, G., Adelstein, M., Bulusu, L., & OPCS. (1984). *Immigrant mortality in England and Wales 1970–78: Causes of death by country of birth.* London: HMSO.

Migge, B., & Gilmartin, M. (2011). Migrants and healthcare: Investigating patient mobility among migrants in Ireland. *Health and Place, 17*(5), 1144–1149.

Nazroo, J. Y. (1997). *The health of Britain's ethnic minorities. Findings from a national survey.* London: Policy Institute.

Peel, A., & Clarke, M. (1990). Pregnant women at work: A study of ethnic minority risk in Leicestershire. *British Journal of Industrial Medicine, 47*(10), 649–655.

Pemberton, S., Phillimore, J., & Robinson, D. (2014). Causes and experiences of poverty among economic migrants in the UK. *University of Birmingham IriS WP 4-2014.* Retrieved from http://www.birmingham.ac.uk/research/activity/superdiversity-institute/publications/working-paper-series.aspx

Phillimore, J. (2011). Approaches to health provision in the age of super-diversity: Accessing the NHS in Britain's most diverse city. *Critical Social Policy, 31*(1), 5–29.

Phillimore, J. (2015). Delivering maternity services in an era of superdiversity: The challenges of novelty and newness. *Ethnic and Racial Studies, 38*(4), 568–582.

Phillimore, J., Thornhill, J., Latif, Z., Uwimana, M., & Goodson, L. (2010). *Delivering in an age of super-diversity. West Midlands review of maternity services for migrant women.* Department of Health, Applied Social Studies, University of Birmingham. Retrieved from http://www.wmemployers.org.uk/media/upload/Library/Migration%20Documents/Publications/Delivering%20in%20an%20Age%20of%20Super-diversity%20v5.pdf

Phillips, D. (2006). Moving towards integration: The housing of asylum seekers and refugees in Britain. *Housing Studies, 21*(4), 539–553.

Randhawa, K. (2014). *Illness and healthcare experiences of recent low income international migrants in a UK city.* Brighton, UK: University of Sussex. Retrieved from http://sro.sussex.ac.uk/

Rex, J. (1991). *Ethnic identity and ethnic mobilisation in Britain.* Warwick, UK: Centre for Research in Ethnic Relations.

Rienzo, C. (2013). Migrants in the UK labour market: An overview. *Migration Observatory Briefing, COMPAS.* Oxford: University of Oxford.

Rocheron, Y. (1988). The Asian mother and baby campaign: The construction of ethnic minorities' health needs. *Critical Social Policy, 8*(22), 4–23.

Rogers, A., & Pilgrim, D. (2010). *A sociology of mental health and illness.* Buckingham: Open University Press.

Smaje, C., & Le Grand, J. (1997). Ethnicity, equity, and the use of health services in the British NHS. *Social Science and Medicine, 45*(3), 485–496.

Urry, J. (2007). *Mobilities.* Cambridge: Polity.

Vertovec, S. (2007). Super-diversity and its implications. *Ethnic and Racial Studies, 30*(6), 1024–1054.

Werbner, P. (1990). *The migration process: Capital, gifts, and offerings among overseas Pakistanis.* Explorations in Anthropology Series, New York: Berg.

Woodhead, M. (2013, January 17). NHS provision for migrants is "too generous," say majority of GPs. *Pulse Today.* Retrieved from http://www.pulsetoday.co.uk/news/practice-news/nhs-provision-for-migrants-is-too-generous-say-majority-of-gps/20001524.article

Continental Nations: Clash of Cultures?

CHAPTER 6

Public Policy, Immigrant Experiences, and Health Outcomes in Austria

Ursula Trummer and Ina Wilczewska

Chapter Objectives

This chapter focuses on Austria as a country with a high standard of social security and a long-standing yet remarkably neglected tradition of immigration. The objectives are:

- to review the main features of immigration history and recent immigration patterns to Austria, including legislative frameworks and political aims;
- to consider the system of welfare in Austria and how immigrants are included or excluded from this system, both at the levels of legislation and observable practice;
- to review available evidence on health status and health perceptions of immigrants living in Austria; and
- to discuss possible interrelationships between immigration policies and regulations, social determinants of health, and migrant health, with a focus on mental health outcomes.

Introduction

Austria is a small, landlocked country in the very heart of Europe, with a geographical territory of 83,878 km^2, and a total population of 8,579,747 inhabitants as of 2015. It bears the history of a large Austro-Hungarian Empire that was reduced to a small republic after the First World War. Following annexation of the so-called "First Republic" by Nazi Germany in 1938 and subsequent occupation by the victorious

Allies in 1945, a state treaty signed in 1955 recognized Austria's independence, making the so-called "Second Republic" a constitutional democracy with a federal parliamentary form of government and nine provinces. A constitutional law that same year declared the country's "perpetual neutrality" as a condition for Soviet military withdrawal. Austria became a member state of the United Nations in December 1955 and a member state of the Council of Europe in April 1956.

Austria took its place in the economy of Western Europe and shared in the prosperity of the postwar period. It became a country characterized by a well-developed market economy, a skilled labour force, a high standard of living, and a comprehensive system of social security and welfare schemes, with close ties to other EU economies, especially Germany's. It became a participating state in the Organization for Security and Co-operation in Europe (OSCE) in June 1973; since January 1, 1995, Austria has been a member state of the European Union, entering the EU Economic and Monetary Union in 1999. Today, Austria's economy is among the wealthiest not only within the EU, but worldwide.

It is argued that Austria has always been a country of immigration, even if public opinion somehow seems to neglect this fact (Jandl & Kraler 2003). Similar to other European countries, its demographic development is that of an aging and shrinking population, with positive net immigration being the only demographic driver of population growth. The total fertility rate was 1.44 children per woman in 2013, measured by the net reproduction rate such that the current generation of reproductive age will numerically reproduce itself by only 69 percent. Life expectancy at birth is 81 years on average (2012), with a considerable difference between men and women of nearly five years (78.4 for men versus 83.6 for women). Population forecasts based on 2013 data see 28 percent of the population being 65 and older in the year 2050 (Statistik Austria, 2014).

Overview of Immigration-Related Public Policy

Regulations on Immigration

According to the OSCE online legislative database (www.legislationline.org), Austria has a strict immigration control system. Indeed, contemporary immigration regulations concerning access to the Austrian labour market as well as to Austrian territory are increasingly tightened. A key feature is the orientation of immigration policies designed to meet the demands of the Austrian labour market and linking labour contracts with residence permits (IOM/EMN, 2014).

Regulations on Labour Immigration

The Austrian Aliens' Act (Fremdengesetz, FrG) of 1997 regulates short stays, long-term residence, and employment immigration in combination with the Foreigners'

Employment Act (Ausländerbeschäftigungsgesetz, AuslBG) of 1975. Both acts were revised in a comprehensive way on July 9, 2002, with further amendments in 2011. They provide for a strict immigration control system by requiring the prospective immigrant to apply for an immigration visa from abroad and subjecting would-be immigrants to a tight quota system.

European Union nationals can take up residence in Austria by (a) pursuing employment as an employee or self-employed person, (b) proving they have sufficient resources and comprehensive health insurance for their family and themselves, or (c) studying in Austria with sufficient resources and comprehensive health insurance for their family and themselves.

In 2011, Austria introduced the so-called "Red-White-Red Card" (colours of the Austrian national flag), a criteria-based immigration scheme that regulates immigration of qualified third-country workers and their families with a view to permanent settlement in Austria. Based on personal and labour market–related criteria, it applies to very highly qualified workers, skilled workers in shortage occupations, other key workers, graduates of Austrian universities, and self-employed key workers.

In order to receive a Red-White-Red Card, the applicant has to achieve a sufficient amount of points (e.g., for education, professional experience, age, language skills). Young migrants are prioritized by the points given for age when they apply for the Red-White-Red Card: 20 points for those under 35, 15 points for those up to 40, and 10 up to 45; no points are given if the applicant is older than 45.

Apart from participation in the labour market, granting of any residence title is based on three general requirements:

1. *Adequate means of subsistence:* Applicants must have fixed and regular incomes enabling them to cover their living costs without resorting to welfare aid from local authorities. At the time of application, the regular monthly income must be equal to the amount of the standard rates of the General Social Insurance Act (ASVG).
2. *Health insurance coverage:* Applicants must have health insurance coverage that provides benefits in Austria.
3. *Adequate accommodation according to local standards:* Applicants must provide evidence of a legal title to an accommodation (e.g., by providing a lease contract) considered adequate for their family size, according to local standards.

Regulations on Asylum/Immigration for Humanitarian Reasons

The Asylum Act of 2005 (Asylgesetz, AsylG) is part of the so-called "alien law package" (*Fremdenrechtspaket*), and is reformed quite regularly (e.g., Fremdenrechtsänderungsgesetz 2009 and 2011, FrÄG). It regulates the conditions and procedures for granting or refusing asylum and subsidiary protection in Austria. In its content it refers to the Geneva Refugee Convention, which was ratified by Austria in August 1953 (UN High Commissioner for Refugees, 1990). It further specifies the rights and responsibilities and different residence possibilities of **asylum-seekers**.

If an application is declared admissible in accordance with the Dublin regulations[1] the asylum-seeker is accommodated in a care institution or facility in one of the federal provinces and this province becomes responsible for supplying the asylum-seeker's basic needs (*Grundversorgung*). Besides granting **refugee** status, a subsidiary protection can be granted in cases where the Geneva Refugee Convention conditions are not met, but the asylum-seeker would still not be safe in his or her country of origin.

According to the United Nations High Commissioner for Refugees (UNHCR, 2013), 52,000 refugees and beneficiaries of the subsidiary protections lived in Austria at the beginning of 2013. According to the data for 2010–2014, Austria was ranked eighth within the 44 industrialized countries included in the UNHCR report (2015) on asylum trends. Regarding the proportion of asylum-seekers to the country population, it had 10.4 asylum-seekers per 1,000 inhabitants. Within the EU, Austria was ranked fourth. In the year 2014, the number of asylum requests amounted to 28,027 (76 percent of whom were men). This figure was 60 percent higher than in 2013. In the first three months of 2015 the number of asylum requests was 150 percent higher than in the same months of the previous year. The majority of asylum-seekers came from Syria (7,754) and Afghanistan (5,070). Asylum-seekers from the Russian Federation (especially from Chechnya) were the third largest group in 2014, in contrast to the previous years when they predominated.

Undocumented/Irregular Migrants

Information on numbers of **undocumented/irregular migrants**[2] is scarce. The latest estimations date from 2008 and give a possible range from a minimum of 18,439 people to a maximum of 54,064 people, with an average estimate of 36,252 (Kraler et al., 2008). The yearly report on organized human smuggling gives numbers of people intercepted on Austrian territory (BK/Bundeskriminalamt, 2014). For 2014, it reports a total of 34,070 people who were intercepted, which represents an increase of about 24 percent as compared to 2013 (27,486 people). It further reports an increased number of alien smugglers (from 352 in 2013 to 511 in 2014) and smuggled aliens (from 12,323 in 2013 to 20,768 in 2014). Most of these smuggled people came from Syria (2014: 6,510; 2013: 1,951), Afghanistan (2014: 4,069; 2013: 1,632), Kosovo (2014: 1,429; 2013: 690), Iraq (2014: 925; 2013: 256), and the Russian Federation (2014: 897; 2013: 1,661). The number of people who entered illegally and stayed decreased from 14,811 in 2013 to 12,791 in 2014. Most of them come from Syria (2014: 2,539; 2013: 992), Eritrea (2014: 1,732; 2013: 152), Nigeria (2014: 726; 2013: 1,181), India (2014: 720; 2013: 1,790), and Somalia (2014: 598; 2013: 202).

These numbers provide evidence about the growing refugee movements related to the wars in Syria and Iraq and the destabilization of Libya, which has resulted in an increase in human smuggling. The decrease in the number of people who entered illegally and stayed on Austrian territory may be a result of stronger control efforts.

Immigration-Related Public Policy

As will be outlined later, meeting labour market demands has been the main focus of Austrian migration policy. With the beginning of labour migration in the 1960s, public policy was dominated by the idea of temporary immigration of "**guest workers**" (***Gastarbeiter***), who while being employed under the same wage and working conditions as Austrian nationals, would be dismissed before them and leave the country after a period of one year (Fassmann & Reeger, 2008). The question of integration came up only about 30 years later when the term was used in federal laws on migration in the Residence Law of 1992, and integration support was mentioned as something to be provided to migrant workers, their families, and recognized refugees. In the years that followed, integration policy took the position that integration of those immigrants already in the country should be given priority over new immigrants.

National Action Plan for Integration

In January 2010, the Austrian federal government adopted the National Action Plan for Integration (NAP.I). The Action Plan was launched as the new foundation of integration policy, combining "challenges, principles and objectives" in seven key action fields:

- Language and Education
- Work and Employment
- Rule of Law and Values
- Health and Social Issues
- Intercultural Dialogue
- Sports and Recreation
- Living and the Regional Dimension of Integration

Among the listed action fields, language is seen as a priority issue. In the NAP.I, the acquisition of German language skills is emphasized as a prerequisite for participation in economic and social life in Austria. Pre-entry language tests for immigrants from third countries were introduced in 2011.

In April 2011, a state secretary on integration was established within the Ministry of Interior, with Sebastian Kurz being appointed to the newly created post. The State

Secretariat moved with Kurz to this ministry when he was appointed as minister for Europe, Integration, and Foreign Affairs in December 2013.

Since 2011, annual Integration Reports and statistical yearbooks on migration and integration are published. In the first Integration Report in 2011, the State Secretariat introduced the policy motto "Integration Based on Merit," promoting the idea that people should not be judged on grounds of their origin, but according to their effort and achievements. The established Expert Council formulated the core of integration policy as being guided by regulated immigration,

> which provides an economic and demographic benefit. It views immigration as a necessity within a demographically shrinking but economically expanding country. For this, the Expert Council supports the commitment towards encouraging the immigration of qualified and highly qualified individuals without putting in question the asylum system guaranteed under human rights regulations or the possibility of family reunification in connection with immigration. (Government of Austria, 2011, p. 9)

The first Integration Report stresses the reciprocal nature of integration: "For successful integration, the accommodating population is just as responsible as the immigrants themselves. ... The required adjustment efforts are not divided equally and following the logic of the quantity they take a higher toll on the immigration population than the receiving society. Still, the latter also have to keep in mind that taking a seat requires being offered one in the first place" (Government of Austria, 2011, p. 9).

Recent Immigration Patterns

A report on Austria in the framework of a European project (Fassmann & Reeger, 2008) distinguishes three phases of immigration, public perception, and political reactions for post–Second World War Austria, defined as (1) an Initial phase, lasting from 1960 until 1973, (2) an Intermediate phase from 1973 to 1993, and (3) a new Stable phase from 1994 until the present.

The Initial phase is characterized by emerging immigration of mainly young, single males driven by the labour market demands of a booming economy. Austria started to recruit labour migrants and set up recruitment agreements[3] with Turkey in 1964 and Yugoslavia in 1966. The policy intention was to fill the gaps in the labour market with so-called "guest workers," who were not considered to be part of Austrian society but rather only temporary residents on Austrian territory. This concept turned out to be a failure.

In the Intermediate phase, there is a shift from male-dominated immigration to family immigration for family reunification. This phase is marked by a considerable change in the economic situation after the first oil price shock in 1973. The arrival of the baby-boom cohorts into the labour market marked the end of the labour shortage. Official recruitment ended completely, and in 1976, the Aliens' Employment Act, which determined the primacy of Austrian nationals in the labour market, became operative. Still, immigration was considered only temporary.

The new Stable phase, then, is characterized by immigration as a constant phenomenon with immigration of young male and female employees. The accession to EU internal migration becomes especially important. The beginning of this phase is marked by the enforcement of the so-called Residence Law in 1993, which regulates new immigration through annual quotas and specific criteria that had to be met—for example, proof of means of subsistence and a place to stay—in order for immigrants to gain a residence permit.

Composition of Migrant Population by Countries of Origin

In 2013, 12.5 percent or 1,000,007 people living in Austria were foreign nationals. The largest group of foreign nationals are immigrants from Germany (157,793), followed by Turkey (113,670) and Serbia (111,280). If second-generation migrants are taken into account, in statistics referred to as "with migration background" (i.e., both parents were born abroad), the share is 19.4 percent or 1,625,000 people. In Vienna, the capital city of Austria and its main urban region, the share of people with migration background is almost 40 percent.

People from the traditional guest worker countries still compose one of the largest groups of individuals in Austria who have a migration background. Immigrants from the former Yugoslavia (counting only countries outside the EU) and their children living in Austria constitute almost one-third (29.3 percent) of all people with migration background in Austria. Around 17 percent of people with migration background originate from Turkey.

Immigrants from the EU reflect the newer phase of immigration and are currently the largest group among people with migration background living in Austria (38.3 percent). Immigrants from countries that joined the EU as of 2004 predominate and amount to 25 percent of all people with migration background. However, some of these people came to Austria as asylum-seekers before their country became a member of the EU, as in the case of Hungary and Poland.

In 2013, the net migration to Austria amounted to 54,700 immigrants, 25 percent higher than in 2012. It has been rising continuously since 2010. This increase is due to, among other factors, the greater number of asylum requests and the growing number of international students at Austrian universities. In any case, more than half of new immigrants came from the EU countries. It might be surprising that almost 12 percent of all people who arrived in Austria in 2013 came from Germany. Germans constitute by far the largest group of foreign nationals in Austria. Reasons for their immigration are mainly related to job and study possibilities. In the winter semester of 2012/2013, Germans constituted around 38 percent of all foreign students in Austria. The next largest groups of immigrants arriving recently in Austria are citizens of countries of the former Yugoslavia (outside the EU), Hungary, Romania, and Poland.

Evidence Concerning the Integration of Immigrants into Society

According to the Migration Integration Policy Index (MIPEX), an interactive tool and reference guide for assessing, comparing, and improving integration policies (www.mipex.eu), Austria is a country where provisions for integration of immigrants show room for improvements. MIPEX measures integration policies in seven domains: (1) labour market mobility, (2) family unification, (3) education, (4) political participation, (5) long-term residence, (6) access to nationality (i.e., citizenship), and (7) anti-discrimination. An eighth domain, health, was introduced in 2015.

The third edition of the MIPEX, conducted in 2011, ranked Austria twenty-fourth of 31 countries with a total score of 42 (of a possible 100). It described the country as having some of the most restrictive eligibility and conditions for family reunion (e.g., age limits, tests abroad), few opportunities in democratic life, and naturalization being "one of the riskiest and most expensive gambles in EU" (MIPEX, 2015a).

In the 2015 edition of MIPEX released on April 30, 2015, Austria was ranked twentieth of 38 countries—integration policy has made progress, but policies still "create as many opportunities as obstacles for non-EU immigrants to fully participate in society" (MIPEX, 2015a). In the newly developed domain of health, however, Austria is described as a country favourable toward the health of its immigrants (MIPEX, 2015b). Out of the eight policy domains, the highest scores are given in the domains of labour market mobility (64) and health (63).

General Social Policy

Austria provides a comprehensive system of social security and welfare schemes. It operates on the principle of social insurance, which provides coverage for all gainfully employed people and, to a large extent, their dependants in cases of sickness, accident, unemployment, parental leave, and pensions. Public welfare benefits are made available by the federal, provincial, and municipal authorities to citizens in need who are not covered by the insurance system. Three components constitute this system: social insurance, public assistance, and social welfare.

- Social insurance includes health, accident, pension, and unemployment insurance.
- Public assistance is provided to families and certain groups and includes, for example, family benefits and long-term care benefits.
- Social welfare provides for those in need and includes, for instance, needs-based guaranteed minimum resources. This so-called *Mindestsicherung*, a needs-based minimum benefit or income, was introduced in 2010 and also includes access to health insurance coverage. (IOM/EMN, 2014)

Access to this system of welfare and social protection for non-Austrian citizens has two gateways. One is employment, following the general rule that social insurance, the core of the social security system in Austria, is based on employment. The other one is constituted through long-term residence, which in general has as a prerequisite of legal and continuous residence of five years in Austria for third-country nationals. Without proof of long-term residence, benefits such as family allowance and child care allowance are not granted.

Labour Market

In general, employment rates among people with a migration background are lower than among Austrians. The employment rate of 15- to 64-year-old people with immigration background in 2013 was 65 percent as compared to 74 percent of people without immigration background. This difference can be explained by the comparatively lower employment rate of immigrant women: 58 percent versus 70 percent of women without migration background (Statistik Austria, 2014).

Migrants are more affected by the moderate but steady rise of unemployment rates since the economic crisis. In January 2015, of the 406,239 (10.5 percent) unemployed people in Austria, 108,193 were migrants. The highest unemployment rates, according to citizenship, are among those from Turkey, Serbia, Bosnia-Herzegovina, Germany, and Romania (ÖIF Monitor Integration & Migration, 2015). Asylum-seekers are not allowed to work in Austria.

Education

People with immigration background living in Austria have significantly different educational profiles than the population without migration background. There is an overrepresentation of immigrants at the highest and the lowest educational levels. Data for 2013 show that 18 percent of all immigrants in Austria have a university or academy diploma compared to 16 percent of people without migration background. This can be explained mostly by the immigration of a highly qualified labour force from other EU countries: while very few people from former Yugoslavia or Turkey have completed higher education, people from other EU, European Economic Area countries and Switzerland have an especially high percentage (26 percent) of university graduates. On the other hand, the highest completed educational level for 62 percent of immigrants from Turkey and 38 percent from the former Yugoslavia aged 25 to 64 is only compulsory schooling (Statistik Austria, 2014).

Income and Poverty

On a general basis, foreign nationals living in Austria have lower incomes than Austrian citizens. Their average annual income of €18,808 in 2012 is approximately 83 percent of the median annual income in Austria. Also, the percentage of employees in the lowest earnings decile (net annual income lower than €9,795 in 2012) amounted to 14.7 percent in the case of foreign nationals, compared to 9.4 percent in the case of Austrian nationals (Statistik Austria, 2014). Yet, not all migrant groups are affected by this disadvantage in income. It is mainly citizens of countries that have joined the EU since 2004 who are affected, as well as people of Turkish origin.

Concerning poverty risks, again immigrant populations are at higher risk than Austrian citizens. In 2012, decidedly more foreign nationals were **at risk of poverty** (31 percent) as compared to Austrian citizens (12 percent). Additionally, the percentage of people living in **manifest poverty** in 2012 and 2013, as measured by an index of deprivation and meeting basic needs, was four times higher for migrants (16 percent) than for people with Austrian citizenship (4 percent).

Racism/Discrimination

Austria has a federal law against discrimination (GlBG, StF: BGBl. I Nr. 66/2004). The Ombud for Equal Treatment is an independent state agency that enforces the right to equality and equal opportunities and combats discrimination. If somebody feels discriminated at work or in other areas of life because of his or her sex, ethnic origin, religion or belief, age, or sexual orientation, the person can get advice, support, and information on equality issues confidentially and free of charge at the Ombud. In 2015, a hotline for incidents of discrimination due to ethnic origin was established as part of the integration policy measures (http://www.bmeia.gv.at/integration/hotline-gegen-diskriminierung). In co-operation with Zivilcourage und Anti-Rassismus-Arbeit (ZARA), an NGO founded in 1999 to combat racism and support people who are affected by racist behaviour, counselling for and support of victims of racism and/or discrimination are offered. In the annual reports of the Ombud for Equal Treatment and ZARA, discrimination because of ethnic origin, religion—especially concerning visual statements like wearing a veil—and/or skin colour occurs frequently.

A qualitative study analyzing the integration of EU citizens in Austria showed that the great majority of them feel a high level of satisfaction and well-being in Austria, and discrimination has been rarely experienced (GFK, 2014). On the contrary, the majority (almost 60 percent) of immigrants from Turkey feel disadvantaged in Austria and report negative experiences with the majority population (Ulram, 2009). "Other people look at me in a strange way" is the most often reported negative experience. Other frequent experiences include, among others, confrontation with people who make demeaning statements about foreigners/migrants, unfriendly treatment while shopping, being disadvantaged by authorities, or being intentionally offended or mobbed (Ulram, 2009).

Access to Health Care

Austria has an insurance-based health care system with compulsory health insurance related to employment and income. Virtually all (99.9 percent) of the population is insured (Hofmarcher, 2013) and has access to a broad range of services. Austria has a health care system that provides a wide range of high-quality services, with costs above the EU average: health expenditure is 11 percent of GDP compared to 9.5 percent in the EU.

Austria has the second highest physician density (after Greece) in the EU (4.8 doctors per 1,000 inhabitants; the EU average is 3.3), and the second highest bed density (after Germany) in the EU (763 hospital beds per 100,000 inhabitants in total). Nurse density is below the EU average (7.7 nurses per 1,000 inhabitants; the EU is 8.9)

Through insurance, labour migrants and their dependants are fully entitled to health care services. Refugees (*Asylberechtigte/Subsidiär Schutzberechtigte*) are also provided with insurance, either through work or by being integrated into the needs-based minimum income (*Mindestsicherung*) program that provides social assistance.

Asylum-Seekers and Unaccompanied Minors

Asylum-seekers in general have restricted entitlement based on federal-level care (*Grundversorgung*, basic care), including general state subsidies for health insurance fees, and, in particular cases, specific services that are not covered by health insurance and nursery care. This also applies to unaccompanied minors. Responsibility for their health is with those who are assigned custody by social welfare services.

Undocumented/Irregular Immigrants

As in most European countries, undocumented or irregular migrants have no access to any kind of social protection. This has recently been discussed as problematic not only for humanitarian but also for economic reasons (Trummer et al., 2014). Concerning access to health care, undocumented migrants are granted coverage only for emergency care, TB treatments, and prenatal and perinatal care (known as "anonymous delivery").

The main policy concerning access to health care for irregular migrants is functional ignorance, meaning that there are no specific regulations on access to health care for irregular migrants, but NGOs that provide health care for this group are subsidized with tax money (Karl-Trummer et al., 2009a, b).

Within these regulations, immigrants who are part of the workforce are being integrated in social welfare measures such as the basic minimum income. Recognized asylum applicants have full access to the health care system. Also, the health care system in Austria is quite sensitive to socio-economic disadvantages, and poverty does not constitute an obstacle to accessing health care (Bachner et al., 2013). In fact, Austria shows the lowest levels of unmet need for health care by income quartiles among the EU countries (GÖG/Gesundheit Österreich GmbH, 2013). However, other factors come into play, above all, factors of ethnocultural and communication-related sensitivities of health care providers.

General Considerations

There are few policies to integrate migrants who have a low command of the German language or different expectations and orientations toward health care organizations and professionals. Implementation of diversity management and especially services to foster understanding—such as interpreting services or mediation services—appears to be insufficient (Karl-Trummer, 2010). Initiatives toward the development of immigrant-sensitive health services are in place, but primarily on the basis of specific programs or actors than on a broader, structural approach to implementation.

To date, the Austrian health care system has no explicit rules on how to deal with immigrant patients who have insufficient command of the German language. The use of professional interpreting services is not mandatory. Although in 2013 a pilot project implemented video interpreting in several hospitals (http://www.videodolmetschen.at/), the availability of professional interpreters for patients with low or no command of the German language are still more an exception than a rule in most Austrian health care facilities. There are no obligatory standards on how to ensure communication or regulations on responsibilities. Also, there is no federal-level code of conduct for medical personnel that would regulate issues of how to deal with patients who have little command of the German language or who have a different cultural background that impacts their health perceptions and needs.

Evidence Concerning the Day-to Day Lived Experiences of Immigrants

What can happen in a health care system that is inclusive and comprehensive but not sensitive to communication issues shall be demonstrated with two cases from two care settings: a hospital and a primary-care surgery.

Case 1: A Hospital Care Incident

The case happened in June 2004 and was widely discussed by the public.

Two Turkish women share a room in the maternity ward of a university clinic. One is in her fortieth week of pregnancy and scheduled for a Caesarean; the other, in her twenty-eighth week of pregnancy, is scheduled for an ultrasound. Both women have a low command of the German language. Through the loudspeaker, the woman scheduled for a Caesarean is asked to go to the labour ward; the one scheduled for an ultrasound responds instead and is sent to the labour ward, carrying the wrong patient record. Due to language problems and maybe also cultural misunderstanding, the upset claims of family members and the remaining woman are not understood or responded to. Only after some time is it discovered that the patients were misidentified. During that time, in the labour ward, the medical and nursery team have already prepared the wrong woman and performed a Caesarean; the birth weight of the baby daughter is 1,200 grams.

Case 2: A Primary Health Care Incident

Case 2 is from the Austrian Critical Incidence Reporting System (CIRS, N110242, http://www.cirsmedical.at/), and dated March 2, 2015. This system enables health care professionals to anonymously report incidents for the purpose of quality development. The report is made by a GP. In his surgery, he encounters a couple from an Arab country, both asylum-seekers. They have no command of the local spoken and written language. Patient records are available to the GP, but he does not know which record belongs to which patient, as he cannot use the names as indicator for sex, and he cannot ask the patients due to their low command of the language. Both patients have an electronic health insurance card as they are in the process of asylum-seeking and as such are eligible for health insurance coverage provided by the state. Due to technical problems, the electronic system assigns the male patient's record to the female patient and vice versa. During the consultation, the GP explains a diagnosis, necessary therapy and medication, issues a prescription and a referral—all to the wrong patient. It is only through the patient's persistent efforts that everything is eventually put in order. The protocol reads that severe damage was prevented because of the patient's "sufficient education and language competence to inform me about my mistake—he could read our letters and at least speak a few words [of] English."

Day-to-Day Living Conditions in Relation to Other Social Determinants of Health

There is little research concerning the day-to-day living conditions of different immigrant groups in Austria. Some evidence is available on immigrants from Turkey and the former Yugoslavia, while there is only limited knowledge for migrants from Asia (who have doubled in numbers from 2000 to 2010) or for migrants from Germany (who constitute the biggest migrant group).

Still, some data are available about the perceptions of migrant groups concerning their living and working conditions and integration into Austrian society. Studies show that immigrants highly value the social security system, especially the health care system and the stable political situation in Austria, as well as good education opportunities and career prospects (Ulram, 2009). They also point to a more positive general mood in society than in their countries of origin (GFK, 2014).

On the other hand, not all immigrants feel their living situation has changed for the better over time. In a survey from 2014, immigrants were asked whether their living situation has changed for the better, the worse, or has stayed the same in the last five years or, if more recent, since they immigrated to Austria. Of Turkish immigrants under study, 43.7 percent said their living situation has changed for the worse, 35.7 percent said it has not changed, and a remaining 20.5 percent stated that it changed for the better. For the migrant population from the former Yugoslavia, 13.2 percent said it changed for the worse, 51.1 percent said it had not changed, and 35.7 percent said it changed for the better (Statistik Austria, 2014).

A qualitative study concerning the experiences of Turkish women living in Vienna points out that their lives are characterized by emotional stress resulting from the contradicting cultural norms and values and from conflicting expectations. The way of living in Austria has led to questioning and sometimes rejecting traditions from their country of origin. On the other hand, women are faced with discrimination in Austria, for example, while visiting the doctor. This leads them to feel that they do not belong anywhere: "We can't live neither here nor there, we are foreigners everywhere" (Trummer et al., 2013).

Evidence Concerning Health Outcomes among Immigrants

Regarding life expectancy, differences between migrants and Austrians are minimal (Statistik Austria, 2014). Still, studies show that holding Turkish or former Yugoslavian citizenship entails a significantly higher risk of having poor self-rated health for women, but not for men, when controlled for socio-economic status (Karl-Trummer et al., 2012).

Self-rated health reveals the heterogeneity of migrant groups in Austria. Fifteen percent of immigrants from Turkey and 11 percent of immigrants from the former

Yugoslavia assess their personal health status as poor or very poor. On the other hand, 6 percent of people from EU/EEA and Switzerland living in Austria evaluate their health as poor or very poor. Austrian nationals score somewhat in the middle with 8 percent. There is an overrepresentation of individuals with migration background among people of working age (15–64 years old) who suffer from chronic health problems. Immigrants from former Yugoslavia and Turkey (51 percent and 48 percent, respectively) report these kinds of health problems compared to 42 percent in the whole working-age population (Statistik Austria, 2014). An Austrian health survey conducted in 2006/2007 compares population with and without immigration background, taking as a reference migrant groups originating from the former Yugoslavia and Turkey. The gathered data show that when considering specific chronic diseases, women from the former Yugoslavia and Turkey have a 3.4 times higher risk of diabetes than women without migration background. The risk of suffering from migraine and headaches or shoulder pains is twice as high for women with migration background living in Austria than for women without migration background (Statistik Austria, 2008).

Mental Health

The evidence base on mental health of migrants in Austria is scarce. On a general level, data show that migrants from Turkey and the former Yugoslavia in particular have a worse assessment of their quality of life regarding vitality and psychological well-being than non-migrants. The same is true for the assessment of the general quality of life. People with migration background have a higher risk of suffering from depression and chronic anxiety. This increased risk amounts to 2.6 times for women and 1.7 times for men (Statistik Austria, 2008).

More recent data from the Trans-cultural Ambulance of Vienna University Clinic for Psychiatry and Psychotherapy provide a first analysis of all patients treated there from 1994 until 2007. The study analyzes data from 1,771 patients, mainly from non-EU countries. In general, the most common main diagnoses are disorders related to neurosis and stress-related spectrum (64 percent), and in second place are affective disorders (14 percent). In third place are schizophrenia and related disorders (9 percent).

The study differentiated between voluntary and involuntary migration, and traumatized and non-traumatized patients, and found considerable differences between voluntary and involuntary immigrants. Neurotic, stress-related, and somatoform disorders are most frequent among patients from war/crisis areas in the former Soviet Union, Asia, or Africa. By contrast, patients diagnosed with schizophrenia spectrum disorders and personality disorders are more often economic migrants from the European Union or the United States. Depression is diagnosed predominantly among immigrants who are long-term residents in Austria while adjustment disorders often appear during the first months of arrival (Holzer & Stompe, 2011).

NGOs working in the field of psychosocial support for immigrants report an immense and increasing need for psychotherapy and psychiatric treatment, especially for asylum-seekers. They also report a recent phenomenon where elderly immigrants who came as *Gastarbeiter* in the 1960s and entered the workforce now experience severe symptoms of depression. "They have spent their working life in Austria, they never learned German properly because at work they did not need it—they dreamed of having a better life going back home in their pension. Now they see their sacrifices good for nothing."[4]

Analysis of the Interrelationship between Public Policy, Living Conditions and Experiences of Immigrants, and Health Outcomes

The current immigration policy focuses on integration of young and skilled migrants, preferably from EU countries, who demonstrate command of the German language before entering the country and who can quickly integrate into the labour market and contribute to the economic success of the country. Today, people from Germany are the largest immigrant group in Austria. Little is known about their living conditions, experiences, and health outcomes, though it may be hypothesized that it will not be very different from those of Austrians with similar socio-economic status.

There is, however, a large group of people with migration background who came during earlier immigration phases when the market demands were different and who do not fit the current desired profile. The socio-economic status, as well as the self-reported and diagnosed health status of immigrants from Turkey and the former Yugoslavia (being the second and third largest immigrant group in Austria, respectively), are disadvantaged compared to the population without immigration background. Turkish immigrants are especially less satisfied with their situation in Austria over past few years, and report feeling disadvantaged and having negative experiences with the majority population. As there are few new immigrants from Turkey to Austria (less than 3 percent in 2013), current integration programs for prospective immigrants before they come to Austria or soon after their arrival will not affect this group.

Concerning public health policy, the inclusiveness of the established system may paradoxically lead to disadvantages for migrant groups. Labour migrants as well as asylum-seekers have legal access to a wide range of services. As shown in the two cases, problems arise when patients enter the system, where a lack of services that ensure communication and understanding can lead to errors and frustrations for both providers as well as patients.

Studies show that immigrants see language acquisition as a priority (GFK, 2014). Still, they may encounter practical and culturally motivated obstacles to learning the language in a timely fashion. Practice shows that at least in the health sector, the expectation that immigrants have language proficiency results in poorly developed interpreting services and endangers the quality of health care for migrants. It seems that such barriers can prevent regular migrants from receiving health care.

Implications for Immigration and Other Public Policy

Since the formulation of a NAP.I in 2010, Austria's immigration policy has been increasingly concerned with integration. Priority is being given to the action fields of language and education, and work and employment, which is apparent in the growing body of regulations concerning language acquisition and access to the labour market. In comparison, regulations that could support the development of diversity management structures within the health care system are missing and need to be developed, taking into account those vulnerable migrant groups who do not fit into the defined integration model.

Conclusions

Contemporary Austria depends on immigration and integration of migrants to compensate for an aging and shrinking population. Immigration policy has set a strict regime that favours young and skilled EU migrants and that focuses on integration. A National Action Plan on Integration (NAP.I) was formulated and has been implemented since 2010. Still, this policy seems to turn a blind eye to those immigrant groups who do not fit into this scheme.

Though part of the NAP.I, the development of a health care system that is responsive to the needs of a heterogeneous migrant population has not yet been tackled systematically. Available data on the health of immigrant groups provide evidence of disadvantage, especially for those who arrived before the strict selective policy framework was implemented—immigrants from Turkey and the former Yugoslavia. In addition, an increasing influx of asylum-seekers increases the demand for mental health care provision for traumatized and vulnerable groups. For these groups in particular, integration policies need to be developed in greater detail and implemented into practices of migrant-sensitive health care provision.

Recalling the reciprocal nature of integration as defined in the NAP.I, it also might be of interest to investigate concepts of integration among immigrant populations in Austria. What does "integration" mean from an immigrant's perspective? To the authors' knowledge, there are no systematic studies on this topic.

Critical Thinking Questions

1. Which factors may contribute to the disadvantaged socio-economic position of migrants from Turkey and the former Yugoslavia?
2. How may those disadvantages be related to their mental health?

3. How can integration policies address the *Gastarbeiter* who immigrated to Austria in the postwar economic boom?
4. What could be incentives for health care organizations to develop migrant-friendly services?
5. Austria's public health system excludes undocumented/irregular immigrants from access to regular health care. What public health risks could this approach entail?

Glossary

Asylum-seekers are people who ask (file an official application) for asylum (i.e., for admission and protection from persecution) in a country other than his or her own and whose asylum application is not yet completed. When granted asylum, these people gain the status of recognized refugees and can stay in the country. If an application is denied, the person must leave the country and may be expelled, as may any non-national in an irregular or unlawful situation, unless permission to stay is provided on humanitarian or other related grounds.

At risk of poverty, one of the national indicators for poverty in Austria, is calculated on the basis of the available household income divided by the number of consumption equivalents in the household. People are considered to be at risk of poverty if their equivalized household income is below an at-risk-of-poverty threshold of 60 percent of the national median household income. In 2014, the equivalized income median was €23,211. The at-risk-of-poverty threshold was therefore €13,926 for a single-person household—approximately €1,161 a month (Statistik Austria, 2008, 2014).

Guest worker (*Gastarbeiter*) is a foreign national who is permitted to live and work temporarily in a host country. After the Second World War, Austria, as well as some other countries (e.g. Germany, Switzerland), started to recruit labour migrants to help rebuild the country's infrastructure. The recruitment agreements were signed with Spain (1962), Turkey (1964), and Yugoslavia (1966). Many of the guest workers who arrived then became permanent residents in Austria, and now they and their descendants constitute some of the largest ethnic groups in the country.

Manifest poverty refers to people who show visible evidence of poverty and who indicate that they cannot afford two or more essential things of daily life (e.g. adequate heating, regular payment of rent and operating expenses, necessary medical and dental visits, payment of unexpected expenses, clothing, food) (Statistik Austria, 2008, 2014).

Refugee is defined as someone who "owing to a well-founded fear of being persecuted for reasons of race, religion, nationality, membership of a particular social group or political opinion, is outside the country of his nationality, and is unable to, or owing to such fear, is unwilling to avail himself of the protection of that country." Austria ratified the Geneva Refugee Convention in 1953 and adopted the official definition of a refugee provided in the Convention.

Undocumented/irregular migrant, according to the definition provided by International Organization for Migration, is a person who, owing to unauthorized entry, breach of a condition of entry, or the expiry of his or her visa, lacks legal status in a transit or host country. The definition covers inter alia those who have entered a transit or host country lawfully but have stayed for a longer period than authorized or subsequently taken up unauthorized employment (also called clandestine or migrant in an irregular situation). The term "irregular" is preferable to "illegal" because the latter carries a criminal connotation and is seen as denying migrants' humanity.

Recommended Readings

European Migration Network (EMN), & Koppenberg, S. (2014). *Austria: Annual policy report 2013*. Vienna: International Organization for Migration.

This report outlines the Austrian legislation, policy, and administrative practices that shape third-country nationals' access to social security. It is the Austrian contribution to a European Migration Network (EMN) study, conducted by the National Contact Point (NCP) Austria within the EMN in the framework of the EMN's Annual Work Programme 2013. Retrieved from http://www.emn.at/de/publikationen/studien

Fassmann, H., & Reeger, U. (2008). *Austria: From guest worker migration to a country of immigration*. IDEA Working Paper no. 1. Retrieved from http://www.idea6fp.uw.edu.pl/pliki/WP1_Austria.pdf

An overview on the Austrian postwar immigration policy that traces Austria's development from a country of emigration to a country of immigration.

Hofmarcher, M., & Quentin, W. (2013). Austria: Health system review. *Health Systems in Transition, 15*(7), 1–291.

Report on the Austrian health care system from the European Observatory on Health Systems and Policies in its Health Systems in Transition (HiT) series. It provides a detailed description of the health system and of reform and policy initiatives in progress or under development.

Hollomey, C., Wöger, A., & Kraler, A. (2011). *The National Policy Frame for the integration of newcomers in Austria: Promoting sustainable policies for integration* (PROSINT). Vienna: ICMPD.

This overview of integration policy in Austria is compiled in the framework of a European study, "Promoting Sustainable Policies for Integration (PROSINT)," which covers nine countries (Austria, Switzerland, Czech Republic, Denmark, Spain, Italy, Netherlands, Sweden, and the United Kingdom). Reports are available online at http://research.icmpd.org/1428.html

Trummer, U., Novak-Zezula, S., Phua, K. H., Griffiths, S., Chung, R., & Yi, H. (2014). *Migrants and healthcare: Social and economic approaches.* ASEF Public Health Network.

Comparative country studies (Austria, Italy, Singapore, and Hong Kong) on exclusion of (undocumented) migrants from health care and its implications.

Related Websites

The Federal Government's Official Information Website on Migration to Austria—www.migration.gv.at/

Austria recently introduced a flexible new immigration model: the Red-White-Red Card offers qualified third-country workers and their family members a new single permit for working and settling permanently in Austria.

Legislation on Line—www.legislationline.org

Established in 2002 to serve as a reference tool and comprehensive database on legislation related to issues such as human trafficking, elections, and citizenship, Legislation on Line provides direct access to international norms and standards relating to specific human dimension issues, and can be searched by topic (e.g., migration) and country (e.g., Austria).

Migrant Integration Policy Index (MIPEX) 2015—www.mipex.eu/

This instrument provides a comparative look at integration policies, measuring policies with 144 policy indicators in all EU member states, Australia, Canada, Iceland, Japan, Korea, New Zealand, Norway, Switzerland, Turkey, and the United States.

Point Calculator for Eligibility to Temporary Residence in Austria—www.migration.gv.at/en/service-and-links/points-calculator.html

The Red-White-Red Card scheme regulates the immigration of qualified third-country nationals to Austria according to a criteria-based model. In order to receive a Red-White-Red Card, the applicant has to achieve a sufficient amount of points (e.g., for education, professional experience, age, and language skills).

Statistics Austria: Migration—www.statistik.at/web_en/statistics/population/migration/

Migration statistics for Austria provided by the National Statistics Institute.

Notes

1. http://ec.europa.eu/dgs/home-affairs/what-we-do/policies/asylum/examination-of-applicants/index_en.htm, June 5, 2015.
2. The terms "undocumented migrant" and "irregular migrant" are used synonymously and refer to a person who, owing to unauthorized entry, breach of a condition of entry, or the expiry of his or her visa, lacks legal status in a transit or receiving country.
3. In 1962 Austria set up the first intergovernmental agreement with Spain, but this remained irrelevant for the most part (Fassmann & Reeger, 2008).
4. Personal communication from an NGO director to the authors.

References

Bachner, F., Ladurner, J., Habimana, K., Ostermann, H., Stadler, I., & Habl, C. (2013). *Das österreichische Gesundheitswesen im internationalen Vergleich.* Ausgabe 2012. Wien: Bundesministerium für Gesundheit.

BK/Bundeskriminalamt. (2014). *Schlepperbericht 2014; Report from the Criminal Intelligence Service Austria on organised human smuggling* [includes an English summary]. Vienna: Author.

Fassmann, H., & Reeger, U. (2008). *Austria: From guest worker migration to a country of immigration.* IDEA Working Papers no. 1 (December).

GFK. (2014). *Integration und EU-Bürger—Ergebnisse der Fokusgruppen.* Retrieved from http://www.bmeia.gv.at/fileadmin/user_upload/bmeia/media/Integration/Studien/GfK_Ergebnisse_der_Fokusgruppen_-_Integration_und_EU-Buerger.pdf

GÖG/Gesundheit Österreich GmbH. (2013). *Das österreichische Gesundheitswesen im internationalen Vergleich.* Wien: Author.

Government of Austria. (2011). *Integration report.* Retrieved from https://www.bmeia.gv.at/en/integration/integration-report/

Hofmarcher, M. (2013). Das österreichische Gesundheitssystem. Akteure. Daten. Analysen. Medizinisch Wissenschaftliche Verlagsgesellschaft.

Holzer, D., & Stompe, H. (2011). Prävalenz psychischer Erkrankungen bei Migranten. *Spectrum Psychiatrie,* March 25, n.p.

IOM/EMN. (2014). *Access to social security for third-country nationals—policies and practice in Austria.* Vienna: National Contact Point Austria in the European Migration Network, IOM Office.

Jandl, M., & Kraler, A. (2003). Austria—a country of immigration. *Online Journal of the Migration Policy Institute.* Retrieved from http://www.migrationpolicy.org/article/austria-country-immigration

Karl-Trummer, U. (2010). *Where evidence meets reality: Views on ethno-cultural diversity management for health care organisations.* Vienna: ARGE Bildungsmanagement- Sigmund Freud University.

Karl-Trummer, U., Metzler, B., & Novak-Zezula, S. (2009a). Health care for undocumented migrants in the EU: Concepts and cases. Background paper developed within the framework of the IOM project "Assisting Migrants and Communities (AMAC): Analysis of Social Determinants of Health and Health Inequalities." Brussels: IOM.

Karl-Trummer, U., Novak-Zezula, S., & Metzler, B. (2009b). Managing a paradox: Health care for undocumented migrants in the EU. *Finnish Journal of Ethnicity and Migration* 4(2), 53–60.

Karl-Trummer, U., Novak-Zezula, S., & Sardadvar, S. (2012). *Gesundheit im urbanen Raum. Die Bedeutung von sozioökonomischer Position und Migrationsstatus als Einflussfaktoren auf die Gesundheit der Wiener Bevölkerung.* Fact Sheet. Center for Health and Migration & Institiut für Wirtschaftsgeographie und Geoinformatik der Wirtschaftsuniversität Wien. Retrieved from http://c-hm.com/Fact_Sheet_Gurr.pdf

Kraler, A., Reichel, D. & Hollomey, C. (2008, November). *Clandestino. Undocumented migration counting the uncountable. Data and trends across Europe. Country report Austria.* (Updated and revised October 2009.) Vienna: ICMPD.

MIPEX. (2015a). *Austria 2014 report. Migrant integration policy index.* Retrieved from http://www.mipex.eu/austria

MIPEX. (2015b). Health. *Migrant Integration Policy Index.* Retrieved from http://www.mipex.eu/taxonomy/term/67

ÖIF Monitor Integration & Migration. (2015, February). Vienna: Author.

Ombud for Equal Treatment. (2015). *Activities and recommendations 2012/2013 at a glance.* Vienna: Ombud for Equal Treatment.

Statistik Austria. (2008). *Sozio-demographische und sozio-ökonomische Determinanten von Gesundheit. Auswertungen der Daten aus der Österreichischen Gesundheitsbefragung 2006/2007.* Retrieved from http://www.statistik.at/web_de/dynamic/statistiken/gesundheit/gesundheitsversorgung/publdetail?id=88&listid=88&detail=458

Statistik Austria. (2014). *Migration & Integration. Zahlen. Daten. Indikatoren 2014.* Wien: Author.

Trummer, U., Novak-Zezula, S., & Cigirli, Z. (2013). *Interkulturelle Lebenswelt und Gesundheit von türkischen Frauen in Wien.* Fact Sheet. Center for Health and Migration & Institiut für Wirtschaftsgeographie und Geoinformatik der Wirtschaftsuniversität Wien. Retrieved from http://c-hm.com/Fact_Sheet_IKL_final.pdf

Trummer, U., Novak-Zezula, S., Phua, K. H., Griffiths, S., Chung, R., & Yi, H. (2014). *Migrants and healthcare. Social and economic approaches.* Singapore: ASEF Public Health Network.

Ulram, P. (2009). *Integration in Österreich. Einstellungen, Orientierungen und Erfahrungen von MigrantInnen und Angehörigen der Mehrheitsbevölkerung.* Wien: GfK/BMI.

UN High Commissioner for Refugees (UNHCR). (1990). *The Refugee Convention, 1951: The Travaux préparatoires analysed with a commentary by Dr. Paul Weis.* Geneva: Author.

UN High Commissioner for Refugees (UNHCR). (2013). *Flucht und Asyl in Österreich—die häufigsten Fragen und Antworten.* Retrieved from http://www.unhcr.at/fileadmin/user_upload/dokumente/02_unhcr/in_oesterreich/Questions_Answers_2013.pdf

UN High Commissioner for Refugees (UNHCR). (2015). *Asylum trends 2014.* Geneva: Author.

CHAPTER 7

Public Policy, Immigrant Experiences, and Health Outcomes in Belgium

Marie Dauvrin

Chapter Objectives

This chapter focuses on Belgium and its experience with immigrants and ethnic minorities. The objectives of this chapter are:

- to describe the evolution of migration in Belgium and its consequences for Belgian society;
- to review specific initiatives aimed at improving the integration of immigrants in society and the health care system;
- to present data on the health status of immigrants and ethnic minorities in Belgium, with a specific focus on data collection issues; and
- to analyze how the complexity of the Belgian health care system impacts the health experiences of immigrants.

Introduction

The issue of immigration in Belgium presents a paradox. On the one hand, Belgium proudly affirms its diversity and celebrates it. For example, in 2014, several events commemorated the fiftieth anniversary of Moroccan and Turkish labour migration conventions. During the 2014 Football World Cup in Brazil, the Red Devils, the national soccer team, became the calling card of multicultural Belgium, supported by the whole country in spite of regional, communitarian, and cultural differences. On the other hand, a growing number of Belgians[1] express negative opinions toward immigration, which has led to modifications in the Code of Nationality as well as asylum policies. Nationalist political groups are now represented in the federal government and hold strategic positions such as the state secretary for asylum and migration. Families are again detained in reception centres, although this has been condemned by the European Union. In such context, attention to diversity and immigration issues in health care remains sparse and may lead to inequities in health care.

Independent since 1830 and a founding member of the European Union, Belgium is a federal state with a parliamentary democracy. It is also a member of NATO. The federal organization consists of three levels of **governance**: the federal state, the federated entities, and local governments (provinces and municipalities). The federated entities are the three regions (Brussels-Capital, Flanders, and Wallonia) and the three communities (French, Flemish, and German). Each entity has its own government and parliament and has complete sovereignty in specific matters. The federal state is responsible for immigration policies (including health care for asylum-seekers) and financing and organization of the **social security system**. Regions are in charge of integration policies. At the lowest level, municipalities play a role in delivering social assistance and promoting social cohesion.

Regarding the welfare system, Belgium's national social security system is based on a **Bismarckian model** and is funded by compulsory social insurance taxes. The social security system provides access to and coverage for health care, and allocations for retirement, unemployment, disability, incapacity, and family support. Other supports are assumed by different actors, but this is beyond the scope of this chapter.

This chapter presents the complex situation of Belgium and how the lack of clear governance is likely to undermine the goal of **equity** for migrants and ethnic minorities. First, the evolution of immigration in Belgium and its specifics will be presented. Second, although immigration issues are unevenly integrated in public policies, this chapter will present some specific initiatives aimed at improving the integration of immigrants, namely, the integration course and the intercultural mediation in health services. It will then present their health outcomes and conclude by analyzing how a variety of complex interactions impact the health experiences of immigrants.

The Migration Landscape in Belgium

Ethnic Census

Before describing the immigrant population in Belgium, it is worth noting that there is no explicit ethnic census in Belgium. Consequently, the two variables for assessing immigration are nationality and country of birth (Hanquinet, Vandezande, Jacobs, & Swyngedouw, 2006). This absence of an ethnic census is explained by historical and political reasons (Jacobs & Réa, 2012). During the Second World War, the absence of accurate ethnic data prevented the Nazis' armies from identifying and deporting

Belgian Jews. After the Second World War, Belgian authorities decided to continue this approach. The motivation is also political because linguistic issues raise other contentious issues among the Belgian population.

In 1921, a linguistic and administrative border divided Belgium into two communities: the Flemish-speaking community in northern Belgium and the French-speaking community in the south. A third community was added in the Eastern cantons: the German-speaking community. These administrative and linguistic borders grant specific rights to citizens, such as being served in their mother tongue in public services. Until 1963, a census determined the border with some municipalities moving from one linguistic regimen to another with consequences for minorities. This led to many conflicts at the population and political levels and the borders were definitively fixed in 1963. However, dissensions still exist about "correct" placements. Conducting an ethnic census, including language preferences, could lead to new tensions and discussions about the so-called "linguistic" rights. Even now, in "bilingual" municipalities, despite victories in municipal elections, some mayors are not officially installed because of linguistic issues (Van Den Wijngaert, 2011).

Legal issues also prevent ethnic data collection. The legislation related to privacy and the treatment of personal data stipulates that data collection related to ethnicity and culture is sensitive and therefore forbidden. However, recent judicial opinions allow the collection of ethnic data under certain conditions: If their value is explicit and legitimate (e.g., for research or public health purposes); if the data are treated anonymously and confidentially; and if the data are relevant, accurate, and kept up-to-date (Ringelheim, 2010). Some exceptions exist in public health: Some contagious diseases are submitted to non-anonymous reporting in order to protect the population (e.g., Creutzfeldt-Jakob disease). Health professionals are required to report specific diseases to the public authorities. Depending on the severity and the contagion risk of the disease, this declaration may not be kept anonymous (Scientific Institute of Public Health, 2015).

This absence of official data on the ethnic diversity or the migrant structure of the Belgian population has impeded the development of specific policies targeted at promoting the integration of immigrants. Belgians with an immigrant background are not distinguished from the rest of the population and no specific protection is granted to ethnic minorities (Hanquinet et al., 2006). Recognition of ethnic minorities is not enacted in Belgian policies at the federal level, with the exception of the community of Roma people; this is an obligation from the European Union (EU). A national integration strategy for Roma was developed by the federal government (European Commission, 2012). At the regional level, ethnic minorities and migrants are recognized in differing terms and in importance, leading to different regional integration policies.

Legal Immigration

Until the 19th century, Belgium was mainly an emigration country, with many leaving for Canada or the United States. Although foreigner immigration is now the main source of immigrants, there are still both immigration and emigration flows among the Belgian population. Since the First World War, there have been more Belgians leaving Belgium than Belgians coming back to the country, with the exception of the economic crisis of the 1930s and the independence of the Congo in 1960, when around 16,000 Belgians returned to Belgium (Perrin, 2006). In 2011, Belgian nationals represented around 15 percent of immigrants and almost 34 percent of emigrants (Ministry of Economy, 2011).

Belgian nationality is obtained through *jus sanguinis* (ancestry) (Lorant & Bhopal, 2010). Only minor grandchildren (less than 18 years of age) of immigrants are automatically granted Belgian nationality according to place of birth. Belgian nationality can also be obtained through a procedure of naturalization or a procedure of declaration: according to the selected procedure, the applicant has to comply with several criteria. Other specific dispositions exist for children under 18 years old (Ministry of Justice, 1984).

The strategic position of Belgium in Europe and its immigrant history have shaped the diversity of the Belgian population. Broadly speaking, international mobility in Belgium remains important and is still increasing: around 160,000 immigrants were registered annually in 2009, 2010, and 2011. The current increase in immigration flows is illustrated by the trend observed since the mid-1980s. In 2011, the resident foreign population was 10.2 percent of the entire population of Belgium, while 12.1 percent of Belgian citizens were born abroad. Among the foreign-born population, almost 70 percent of legal immigrants in Belgium are European citizens from the EU-28 (Ministry of Economy, 2011). The presence of many European institutions and agencies, NATO headquarters, and other international organizations partly explain this European immigration, but other factors, such as fiscal advantages and cheaper real estate opportunities, have stimulated the immigration of French and Dutch citizens to Belgium. An important fact is that the distribution of immigrants is unequal between the three Belgian regions: people without Belgian nationality make up nearly half the population (46 percent) in Brussels, 10 percent in Wallonia, and 7.3 percent in Flanders (Perrin, 2006).

The three main reasons for legal migration to Belgium include labour, studies, and family reunification (Perrin, 2006). In Belgium, the main labour migration flows began in the early 20th century. At this time, foreigners constituted about 3 percent of the total population of Belgium and 90 percent of these came from bordering countries. Between the two world wars, this proportion rose to 4 percent, mainly due to migration flows from Italy and Eastern Europe. Belgium's immigration policy in the

1930s restricted immigrants to working for at least three years in the same economic area. This constraint has shaped the distribution of migrant populations in Belgium. During the 1960s, the extension of immigration permits to all industrial sectors and services led to increased numbers of foreign workers coming to Belgium's main cities. These were mainly Italian, Spanish, and Greek immigrants at first, followed by Moroccans and Turks.

Specific conventions were made between Belgium and third countries, such as Italy (the so-called "Coal Accords"), Morocco, and Turkey. The first Italians arrived in Belgium in the 1950s after the Second World War, mainly for labour in the mining industry. Most of their descendants still live in these same areas (Morelli, 1992). The tragic accident of the "Bois du Cazier" in 1956 focused Belgians' attention on the poor living conditions of Italian miners: On August 8, 1956, a fire in the mine on the site "Bois du Cazier" killed 262 men (136 Italian, 95 Belgian, and a mixed group of European workers).

Most of the Italians came from the same villages in Italy and left families without resources, leading to a modification of immigration policy. Families were allowed to join the men working in Belgium. A few years later, Moroccan and Turks came to Belgium to work for some of the main public sites such as the Brussels underground, the junction "North-South," and other infrastructure projects (Réa & Martiniello, 2012). However, there are more Greeks than Turks in Belgium, confirming the view that legal migration to Belgium is mostly European (Ministry of Economy, 2011).

Nowadays, the health sector is particularly concerned with labour immigration. Some health institutions have developed immigration-based recruitment policies in order to combat the shortage of practising health professionals, especially nurses. Immigrant health professionals come mainly from adjacent countries such as France or the Netherlands and from traditional immigration countries such as Italy and Morocco (Pacolet & Merckx, 2006). More recently, Poland, Romania, the Philippines, and Lebanon have been identified as the four main countries of origin for foreign nurses (Wets & de Bruyn, 2011). Although data remain sparse, it appears that the provision of health care for the elderly has become an economic niche occupied by Congolese nurses in urban areas such as Brussels.

After the first petroleum crisis, the Belgian government stopped labour migration in 1974, which led to a decrease in the number of immigrants and to declines in foreign residents in 1982 and 1983. However, since 1984, immigration has increased and this trend is continuing. Among other developments, the successive waves of enlargement of the European Union in 2004 and 2007 contributed to the increase of European migration (the increases of 2004 and 2007 included Cyprus, Czech Republic, Estonia, Hungary, Latvia, Lithuania, Malta, Poland, Slovakia, Slovenia, Bulgaria, and Romania).

International students constitute a separate and growing category distinct from traditional labour migrants. The Bologna Decree defines the rules for students willing to move from one country to another inside 47 European countries. It also reinforced mobility through provision of equivalence between diplomas. A growing number of universities and university colleges are developing specific programs to attract international students. Three situations of student mobility coexist: (1) the migration of students in a strict sense (foreign students beginning a complete curriculum abroad, which is especially the case for French students in health sciences such as dentistry, nursing, midwifery, and physiotherapy); (2) student mobility (short-term education projects such as the "Erasmus" program), and (3) "improvement" migration (students involved in a third cycle of education, such as PhD students). In 2012, most foreigners requesting student visas came from Cameroon. Contrary to labour immigrants, students are less likely to stay in Belgium after completing their courses of study.

Beside labour and student immigrants, since 1974 family reunification has become the most widespread form of legal immigration in Belgium (Lodewyckx, Timmerman, & Wets, 2011). The European Council Directive 2003/86/EC, dated September 22, 2003, on the right to family reunification, states that only "third-country nationals who hold a residence permit valid for at least one year in one of the Member States and who have the genuine option of long-term residence can apply for family reunification" (Council of the European Union, 2003). It does not apply to European Union citizens or third-country nationals awaiting refugee status or under temporary forms of protection. Foreigners recognized as resident in Belgium have the right to bring spouses and underage children and, under certain conditions, other family members to live with them.

This issue is of major importance since growing numbers of young migrants marry people from their country of origin. This rule also applies to Belgians or other Europeans who are married to non-European citizens or are parents of children who are non-EU citizens. Family reunification also applies to elderly relatives of resident migrants, but to a far lesser degree (Lodewyckx et al., 2011). Among migrants applying for family reunification, less than 2 percent were 59 years or over. However, although official data are sparse, a new form of family reunification has recently appeared in Belgium—elderly family members migrating to join their families following the death of their spouse.

Colonial Heritage

From 1885 to 1960, Belgium maintained a colony in Congo. Despite the tumultuous history between the two countries, strong relationships still exist and Belgium hosts an important community of Congolese. In addition, after the First World War, the

League of Nations asked Belgium to take over from Germany the administration of Rwanda and Burundi. Again, this may explain the presence of strong and established communities of Rwandese and Burundi in Belgium.

Asylum-Seekers and Refugees

Many people seek asylum in Belgium for political, economic, medical, or climatic reasons (Home Affairs FPS, 1980). In 2013, asylum-seekers came mostly from Afghanistan (for a third year in a row), Guinea, Democratic Republic of Congo, Russia, and Syria (FEDASIL, 2014). Depending on their motives in applying for asylum and their entry point in Belgium, asylum-seekers are hosted in either open detention centres, closed detention centres, or with friends or family (Belgian Red Cross, 2014; FEDASIL, 2014). These centres are managed either by the Federal Agency for the Reception of Asylum Seekers—FEDASIL (FEDASIL, 2014)—or the Belgian Red Cross (convention with FEDASIL, only open centres). There are also Local Initiatives of Reception managed by municipalities in partnership with FEDASIL. When the application is accepted in the first stage of the procedure, asylum-seekers may benefit from housing within the community, which is often provided by the local public welfare centre.

During 2009–2011, Belgium experienced what was called the "asylum crisis." According to public authorities, an uncontrolled flow of asylum-seekers during this period reached Belgium. Consequently, the federal government struggled to deal with this flow and there were not enough places in reception centres for asylum-seekers. To achieve its goals of providing housing, the federal government was required to place asylum-seekers in hotels to avoid payment of fines imposed by the legal system. Indeed, some asylum-seekers brought suit against FEDASIL because it was not meeting its mission of protecting and receiving the asylum-seekers. At this time, suggested solutions included creating additional spaces in reception centres, restricting the asylum procedure, and accelerating the process to decrease the number of people waiting in reception centres.

During the most recent legislature (2011–2014), the nomination of a liberal state secretary for asylum and migration, Maggie De Block, led to the implementation of some of these measures and modifications in asylum and immigration policies. Procedures have been accelerated; the principle of the "last in, first out" has been applied; the law has been modified (among others, modifying the list of "safe countries" and the regulation regarding multiple asylum applications); the backlog in the processing of applications has been reduced; the coordination and the exchange of information among agencies have been improved; and dissuasion campaigns have been launched outside Belgium, sending an anti-immigration message to potential immigrants. Consequently, the number of asylum-seekers applying in Belgium has decreased in 2013 (–26.2 percent when compared to 2012), reaching the lowest number of applications since 2008 (FEDASIL, 2014).

When compared to other European countries, Belgium is one of the only countries where a decreasing immigration trend is observed. However, a higher number of protections have been granted to asylum-seekers as compared to previous years (6,313 people, including children, received protection in 2013). Despite a hardening of conditions, the objective of the federal authorities remains to grant protection to those who need it. During this current legislature, beginning in October 2014, a new state secretary for asylum and migration, Theo Francken, was designated. His political association with a nationalist Flemish party has already reinforced the hardening of immigration policies. He recently announced the return to a policy of placing families in detention centres, although Belgium has been severely criticized for keeping children within these closed centres.

Irregular Migrants

According to Belgian law, irregular migrants are people without legal authorization to stay on the territory, either because they did not have a permit to enter in Belgium or they overstayed their visa, or they are are not eligible for refugee status (Home Affairs FPS, 1980). During regularization procedures in the early 2000s, around 32,000 claims, representing around 50,000 people and 140 different nationalities, were introduced (FEDASIL, 2014). **Regularization** was a form of amnesty whereby those who did not meet conditions for being recognized as refugees were allowed to apply to receive legal status of residency based on length of stay in Belgium or proof of integration, such as having children regularly attending school.

But, since this campaign, no additional data on illegal immigration have been collected. Estimates report that illegal migration represents around 10 percent of legal migration, which comes out to about 100,000 to 110,000 people in Belgium. This group is highly heterogeneous in terms of country of origin, migration trajectory, socio-economic status, and, more importantly, in health care needs (CLANDESTINO, 2009). There are regular demonstrations in Brussels that aim to bring attention to the specific situations of irregular migrants and call for massive regularization.

Immigration and Social Life

Federal Integration Policies

Integration of immigrants is enshrined in and enacted through the governmental declaration of October 2014 entitled "Equality of Gender, Equality of Opportunities" in the section on "Discriminations, Diversity and Racism." In this section, the federal government acknowledges that:

> Our current society is diversified and based on a mix of different cultures and philosophical convictions. This situation creates opportunities that we have to take. The government will support the different communities of Belgium to share a common basis of common democratic values, and will fight against all forms of political or religious extremism. In the vision of the development of an open and tolerant society, the government will give priority to the fight against all forms of racism and hate incitation against persons with foreign background, anti-Semitism, intolerance, extremism and intercultural violence. (Belgian Government, 2014, p. 222; author's translation)

The purpose of this declaration is to provide better documentation of inequalities and the strategies developed in order to decrease it, especially issues of accessing the labour market in both the public and the private sectors. The federal government also plans an update of the 2007 legislation related to anti-discrimination and anti-racism and to improve execution of Regulation 13/2013, which is related to hate crimes.[2] An evaluation of the national strategy of integration of Roma will be conducted. Specific aspects in immigration issues are targeted such as marriages of convenience, where marriages take place between Belgian citizens and non-Belgians in order for non-Belgians to obtain papers to remain in the country, and in situations where immigrants commit crimes in Belgium.

The current federal government was formed against a context of fear and Islamophobia. Indeed, a terrorist attack against the Jewish Museum in May 2014 killed four people; around 400 young Belgians left to join Syria and other rebel factions in the Middle East; and the group Sharia4Belgium regularly issues threats against Belgian democracy. Consequently, contrary to Italians, Greeks, and other Europeans, integration is more difficult for Moroccans and Turks as most (but not all) of them are Muslims while Belgium is mainly Roman Catholic. Despite the popular view that almost 30 percent of the Belgian population is Muslim, Muslims represent only 6 percent of the Belgian population.

To achieve its objectives of assuring equal opportunities, Belgium had until 2014 the Centre for Equal Opportunities and Opposition to Racism, a governmental agency. In May 2014, it was divided in two distinct and independent centres: the Interfederal Centre for Equal Opportunities and the Federal Migration Centre. The Interfederal Centre for Equal Opportunities aims at providing the competencies of the Centre to the regions and the communities. Consequently, it simplifies procedures for citizens who wish to introduce a complaint or raise issues of discrimination. Citizens may directly contact the central office in Brussels or regional contact points in Flanders (the Meldpunten Discriminatie integrated with the Interfederal Centre since 2014) or in Wallonia (the Espace Wallonie).

The Federal Migration Centre aims at promoting rights for foreigners in Belgium by documenting the nature and the magnitude of migration flows to support political decision making, and struggling against different forms of human trafficking (Chancellery of the Prime Minister, Justice FPS, Personnel & Organisation FPS, Federal Agency for the Reception of Asylum Seekers, 2014). It has mainly a consultative/preventive role rather than a decision/obligation role (Federal Migration Center/Interfederal Center for Equal Opportunities, 2015).

Regional Integration Policies

Alongside the federal centre, social integration of migrants is also a political responsibility devolved to the federal entities, namely the regions (Brussels, Flanders, and Wallonia). Consequently, the objectives, the content, and the resources devoted to social integration of migrants are influenced by the regional context. Traditionally, policies in Flanders are influenced by the Netherlands and the United Kingdom, while policies in Wallonia are more influenced by the political discourse of France (Jacobs & Réa, 2005, 2012). Flemish integration policies aim at promoting integration and assimilation while Wallonia tends to focus on socio-economic issues per se rather than immigration issues.

In Flanders, the *Vlaamse Overheid* (Flemish Authority) requires that all legal immigrants aged 18 and over attend the *inburgeringstraject*, especially if they plan to stay for an extended period (Agentschap voor Binnenlands Bestuur, 2014; Vlaamse Overheid, 2014). The civic integration project encompasses a social orientation course (introduction to Flemish and Belgian society, including use of health services), a basic Dutch-as-second-language course, career orientation, and an individual counselling program. The program is tailored to the needs of the immigrant and is compulsory for some target groups: people who recently immigrated to Belgium and have taken up residence in Flanders, and clergymen from religions recognized by the Flemish authorities (e.g., Belgian imams should attend this *inburgeringstraject*). Other target groups may benefit from the program, such as Belgians born abroad who have at least one parent not born in Belgium.

The program is delivered in Dutch or another language (e.g., French, Arabic, or Chinese). Specific programs exist for children, delivered in schools. Migrants living in Brussels may attend the civic integration program organized by the Vlaamse Overheid (Agentschap voor Binnenlands Bestuur, 2014; Vlaamse Overheid, 2014). Before the civic integration project, some forms of social aid (e.g., social housing) were available only if the immigrant spoke Flemish. This was called the *Wooncode* and was aimed at privileging immigrants showing a desire for integration (Jacobs & Réa, 2012). At the same time, the Flemish authorities financially supported cultural immigrant associations to help people preserve their cultural identity. This second measure was strongly curtailed after the assassinations of the extreme-right leader Pim Fortuyn (1948–2002) and the filmmaker Theo Van Gogh (1957–2004) in the Netherlands, against the context of rising Islamophobia after the attacks of September 2001.

In Wallonia and the French part of Brussels, the two regional governments agreed in February 2014 on the development of a civic integration program with content similar to the Flemish program. In July 2014, the new Walloon government decided to include basic French courses in the program (Gouvernement Wallon, 2014). The official civic integration program is currently being implemented (Communauté Française de Belgique, 2015). These programs will be organized by associations with a specific convention with the governments, such as the Centre d'Action Interculturelle de Namur (CAI) or the Centre Régional d'Intégration de Charleroi (CRIC). Differences in implementation of the social integration policies among agencies are likely to produce inequalities among immigrants according to place of residence. However, data lack evidence to support this hypothesis.

Education

All children are obliged at attend school from six to 18 years of age, whatever their legal status in Belgium (Home Affairs, 1983). Consequently, irregular children and children in open detention centres for asylum-seekers have full access to the national school system, either in French-speaking or Dutch-speaking schools (Social Integration, Fight against Poverty and Social Economy PPS, 2007). Some schools have specific classrooms for these children in order to improve their language skills. In addition, these children benefit from school health and psychological services (Ministry of the French Community, 2001; Ministry of the Flemish Community, 2006). School attendance plays a major role in integration of children and their families.

As the process of being recognized as a refugee may take years, participation of children in social life is often a protective factor against deportation of the whole family. Similar situations have been observed with irregular migrants' children who attend school: Integration of the children into the educational system has a protective effect on the parents. This may lead to uncomfortable situations for these children, as they carry the responsibility for their families' integration and receiving permanent residency in Belgium. Depending on the awareness of the educational staff, specific attention will be paid to these children in order to prevent mental health problems and other harmful conditions.

For Belgian children with an immigrant background, the situation is somewhat more complicated.[1] They have the same access to the educational system as other children, but implicit discrimination is likely occurring for these children. The results from the Programme for International Student Assessment (PISA) surveys from the OECD showed a considerable gap between immigrants and Belgian children in terms of educational outcomes (OECD, 2013). The proportion of immigrants and ethnic minorities obtaining a secondary education degree is on the rise, but studies show that Moroccan and Turkish children are more likely to attend the vocational track than other students (Lorant & Dauvrin, 2012). Moreover, the PISA surveys highlighted that immigrant children are more likely to enroll in professional secondary schools, rather than academic schools, or the special education system (for children with physical, mental, or learning disabilities) than Belgian-born children (OECD, 2013).

This is partly explained by the low socio-economic status of the parents and/or the language spoken at home. Moreover, the low number of teachers and educators from immigrant backgrounds has been identified as a potential barrier to integration. Stigmatization of migrant students and pupils increases the risk of school dropout with negative consequences for their future. Positive role models are needed to support the ideal of a multicultural society for youth and children (Centre Interfédéral pour l'Egalité des Chances et la Lutte contre le Racisme et les Discriminations, 2014).

Political Participation

The political career of the former Belgian Prime Minister Elio Di Rupo (2011–2014) is an example of immigrants' successful participation in political life. Born as a second-generation immigrant, Di Rupo's parents came from Italy in the 1950s. After receiving a PhD in sciences, he began a successful political career as a member of the socialist coalition. Despite this success story, there were incidents such as the controversy about a Belgian Muslim deputy who took the oath while wearing her Muslim veil, reinforcing the view that not all immigrants or ethnic minorities are able to express their own identities or opinions. The 2014 federal government has unofficial data showing that 10 of 150 members of the Chamber of Representatives and six of 60 members of the Senate have an immigrant background.

As members of the EU-28, European citizens are granted political participation in Belgium according to European directives. Non-European legal citizens may vote and are eligible for election at the municipal level if they have been legally living in Belgium for at least five years and are still granted their civic rights, but lose these rights if they have a criminal conviction (Milquet, 2012). Again, there are no recent data, but the participation of immigrants appears to be increasing at local levels (municipalities), and is associated with an increased sensitivity toward specific issues of importance for immigrant populations. Most visible political actors with immigrant backgrounds are from Morocco, Turkey, and Congo and are representative of the "traditional" immigrant groups in Belgium, apart from European citizens. However, despite increasing participation of immigrants in political life at local and federal levels, many stakeholders still lack commitment to addressing issues of the welfare of immigrants. Currently, the main topics discussed regarding immigration are related to national security, control of the flows of irregular migration, and assimilation policies.

Labour Market

The freedom of movement inside the European Economic Area (EEA) allows immigrants to search for a job in Belgium without a specific permit. In contrast, immigrants from outside the EEA require a work permit, of which there are several varieties based on the type of job and the worker's length of stay. Overall, employment rates between Belgium-born citizens and immigrants from EU countries are quite similar (around 68 percent). However, significant differences exist when considering unemployment rates: 4.7 percent for Belgians, 6.7 percent for EU citizens, and 14.3 percent for non-EU citizens (DeKeyser, Delhez, & Zimmer, 2012). In addition, the unemployment rate is higher among women and especially among women from non-EU backgrounds (37 percent are considered employed, while Belgian and European women have, respectively, an employment rate of 55.2 percent and 58.7 percent). This difference between women is partly explained by the fact that women of non-EU origin have on average more children under 15 years old at home. It has been documented that women are more likely to leave the labour market in order to take care of the household (DeKeyser et al., 2012).

Both immigrant women and men are underrepresented in public administration and educational system employment, although it may be explained by the fact that there are specific requirements related to these kinds of positions, such as nationality and equivalence of degrees and diplomas. Non-EU men are more likely to work in the hospitality industry (pubs, bars, and restaurants) than EU men, who are more represented in the building industry. Non-EU women are overrepresented in housing/cleaning services and in the health/social sector. EU women are well represented in the services area, especially because they are likely to be employed by international institutions. The proportion of short-term contracts is higher among non-EU migrants (16 percent) than among EU citizens (10.7 percent) and those with Belgian nationality (7.3 percent) (DeKeyser et al., 2012).

There is little data regarding the quality and working conditions of irregular migrants. Some jobs—such as domestic work, babysitting, home care for seniors, or long-term care for disabled people—are filled mainly by women who are irregular migrants (Ouali & Cennicola, 2013). Men who are irregular migrants are more likely to work in the building industry, restaurants and bars, and night shops (i.e., stores open during irregular hours). Frequent efforts are organized by the police to track illegal workers, leading, in some circumstances, to their deportation. However, migrants will usually not be (directly) punished for working without authorization: The consequences will fall upon the employer, especially if there is suspicion of human exploitation. As they do not have any social protection, these illegal workers are even more vulnerable. Some tragic situations have occurred in the workplace, as in the case of a Polish man who was left unconscious in front of an emergency department after falling from several floors. He did not have any identity document or insurance coverage. His wife found out what happened 12 hours after the accident, when colleagues of the injured man had gone home.

The integration of immigrants into the labour market has been the focus of numerous political discussions and measures to improve their participation. Three federal laws prevent discrimination in the labour market (Centre Interfédéral pour l'Egalité des Chances et la Lutte contre le Racisme et les Discriminations, 2014). These concern access to the labour market, working conditions, professional relationships between superiors and employees, and the rights and obligations of each party in the private and public sectors. Discrimination is defined as any differences in treatment based on age, sexual orientation, civil status, income, beliefs or ideology, political convictions, language, current or forthcoming health status, disability, physical or genetic characteristics, social origin, gender, nationality, racial background, colour of skin, ancestry, and national or ethnic origin.

The concept of "reasonable accommodation" has been discussed regarding labour market issues. Indeed, legally speaking, the requirements of equality and non-discrimination require that employers, public services, and other economic actors adapt their practices, on the condition that this adaptation is "reasonable," that is to say, without occasioning a disproportionate burden to the one who has to deploy it (Adam et al., 2010). The main question is identifying which groups are targeted and how they represent disadvantaged groups or communities. Importantly, these adaptations should be discussed and consensually accepted by both parties.

Currently, most of the requests for reasonable accommodations are treated on a case-by-case basis. If this system allows the applicant's specific situation to be taken into account, its discretionary application may lead to inequalities among immigrants. Requests generally concern having days off for religious reasons (most of the official holidays are based on the Roman Catholic calendar such as Ascension Day or All Saints Day), adaptation of the work during a fasting period, and adaptation of catering or clothing regulations.

Several studies established the existence of employment discrimination due to the ethnic origin of the applicants. In a study conducted by two universities, almost half of foreign job seekers received unequal treatment during job interviews when compared to Belgians with the same qualifications. Job seekers from immigrant backgrounds are less likely to be invited to a job interview (Centre Interfédéral pour l'Egalité des Chances et la Lutte contre le Racisme et les Discriminations, 2014; Hamzaoui & Krzeslo, 2007). Some analysis has been made of the impact on a prospective employer if a woman applying for a job is wearing a Muslim veil. In public services, the main discourse promotes "neutrality," suggesting that workers should avoid wearing explicit signs of their religious, philosophical, or political convictions.

Partnerships between public services concerned with labour integration and cultural associations are likely to improve access to labour market for immigrants (Hamzaoui & Krzeslo, 2007). The development of interregional co-operation that will exchange best practices is also considered a means of integrating immigrants in the labour market. Further recommendations are to better define target groups and to develop assessment tools for this (Hamzaoui & Krzeslo, 2007). Gender should be included as an issue of concern to prevent discrimination against women.

Income, Poverty, and Housing

There are many overlaps between socio-economic inequalities and ethnic inequalities and distinguishing the relative contribution of socio-economic status and aspects of ethnicity in creating inequalities remains difficult (Lorant & Bhopal, 2011; Tilly, 1998). Overall, non-EU immigrants living in Belgium are more likely to have lower economic status than EU migrants or Belgian nationals. As most EU citizens work in international institutions, they may have special supports for finding housing or accessing other resources. Their average income usually exceeds the average income of Belgians, shielding them from financial troubles. However, large discrepancies exist among nationality groups, complicating the implementation of solutions. For example, French citizens living in Brussels have higher socio-economic status than Belgians living in Brussels, while French citizens living near the borders have lower socio-economic status than Belgians in the same area (Deboosere & Gadeyne, 2005). Migrants from non-EU countries or from Eastern Europe are more likely to be among the lowest socio-economic groups.

Although discrimination in access to proper housing is forbidden by law, immigrants may be impeded by discretionary decisions made by owners based on discrimination. Associations of tenants, unions, and other NGOs often denounce such discriminatory practices. A recent report from the Interfederal Migration Centre highlights the fact that obtaining proof of discrimination is often difficult and that there are no legal sanctions for such discrimination (Centre Interfédéral pour l'Egalité des Chances et la Lutte contre le Racisme et les Discriminations, 2014).

Immigration and Health

In the absence of an ethnic census, information on immigrant health is based either on nationality or country of birth when considered at the national level. It can also be based on more specific measures, but is available only for specific groups or settings, for example, reception centres for asylum-seekers or primary-care services. There is currently not enough data to provide an accurate overview of the health status of immigrants and ethnic minorities in Belgium for specific issues (e.g., for cardiovascular diseases or oral health).

The Belgian Health Care System

Overall, the Belgian health care system has good accessibility and is of high quality. The health system operates through social insurance, combining horizontal equity (between healthy and sick people) and vertical equity (financing is mainly achieved through social security contributions based to a large extent on employment incomes). Almost 99 percent of the population, including irregular immigrants, benefit from a broad health insurance package through the social security system (Gerkens & Merkur, 2010).

Health issues are a responsibility of the federated entities, which are in charge of some aspects of health care provision: "The regulation and financing of the compulsory health insurance; the determination of accreditation criteria; the financing of hospital budgets and heavy medical care units; legislation covering different professional qualifications; and the registration of pharmaceuticals and their price control" (Gerkens & Merkur, 2010, p. 15). Federated entities are in charge of "health promotion and prevention; maternity and child health care and social services; different aspects of community care; coordination and collaboration in primary health care and palliative care; the implementation of accreditation standards and the determination of additional accreditation criteria; and the financing of hospital investment" (Gerkens & Merkur, 2010, p. 32).

Health Status of Immigrants

Because the immigrant population in Belgium is heterogeneous, the overall health status of immigrants and ethnic minorities in Belgium is also heterogeneous. When questions of immigration and health are discussed, it mainly concerns immigrants from Turkish or Moroccan backgrounds rather than European ones. Linguistic issues and cultural differences are commonly reported as main difficulties when caring for these non-European groups (Dauvrin, Geerts, & Lorant, 2010; Scheppers, van Dongen, Dekker, Geertzen, & Dekker, 2006). For European citizens and irregular immigrants, insurance coverage and legal entitlement to health care are of special concern.

Noirhomme-Renard and Deccache (2007) identified a healthy immigrant effect among first-generation youth migrants, but this effect rapidly decreased over time. The same result was found by De Grande et al.: The second-generation of Maghrebins and Turks have worse health status than the first generation of Maghrebins and Turks (De Grande, Vandenheede, Gadeyne, & Deboosere, 2014). On the contrary, similar immigrants from sub-Saharan Africa reported feeling healthier than Belgians. Furthermore, there were no differences between Belgians and the second-generation of sub-Saharan Africans (De Grande et al., 2014).

Surprisingly, immigrant men from Turkey and Morocco have a lower mortality risk than Belgian men (Deboosere & Gadeyne, 2005). Even after controlling for the **salmon bias** (i.e., people returning to their country of origin to die), this advantage persists for men. In this study, only French immigrants have a higher risk of mortality than Belgian men. Women from sub-Saharan Africa have a higher mortality risk than Belgian women, while Spanish women have a lower mortality risk when compared to Belgian women. Again, when socio-economic status is included in the statistical analyses, the relative risk is even smaller for immigrant populations.

The excess mortality risk for women is partly explained by the higher prevalence of infectious diseases. Vandenheede and colleagues also found that North Africans have higher diabetes-related mortality when compared to Belgians (Vandenheede, Lammens, Deboosere, Gadeyne, & De Spiegelaere, 2011). This excessive risk of mortality is partly explained by the differences in educational status and is more likely to affect women.

In Brussels, excessive perinatal mortality has been documented among children with an immigrant background: 6.8 deaths per 1,000 live births among Turkish women, 6.2 per 1,000 live births among sub-Saharan African women, and 3 per 1,000 live births among Belgian women for the period running from 28 weeks of pregnancy until delivery (Haelterman, De Spiegelaere, & Masuy-Stroobant, 2007). It is worth noting that children of mothers from sub-Saharan Africa have a mortality rate of 2.8 per 1,000 live births in the period ranging from 28 days after delivery to 364 days, while children born from other women have mortality rates oscillating between 1.5 and 1.9 deaths per 1,000 live births.

At the national level, premature birth is a risk factor: Children of foreign-born mothers are more at risk of mortality from premature births, at birth, or during the neonatal period (seven days after birth). Premature births are around 31.2 percent of the causes of deaths among children of foreign-born mothers while it accounts for only 12.7 percent among Belgians. Among women from sub-Saharan Africa, the proportion of deaths due to premature birth rises to 2.5 per 1,000 births while it is only 0.9 per 1,000 births among Belgian women (Haelterman et al., 2007). In the perinatal period, genetic abnormalities represent 27.3 percent of the deaths at birth for children of foreign mothers, and 22.7 percent among Belgians; excessive mortality for foreigners at birth is 20.3 percent versus 12.3 percent for Belgian women (Haelterman et al., 2007).

When looking at other health indicators, Turkish and Moroccan immigrants are more likely to experience worse subjective health—the self-reporting of health status—than Belgians (Lorant, Van Oyen, & Thomas, 2008), while Europeans have better subjective health. This worse subjective health is partly explained by contextual factors, such as the highest unemployment rate among Turks and Moroccans. After adjusting for socio-economic and contextual factors, Turks and Moroccans tend to have the same level of subjective health as Belgians. Similar results for irregular immigrants were found by Médecins du Monde. In a sample of 503 people, almost 21 percent reported poor to very poor subjective health (Observatoire Européen de l'Accès aux Soins des Médecins du Monde, 2007).

In terms of mental health issues, Turkish and Moroccan immigrants are more at risk of severe anxiety, depression, and psychosis (Fossion et al., 2002; Fossion et al., 2004; Levecque, Lodewyckx, & Bracke, 2008; Levecque, Lodewyckx, & Vranken, 2007). The psychosis rate among migrants is increasing. Fossion and colleagues identified the socio-demographic characteristics of these patients and found an association between the higher risk of psychosis and their high unemployment rate (Fossion et al., 2002). This study also provided evidence of the ambivalent role of the family—that is, whether a family has a protecting or a threatening role, depending on each patient's situation. They also identified that Turkish and Moroccan immigrants lacked a psychiatrist. This study also highlighted the protective role played by Muslim religious beliefs, which translated into lower alcohol consumption and lower suicide rates.

Levecque found that low educational level, region of origin, and poor participation in the labour market are the three main factors increasing risk of severe depression or chronic anxiety among immigrant Turks and Moroccans (Levecque et al., 2008; Levecque et al., 2007). Due to their particular situations, irregular immigrants and asylum-seekers are even more vulnerable to mental health issues (Croix Rouge de Belgique, 2005; Dogniez & Post, 2003; Observatoire Européen de l'Accès aux Soins des Médecins du Monde, 2007).

Administrative procedures, poor reception conditions, and insufficient training of health care professionals are among the factors increasing the risk of poor mental health among these groups. Keygnaert et al. found that female asylum-seekers, refugees, and irregular migrants are particularly vulnerable to violence, especially sexual violence (including rape and sexual exploitation) (Keygnaert, Vettenburg, & Temmerman, 2012). In a study among first-generation adolescents, Derluyn, Broekaert, and Schuyten (2008) found that these youth experienced more traumatic events and had a higher prevalence of borderline mental health troubles. Noir homme-Renard and Decacche also identified several risk factors for poor mental health among immigrant adolescents—feeling discouragement or sadness, stress, relationship difficulties, depression symptoms or dark thoughts, and concentration difficulties (Noirhomme-Renard & Deccache, 2007).

However, immigration factors should be considered alongside other risk factors and protective factors. Some authors recommend a careful use of "ethno-psychiatry" in order to avoid a biased perspective of the health of migrants. Again, specific attention should be paid to girls, as they are more at risk of traumatic events, human trafficking, human exploitation, forced marriages, and familial and marital violence. Indicators of sexual and reproductive health are also reported as worse among asylum-seekers and irregular immigrants than among the native-born Belgian population. Although women are more at risk, these issues are also important for the male immigrant population (Keygnaert, Vettenburg, Roelens, & Temmerman, 2014).

A gender gradient is also observed regarding chronic diseases. Women from immigrant backgrounds have a higher risk of type 2 diabetes mellitus as compared to men from immigrant backgrounds (Vandenheede & Deboosere, 2009; Vandenheede et al., 2011). Moreover, immigrant women are more at risk for diabetes-related mortality, especially for teenagers' mothers and multiparous women (Vandenheede, Deboosere, Gadeyne, & De Spiegelaere, 2012). Both women and men of immigrant backgrounds are more at risk of having type 2 diabetes mellitus as compared to Belgians (Vandenheede & Deboosere, 2009). For women, this risk remains after controlling for socio-economic status, level of physical activity, and health habits.

Prevalence of tuberculosis, HIV, and sexually transmitted infections is higher among non-Belgians (according to the nationality), but this effect may be underestimated in the absence of accurate data (Fonds des Affections Respiratoires, 2013, 2014; Sasse, Verbrugge, & Van Beckhoven, 2012). Although the epidemic of HIV has remained stable over time in Belgium, most of the newly diagnosed cases are among the foreign-born population. Breastfeeding is the primary source of HIV infection among sub-Saharan children, while drug injection is the leading cause for migrants from North Africa. Regarding tuberculosis, the three regions of Belgium are differently affected by the disease—most of the newly diagnosed cases are in Brussels. Although tuberculosis is more prevalent among refugees, asylum-seekers, and irregular migrants, there is also a risk of contracting it in international institutions because of the mobility of workers in the European Economic Area (EEA). All asylum-seekers are screened for tuberculosis when they apply for asylum (X-ray machines are available at the Foreign Office and in some asylum centres).

Treatment against tuberculosis is free and often provided in closed hospital units to prevent the spread of the disease. Moreover, asylum-seekers may be immunized against specific diseases. Some of these expensive vaccinations are not covered by the national health insurance for Belgians (these vaccinations are not considered as necessary even though they are often required when travelling abroad), but are freely administered to asylum-seekers in order to protect the Belgian population (FEDASIL, 2012, 2014; Flemish Lung and Tuberculosis Association, 2014; FARES, 2014). Cross-contamination between HIV and tuberculosis is more prevalent among young men from sub-Saharan Africa. Systematic testing of HIV for all patients who have tuberculosis has been recommended (FARES, 2013).

Similarly, Belgian studies have shown inequalities in access to, use of, and quality of health care between immigrants and ethnic minorities and the general Belgian population. In primary-care services, when compared to the general Belgian population, migrants from Turkish or Moroccan backgrounds are less likely to have referring GPs, screening, or vaccinations (Anson, 2001; Demarest et al., 2006). Immigrants and ethnic minorities also have less access to specialized medicine in Belgium.

Cultural Competence of Health Care Professionals

Recent research in Belgium identified the three most important intercultural situations encountered by health professionals: The family intervenes in the care of the patient; a migrant patient has more vulnerable socio-economic status; and the patient did not understand her or his health problem (Dauvrin, 2013; Dauvrin & Lorant, 2014b). But although these situations were reported as frequent, they were not reported as difficult. Indeed, the most difficult situation was when the patient did not speak the local language of French or Dutch. Health care professionals pointed out difficulties carrying out administrative procedures, mainly because of the poor socio-economic status of the migrants and their inability to understand procedures, and the need for additional resources to deliver proper care to migrants. Despite the absence of compulsory norms in training and lifelong learning for health professionals, it appears that health professionals somehow manage to care for immigrants even though they displayed lower than average cultural competence scores (Dauvrin & Lorant, 2014b). De Maesschalck also supported the need for additional training of health care professionals to help improve communication (De Maesschalck, 2012).

Integration of Immigrants in the Health Care System

Despite several publicly funded initiatives and local projects, the question of immigration and health remains poorly developed in Belgium. Recent works of the Assises de l'Interculturalité (2010) and the group Tackling Health Inequalities in Belgium (TAHIB, 2010) have both contributed to initiating these debates. From 2008 to 2010, the EUGATE project, funded by the European Commission, synthesized the recommendations of Belgian and European experts on best practices in access and health care delivery, with some specific recommendations for Belgium (Dauvrin & Lorant, 2010;

Deville et al., 2011; Priebe et al., 2013). The main recommendation was improving the conversation around immigration and health as Belgium lags behind neighbouring countries such as the Netherlands, Germany, or the United Kingdom. Lorant and Bophal compared Belgium and Scotland regarding immigration and health, and found more health inequalities among immigrant populations in Belgium than in Scotland, and that norms supporting equity for immigrants are needed (Lorant & Bhopal, 2010).

From 2010 to 2011, the Ministry of Public Health commissioned the ETHEALTH (Ethnicity and Health) expert group to provide recommendations for reducing health inequalities for immigrants and ethnic minorities (Dauvrin, Derluyn, Coune, Verrept, & Lorant, 2012; Derluyn, Lorant, Dauvrin, Coune, & Verrept, 2011a, 2011b; Lorant, Derluyn, Dauvrin, Coune, & Verrept, 2011). This group came up with 46 recommendations ranging from the individual to the macro-political level. At the end of the process, two main lessons emerged: The combination of scientific knowledge and practical expertise helped to provide suitable recommendations, but the low level of commitment at the political level may have jeopardized the implementation of the recommendations. This consultation led Belgium to adopt equity standards in 2014, and a pilot test of the project was conducted in 2015.

Alongside the ETHEALTH project, two initiatives targeting the health of immigrants have been developed in Belgium. The first initiative focuses on access to health, namely, the provision of urgent medical aid for irregular immigrants, while the second initiative focuses on the quality of health care—that is, the intercultural mediation.

Access to Health Care for Irregular Migrants: The Provision of Urgent Medical Aid

For almost two decades, Belgium developed a utilitarian approach to provision of health care for irregular immigrants (Romero-Ortuño, 2004). In utilitarian approaches of health care for irregular migrants, the main objective of the health care delivery is to protect the Belgian population against possible contagious diseases (as opposed to humanitarian approaches, which promote the health of irregular migrants, especially the most vulnerable). The Royal Decree of 1996 for Urgent Medical Aid organizes the entitlement and coverage of health care for undocumented migrants (UMA), which is not to be confused with emergency care, which is always provided regardless of the person's status (Dauvrin, 2012; Home Affairs FPS, 1996, 2003). Three conditions determine entitlement to health care for undocumented immigrants: (1) if the applicant lives in poor socio-economic conditions (e.g., has no regular income); (2) if the applicant has illegal status of residence in Belgium; and (3) if the applicant does not have a fixed address. This last condition is not explicitly required by the Royal Decree but is required by the Public Centre of Social Action (PCAS), which is in charge of the administrative procedure.

In theory, the procedure of UMA offers a wide range of services, offering the same coverage for irregular immigrants and Belgians. UMA can be delivered in inpatient or outpatient services and involves preventive (e.g., vaccinations) and curative health care. It thus theoretically involves all procedures, therapies, and drugs authorized by the Belgian social security system. However, the services covered and/or delivered are at the discretion of physicians (only physicians are allowed to initiate an UMA procedure, not other health professionals) and PCAS (Casman, 2008; Dauvrin, 2012). Indeed, administrative procedures, lack of knowledge of health professionals and patients, implicit selection, and other barriers prevent patients from accessing adequate health care (Derluyn et al., 2011b; Lorant et al., 2011).

Reports from Médecins du Monde showed that, according to the law, the coverage of health care needs for UMA should be 99 percent, but, in fact, this coverage reaches a threshold of 14 percent (Observatoire Européen de l'Accès aux Soins des Médecins du Monde, 2007). Some physicians reported offering free health care to avoid administrative procedures while others confessed that, because of their lack of knowledge of the procedure, they will provide only emergency care (Dauvrin et al., 2010). This arbitrary allocation of resources and health care is likely to increase health inequalities among irregular migrants (Dauvrin, Lorant et al., 2012).

There is no direct payment required during the whole procedure of UMA: everything (or almost everything) is free for patients (MedImmigrant, 2014). The health professionals or the health services will directly bill the **Public Centre of Social Action**. Public Centres of Social Action are in charge of social aid at the local level and are dependent on the municipalities. The PCSA provide assistance for those in poor socio-economic conditions either through income assistance (income of "social integration") provided when the person cannot benefit from unemployment allocations, disability allocations, or retirement allocations; or through material assistance (medical aid, housing facilities, food packs, or second-hand clothing); or through social support (e.g., counselling by social workers).

The PCSA take care of all people who live legally or illegally within the limits of the municipality (Social Integration, Fight against Poverty and Social Economy PPS, 1976). As UMA and, more broadly, social aid are organized at the local level by the PCAS, there are differences between municipalities concerning the coverage, the organization, and the priorities in social aid. For example, a municipality with a high proportion of seniors may prefer investing in nursing homes rather than in health care support for irregular immigrants. In other municipalities, support for irregular migrants may be perceived as a priority and specific staff are designated to assist these people.

The main problem is that these differences between municipalities are also likely to increase inequalities between irregular immigrants and others. At the heart of the situation, it should be noted that UMA is a federal law, but as it is part of social aid, its application is left to the discretion of the municipalities as the organization and delivery of social aid is a municipal responsibility. The federal level may only give advice concerning procedures (to avoid the risk of meddling) (Casman, 2008; Dauvrin, 2012; MedImmigrant, 2014). Consequently, no one could force a municipality to take a fair share in supporting irregular immigrants or other people living in poor socio-economic conditions.

Improving Quality of Care: Intercultural Mediation

In 1990, the General Commissar on Integration Policy reported that integration of non-Belgian citizens was a total failure and that efforts should be made to improve the situation. This report led to several measures on the labour market, the educational system, and the health care system. In 1996, a think tank of the Centre for Equal Opportunities began reflecting on how to improve the quality of care for migrants. This led to the creation of an Intercultural Mediation Cell at the Ministry of Public Health and a pilot test of intercultural mediators in some hospitals, with the support of NGOs that already provide these services on a discretionary basis.

From 1997 to date, the intercultural mediators have been implemented in several general and psychiatric hospitals. The mediators are funded by the Ministry of Public Health, but the hospitals have to prove that they have a real need. Every year, the hospitals must justify the use of the mediators in order to maintain the project. In 1999, the funding of intercultural mediators was officially inscribed in the federal law related to hospital funding. In 2002, Belgium adopted a law related to the rights of the patient. This law states that "information should be provided in a clear language that the patient understands" (Ministry of Public Health and Social Affairs, 2002). Although there is no explicit mention of using interpreters or intercultural mediators, this law identifies the need for specific attention to the linguistic and cultural barriers that may arise between health professionals and patients.

A recent study in Belgium showed that health professionals do feel responsible when it comes to adapting to the communication needs of the patients (Dauvrin & Lorant, 2014a). In 2012 intercultural mediation was deployed through videoconferences in hospitals. In 2014, the first consultations by videoconference were held in primary-care services, expanding the scope of intercultural mediation. In 2015, some federal detention centres for asylum-seekers also benefited from intercultural mediation through videoconferences (Ministry of Public Health, 2011).

Besides liaison interpreting, intercultural mediators have a wide range of activities: culture brokerage, mediation of conflicts, advocacy, patient information, and outreach activities. They play a key role in providing support to the patients as well as to the health professionals, and they may be involved in facilitating lifelong learning for health professionals. However, it appears that intercultural mediators are underused and that some of their competences are never solicited by the health professionals (Verrept, 2008). The introduction of videoconferences decreased some of the barriers to the use of intercultural mediators, leading to a renewed interest among health care professionals in working with intercultural mediators.

Nierkens and colleagues assessed the impact of intercultural mediators on patient satisfaction, supporting the hypothesis that intercultural mediation has a positive impact on the therapeutic relationship. They also reported that the length of stay in the country did not decrease the need for intercultural mediation (Nierkens, Krumeich, di Ridder, & Van Dongen, 2002).

Intercultural mediators are key actors in supporting the integration of immigrants within the health care system and in the rest of society. If they have the opportunity to exert their role as patient educators, intercultural mediators may help patients to better understand how the health system, the social security system, and the municipality function. However, efforts should be made to increase health professionals' knowledge of intercultural mediation. A survey in two Belgian hospitals highlighted that health professionals do not have enough knowledge about intercultural mediation. Indeed, although 80 percent of the respondents acknowledged the existence of the service in their hospital, only 76 percent had heard about the role of intercultural mediators. Only 22 percent reported knowing the names of the mediators but, in reality, only 8 percent reported the correct names of the mediators (Dauvrin & Lorant, 2014b).

Although these two initiatives aim at different objectives, they both illustrate the gap between positive goals and existing practices. Indeed, in these two situations, health professionals seem to lack information about how to use the service or the procedure. Sensitivity education of health professionals and other service providers such as social workers regarding migration and health is still lacking in the attempt to achieve equity in the social security system.

Conclusion

There is an overall reluctance to implement "cultural competence" or "diversity sensitivity," but the municipal level commits itself to reducing health inequities. Indeed, although there is no clear picture of existing actions at the local level, health professionals have proven and are still proving their competence in meeting specific needs of immigrants. Local centres of integration organize activities for immigrants and professionals, some health services involve patients in the design of services or in establishing priorities in health activities, and there is increasing political participation. Recent empirical findings show that leaders are likely to make a difference at the service level, supporting the need of having "champions" in cultural competence (Dauvrin & Lorant, 2015). This is likely to help respond to the overall lack of current leadership and of attention to the voice of immigrants in the health care system. Further efforts should be made to integrate not only the immigrants but all patients in the health system as partners rather than as clients.

The recent trends of moving from intercultural care to equity care seem to be more appropriate to the Belgian context. Indeed, while intercultural care and immigration are likely to raise tensions at political and societal levels, equity care encompasses a broader perspective that integrates the intersectionality of different factors of vulnerability. As we have seen in Belgium, socio-economic status, age, life course trajectories, gender, and other political contexts are strong determinants of health status and the access and quality of health care for migrant populations.

Critical Thinking Questions

1. What are the factors contributing to the health status of immigrants in Belgium?
2. What are the main barriers to implementing immigrant health policies in Belgium?
3. How can health policies include the intersectionality of risks in order to improve health of immigrants?
4. How can health policies improve the health of immigrants in the absence of accurate data?
5. Which factors could prevent the implementation of these policies and legislation?

Glossary

Bismarckian model is one model of funding and delivering health care (and, in Belgium, other social allocations). The entitlement is based on the recipient's contribution status and the funding is based on wages for both employees and employers. The model covers defined benefits with an explicit rationing and implies reimbursement for patients (in Belgium) (Dixon, 2013).

Equity aims to reduce differences in opportunity for different population groups when these differences are systematic, socially produced, and unfair (Whitehead & Dahlgren, 2006).

Governance "is the process by which an organization safeguards the interests of its stakeholders and delivers its objectives through a monitored framework of rules and procedures" (Pearson, 2013, p. 502).

Public Centre of Social Action is the municipal public service in charge of social action at the local level. A PCSA's main purpose is to deliver social services and promote individual well-being. Although the services provided by each PCSA vary from one municipality to another, the following services are likely to be organized: financial assistance, housing, medical assistance, home care, employment support, psychosocial aid, debts mediation, legal assistance, and culture vouchers to support cultural and social participation.

Regularization is an exceptional procedure that grants legal status to undocumented migrants. From time to time, under specific circumstances, the federal state may organize exceptional regularization for undocumented migrants. This could be considered a form of amnesty: people who do not comply at this time with the conditions for being recognized as refugees are allowed to apply for legal status of residency based on their length of stay in Belgium or present proof of their integration (e.g., having children regularly attending school).

Social security system provides access to and coverage for health care, and allocations for retirement, unemployment, disability, incapacity, and family support. Funding is obtained through compulsory social taxes. Allocation of resources to the different functions of social security is made by consensus between social partners (mostly unions) and representatives of the employers.

Recommended Readings

Dauvrin, M., Derluyn, I., Coune, I., Verrept, H., & Lorant, V. (2012). Towards fair health policies for migrants and ethnic minorities: The case-study of ETHEALTH in Belgium. *BMC Public Health, 12*(726).

This open-access publication presents the process and the outcomes of the ETHEALTH group, which provides recommendations in order to improve equity in health.

Gerkens, S., & Merkur, S. (2010). Belgium: Health system review. *Health Systems in Transition, 12*(5), 1–266, xxv.

The Belgian health care system is complex; this extensive review presents different facets of the health care system and will help the reader to understand the challenges in providing health care to a diverse and aging population.

Ingleby, D., Krasnik, A., Lorant, V., & Razum, O. (Eds.). (2012). *Health inequalities and risk factors among migrants and ethnic minorities* (Vol. 1). Antwerpen-Apeldoorn: Garant.

This book reviews the complex interaction between social determinants of health and ethnicity, and provides an overview of the situation in Europe.

Lorant, V., & Bhopal, R. (2010). Comparing policies to tackle ethnic inequalities in health: Belgium 1 Scotland 4. *European Journal of Public Health, 21*(2), 235–240.
By comparing Scotland and Belgium, Lorant and Bhopal highlight the challenges encountered by two European countries when tackling ethnic inequalities. It is an interesting exercise that reviews several aspects of health policies.

Tilly, C. (1998). *Durable inequality*. Berkeley: University of California Press.
In his theory of durable inequality, Charles Tilly explains why ethnic and socio-economic inequalities are co-constructed and sustained over time in societies.

Related Websites

EUGATE Best Practice in Health Services for Immigrants in Europe—www.eugate.org.uk/
This website reports the results and recommendations of the EUGATE project for several European countries.

Federal Migration Center/Interfederal Center for Equal Opportunities—www.diversity belgium.be
These centres are both consultative organs that provide documentation, resources, and legislations regarding discrimination and equal opportunities. Claims can be introduced through the website.

MedImmigrant—www.medimmigrant.be
This NGO provides all information regarding entitlement and access to health care for migrants (all categories of legal and irregular migrants).

MigHealthNet—www.mighealth.net
This Wikipedia-like website contains information regarding health, access to health care, and other topics for various European countries, including Belgium.

Ministry of Public Health—www.health.belgium.be
The official website of the Ministry of Public Health in Belgium, this site has information regarding intercultural mediation, patient rights, and links to other useful resources.

Notes

1. There is some ambiguity in the use of the term "Belgian." In the national health interview survey, Belgians are those whose household members were born in Belgium and whose parents are Belgian. In some studies, one can be defined as Belgian of migrant background if one was born in another country of non-Belgian parents yet has been naturalized as a Belgian citizen. In other studies differences

will only be based on nationality *stricto sensu* where one's background is Belgian French, Flemish, or Belgian German.

2. Loi générale du 10 mai 2007 tendant à remplacer certaines formes de discrimination, remplaçant la loi du 25 février 2003 [General law of May 10, 2007, aiming at replacing some forms of discrimination, replacing the law of February 25, 2003]; Loi du 10 mai 2007 tendant à lutter contre les discriminations entre les hommes et les femmes qui remplace la loi du 7 mai 1999 sur l'égalité de traitement entre les hommes et les femmes [Law of May 10, 2007, aiming at fighting against discrimination between men and women, replacing the law of May 7, 1999, on equal treatment between men and women]; Loi du 30 juillet 1981 tendant à réprimer certains actes inspirés par le racisme et la xénophobie [Law of July 30, 1981, aiming at reducing racism and xenophobia].

References

Adam, I., Rea, A., Coene, G., Crosby, A., Hamdoui, S., Teney, C., & Giladi, M. (2010). *La diversité culturelle sur le lieu de travail. Pratiques d'aménagements raisonnables* (pp. 151). Brussels: Centre pour l'Egalité des Chances et la Lutte contre le Racisme.

Agentschap voor Binnenlands Bestuur. (2014). *Wat is inburgering?* Retrieved from http://www.inburgering.be

Anson, O. (2001). Inequality in the access to preventive health care: The case of immigrants in Belgium. *Archives of Public Health, 59*, 265–279.

Assises de l'Interculturalité. (2010). *Rapport final.* Brussels: Assises de l'Interculturalité,.

Belgian Government. (2014). Website of the Belgian government. Retrieved from http://www.belgium.be

Belgian Red Cross. (2014). *Reception centres for asylum-seekers.* Retrieved from http://www.croix-rouge.be/activites/solidarite/asile-et-migration/les-centres-de28099accueil/

Casman, M. (2008). *Rapport d'observation des pratiques des Centres Publics d'Action Sociale en matière de carte médicale.* Liège, Belgium: Université de Liège.

Centre Interfédéral pour l'Egalité des Chances et la Lutte contre le Racisme et les Discriminations. (2014). *Discrimination-diversité: pour un plan d'action interfédéral contre le racisme. Rapport annuel 2013* (p. 187). Brussels: Centre Interfédéral pour l'Egalité des Chances et la Lutte contre le Racisme et les Discriminations.

CLANDESTINO. (2009). *Undocumented migration: Counting the uncountable. Data and trends across Europe. Final report.* Brussels: European Commission.

Croix Rouge de Belgique. (2005). Projet 2004. Evaluation du projet. Assistance psychosociale et thérapeutique des demandeurs d'asile (p. 90). Brussels: Croix Rouge de Belgique,.

Dauvrin, M. (2012). L'accès aux soins pour les migrants en Belgique. *Revue de Droit Sanitaire et Social, S1*(HS2012), 75–85.

Dauvrin, M. (2013). *Cultural competence in health care: Challenging inequalities, involving institutions.* (Dissertation, Institute of Health and Society, Université catholique de Louvain, Brussels.)

Dauvrin, M., Derluyn, I., Coune, I., Verrept, H., & Lorant, V. (2012). Towards fair health policies for migrants and ethnic minorities: The case-study of ETHEALTH in Belgium. *BMC Public Health, 12*, 726.

Dauvrin, M., Geerts, C., & Lorant, V. (2010). Santé des migrants et bonnes pratiques. Résultats belges du projet EUGATE. *Santé conjuguée, 51*, 19–25.

Dauvrin, M., & Lorant, V. (2010). Bonnes Pratiques dans les Services de Santé pour les Immigrants en Europe: résultats belges du projet EUGATE. Translated by the Institute of Health and Society. *EUGATE project.* Brussels: Université catholique de Louvain.

Dauvrin, M., & Lorant, V. (2014a). Adaptation of health care for migrants: Whose responsibility? *BMC Health Services Research, 14*(1), 294.

Dauvrin, M., & Lorant, V. (2014b). COMETH Compétences en Ethnicité et Santé. Rapport de recherche (pp. 1–76). Brussels: Institut de recherche Santé et Société, Université catholique de Louvain.

Dauvrin, M., & Lorant, V. (2015). Leadership and cultural competence of healthcare professionals: A social network analysis. *Nursing Research, 64*(3), 200–210.

Dauvrin, M., Lorant, V., Sandhu, S., Deville, W., Dia, H., Dias, S., ... Priebe, S. (2012). Health care for irregular migrants: Pragmatism across Europe: A qualitative study. *BMC Research Notes, 5*, 99.

De Grande, H., Vandenheede, H., Gadeyne, S., & Deboosere, P. (2014). Health status and mortality rates of adolescents and young adults in the Brussels-capital region: Differences according to region of origin and migration history. *Ethnicity and Health, 19*(2), 122–143.

De Maesschalck, S. (2012). *Linguistic and cultural diversity in the consultation room: A tango between physicians and their ethnic minority patients.* (Doctor in Medical Sciences thesis, Ghent University, Ghent, Belgium.)

Deboosere, P., & Gadeyne, S. (2005). Adult migrant mortality advantage in Belgium: Evidence using census and register data. *Population, 60*(5–6), 655–698.

DeKeyser, T., Delhez, P., & Zimmer, H. (2012). L'insertion des personnes étrangères sur le marché du travail. *Revue Economique*, December, 25–44.

Demarest, S., Gisle, L., Hesse, E., Miermans, P., Tafforeau, J., & Van der Heyden, J. (2006). *Enquête de Santé par Interview Belgique 2004*. Brussels: Institut Scientifique de Santé Publique.

Derluyn, I., Broekaert, E., & Schuyten, G. (2008). Emotional and behavioural problems in migrant adolescents in Belgium. *European Child and Adult Psychiatry*, 17(1), 54–62.

Derluyn, I., Lorant, V., Dauvrin, M., Coune, I., & Verrept, H. (2011a). Gelijwaardige gezondheid voor migranten en ethnisch-culturele minderheden. In D. Dierckx, J. Vranken, J. Coene, & A. Van Haarlem (Eds.), *Armoede en sociale uitsluiting. Jaarboek* 2011. Leuven, Belgium: Acco.

Derluyn, I., Lorant, V., Dauvrin, M., Coune, I., & Verrept, H. (2011b). *Naar een interculturelegezondheidszorg:* Aanbevelingen van de ETHEALTH-groep voor een gelijkwaardige gezondheid en gezondheidszorg voor migranten en etnische minderheden. Brussels: FOD Volksgezondheid.

Deville, W., Greacen, T., Bogic, M., Dauvrin, M., Dias, S., Gaddini, A., ... Priebe, S. (2011). Health care for immigrants in Europe: Is there still consensus among country experts about principles of good practice? A Delphi study. *BMC Public Health, 11*, 699.

Dixon, A. (2013). Funding and delivering health care. In C. Guest, W. Ricciardi, I. Kawachi, & I. Lang (Eds.), *Oxford handbook of public health practice* (3rd ed., pp. 346–355). Oxford: Oxford University Press.

Dogniez, E., & Post, B. (2003). *Evaluation de l'assistance psychosociale et thérapeutique auprès des demandeurs d'asile. Enquête menée auprès des structures d'accueil et des services de soins en santé mentale présentes en province de Liège et du Luxembourg.* (p. 160). Brussels: Croix-Rouge de Belgique.

European Commission. (2012). *National Roma integration strategy.* Brussels: European Commission.

FEDASIL. (2012). *Rapport annuel 2011* (pp. 1–48). Brussels: FEDASIL.

FEDASIL. (2014). *Agence fédérale pour l'accueil des demandeurs d'asile/Federaal agentschap voor het opvang van azielzoekers.* Retrieved from http://www.fedasil.be

Federal Migration Center/Interfederal Center for Equal Opportunities. (2015). Retrieved from http://www.diversitybelgium.be

Flemish Lung and Tuberculosis Association. (2014). *Vlaamse Vereniging voor Respiratoire Gezondheidszorg en Tuberculosebestrijdding vzw.* Retrieved from http://www.vrgt.be

Fossion, P., Ledoux, Y., Valente, F., Servais, L., Staner, L., Pelc, I., & Minner, P. (2002). Psychiatric disorders and social characteristics among second-generation Moroccan migrants in Belgium: An age-and gender-controlled study conducted in a psychiatric emergency department. *European Psychiatry, 17*(8), 443–450.

Fossion, P., Servais, L., Rejas, M., Ledoux, Y., Pelc, I., & Minner, P. (2004). Psychosis, migration, and social environment: An age-and-gender controlled study. *European Psychiatry, 19*(6), 338–343.

Fonds des Affections Respiratoires/Vlaamse Vereniging voor Respiratoire Gezondheigszorg en Tuberculosebestrijding (FARES/VRGT). (2013). In FARES/VRGT (Ed.), *Registre belge de la tuberculose 2011.* Brussels: Author.

Fonds des Affections Respiratoires/Vlaamse Vereniging voor Respiratoire Gezondheigszorg en Tuberculosebestrijding. (2014). *Fonds des Affections Respiratoires et de l'Education pour la Santé FARES.* Retrieved from http://www.fares.be.

Gerkens, S., & Merkur, S. (2010). Belgium: Health system review. *Health Systems in Transition, 12*(5), 1–266.

Gouvernement Wallon. (2014, July 2). *Le parcours d'intégration des primo-arrivants adopté par le Gouvernement wallon.* Retrieved from http://gouvernement.wallonie.be/le-parcours-d-int-gration-des-primo-arrivants-adopt-par-le-gouvernement-wallon

Haelterman, E., De Spiegelaere, M., & Masuy-Stroobant, G. (2007). *Les indicateurs de santé périnatale en région de Bruxelles-Capitale: 1998–2004.* Brussels: Observatoire de la santé et du social.

Hamzaoui, M., & Krzeslo, E. (2007). Intervention directe sur l'emploi en région Bruxelles-Capitale: Le cas des primo-arrivants de nationalité ou d'origine étrangère. In *Projet FSE*

Insertion socio-professionnelle des primo-arrivants (Vol. 4, pp. 1–65). Brussels: Centre de Sociologie du Travail de l'Emploi et de la Formation-Université Libre de Bruxelles.

Hanquinet, L., Vandezande, V., Jacobs, D., & Swyngedouw, M. (2006). Preparatory study for survey and quantitative research on ethnic minority groups in Belgium (pp. 1–79). Prepared for the Ulens Project in association with the Fondation Roi Baudouin- Koning Boudewijn Stichting. Brussels: ISPO- K.U. Leuven & GERME- ULB.

Jacobs, D., & Réa, A. (2005). Construction et importation des classements ethniques. Allochtones et immigrés aux Pays-Bas et en Belgique. *Revue européenne des migrations internationales, 21*(2), 35–59.

Jacobs, D., & Réa, A. (2012). "Allochthones" in the Netherlands and Belgium. *International Migration, 50*(6), 42–57.

Keygnaert, I., Vettenburg, N., Roelens, K., & Temmerman, M. (2014). Sexual health is dead in my body: Participatory assessment of sexual health determinants by refugees, asylum seekers, and undocumented migrants in Belgium and The Netherlands. *BMC Public Health, 14*, 416.

Keygnaert, I., Vettenburg, N., & Temmerman, M. (2012). Hidden violence is silent rape: Sexual and gender-based violence in refugees, asylum seekers, and undocumented migrants in Belgium and the Netherlands. *Culture, Health and Sexuality, 14*(5), 505–520.

Levecque, K., Lodewyckx, I., & Bracke, P. (2008). Psychological distress, depression, and generalised anxiety in Turkish and Moroccan immigrants in Belgium. A general population study. *Social Psychiatry and Psychiatric Epidemiology 44*(3), 431–441.

Levecque, K., Lodewyckx, I., & Vranken, J. (2007). Depression and generalised anxiety in the general population in Belgium: A comparison between native and immigrant groups. *Journal of Affective Disorders, 97*(1–3), 229–239.

Lodewyckx, I., Timmerman, C., & Wets, J. (2011). *Le regroupement familial en Belgique: les chiffres derrière le mythe.* Brussels: Fondation Roi Baudouin.

Lorant, V., & Bhopal, R. (2010). Comparing policies to tackle ethnic inequalities in health: Belgium 1 Scotland 4. *European Journal of Public Health, 21*(2), 235–240.

Lorant, V., & Bhopal, R. S. (2011). Ethnicity, socio-economic status, and health research: Insights from and implications of Charles Tilly's theory of durable inequality. *Journal of Epidemiology and Community Health, 65*(8), 671–675.

Lorant, V., & Dauvrin, M. (2012). Ethnicity and socioeconomic status as determinants of health. In D. Ingleby, A. Krasnik, V. Lorant, & O. Razum (Eds.), *Health inequalities and risk factors among migrants and ethnic minorities* (Vol. 1, pp. 69–78). Antwerpen-Apeldoorn: Garant.

Lorant, V., Derluyn, I., Dauvrin, M., Coune, I., & Verrept, H. (2011). *Vers des soins de santé interculturels: Recommandations du groupe ETHEALTH en faveur de la réduction des inégalités de santé parmi les migrants et minorités ethniques.* Bruxelles: SPF Santé Publique Environnement et Sécurité de la Chaine Alimentaire.

Lorant, V., Van Oyen, H., & Thomas, I. (2008). Contextual factors and immigrants' health status: Double jeopardy. *Health and Place, 14*(4), 678–692.

MedImmigrant. (2014). Retrieved from http://www.medimmigrant.be

Milquet, J. (2012). *Droit de vote des étrangers non belges aux élections municipales du 14 octobre 2012: deux mois encore pour s'inscrire.* Retrieved from http://www.elections.fgov.be/fileadmin/user_upload/Elections/20120531-Vote-des-etrangers-elections-communales.pdf

Ministry of Economy. (2011). *Population par nationalité, sexe, groupe et classe d'âges au 1er janvier 2008.* Retrieved from http://statbel.fgov.be/fr/statistiques/chiffres/population/structure/natact/index.jsp

Ministry of Public Health. (2011, February 2). *Cellule de Médiation Interculturelle.* Retrieved from http://www.health.belgium.be/eportal/Myhealth/PatientrightsandInterculturalm/Interculturalmediation/index.htm?fodnlang=fr#.Ugefxaz-Qtc

Morelli, A. (1992). *Histoire des étrangers et des émigrants en Belgique* (p. 331). Bruxelles: Editions Vie ouvrière.

Nierkens, V., Krumeich, A., di Ridder, R., & Van Dongen, M. (2002). The future of intercultural mediation in Belgium. *Patient Education and Counseling, 46*(4), 253–259.

Noirhomme-Renard, F., & Deccache, A. (2007). La sante physique, mentale et les comportements de sante des adolescents immigrants de premiere generation. *Archives de Pédiatrie, 14*(8), 1020–1027.

Observatoire Européen de l'Accès aux Soins des Médecins du Monde. (2007). *Enquête européenne sur l'accès aux soins des personnes en situation irrégulière.* Brussels: Médecins du Monde.

OECD. (2013). *Programme for International Student Assessment PISA. Results 2012. Belgium* (p. 8). Paris: OECD.

Ouali, N., & Cennicola, P. (2013). Etude de la discrimination en Belgique et en Wallonie: analyse des positions sur le marché du travail selon le genre et la nationalité (pp. 1–152). Namur, Belgium: Institut wallon de l'évaluation de la prospective et de la statistique.

Pacolet, J., & Merckx, S. (2006). *Managed migration and the labour market: The health sector, the Belgian case.* Report prepared for the European Migration Network. Leuven, Belgium: Katholieke Universiteit Leuven.

Pearson, V. (2013). Governance and accountability. In C. Guest, W. Ricciardi, I. Kawachi, & I. Lang (Eds.), *Oxford handbook of public health practice* (3rd ed., pp. 502–511). Oxford: Oxford University Press.

Perrin, N. (2006). *L'évolution du nombre d'étrangers en Belgique* (pp. 1–15). Louvain-la-Neuve, Belgium: UCL-Groupe de démographie appliquée.

Priebe, S., Bogic, M., Adany, R., Bjerre, N. V., Dauvrin, M., Deville, W., ... McCabe, R. (2013). Good practice in emergency care: Views from practitioners. In B. Rechel, P. Mladovsky, W. Deville, B. Rijks, R. Petro-Benedict, & M. McKee (Eds.), *Migration and health in the European Union* (pp. 213–226). Maidenhead, Berkshire: Open University Press McGraw-Hill Education.

Réa, A., & Martiniello, M. (2012). *Une brève histoire de l'immigration en Belgique* (p. 68). Brussels: Fédération Wallonie-Bruxelles.

Ringelheim, J. (2010). Recueil de données, catégories ethniques et mesure de discrimination: un débat Européen. *Revue trimestrielle des Droits de l'Homme, 82*, 269–313.

Romero-Ortuño, R. (2004). Access to health care for illegal immigrants in the EU: Should we be concerned? *European Journal of Health Law, 11*(3), 245–272. doi: 10.1163/1571809042388572.

Sasse, A., Verbrugge, R., & Van Beckhoven, D. (2012). *Épidemiologie du SIDA et de l'infection à VIH en Belgique. Situation au 31 décembre 2011.* Brussels: Institut Scientifique de Santé Publique, Wetenschappeliijke Instituut Volksgezondheid.

Scheppers, E., van Dongen, E., Dekker, J., Geertzen, J., & Dekker, J. (2006). Potential barriers to the use of health services among ethnic minorities: A review. *Family practice, 23*(3), 325–348.

Scientific Institute of Public Health. (2015). *Déclaration des maladies transmissibles.* Retrieved from https://www.wiv-isp.be/matra/cf/connexion.aspx

TAHIB, T. H. I. i. B. (2010). *L'inégalité sociale en matière de santé reste tenace en Belgique.* Brussels: TAHIB.

Tilly, C. (1998). *Durable inequality.* Berkeley: University of California Press.

Van Den Wijngaert, M. (2011). *D'une Belgique Unitaire à une Belgique fédérale. 40 ans d'évolution politique des communautés et des régions (1971–2011).* Brussels: Vlaams Parlement/Academic Scientific Publisher.

Vandenheede, H., & Deboosere, P. (2009). Type 2 diabetes in Belgians of Turkish and Moroccan origin. *Archives of Public Health, 67*(2), 62–87.

Vandenheede, H., Deboosere, P., Gadeyne, S., & De Spiegelaere, M. (2012). The associations between nationality, fertility history, and diabetes-related mortality: A retrospective cohort study in the Brussels-Capital Region (2001–2005). *Journal of Public Health, 34*(1), 100–107.

Vandenheede, H., Lammens, L., Deboosere, P., Gadeyne, S., & De Spiegelaere, M. (2011). Ethnic differences in diabetes-related mortality in the Brussels-Capital Region (2001–05): The role of socioeconomic position. *International Journal of Public Health, 56*(5), 533–539.

Verrept, H. (2008). Intercultural mediation: An answer to health care disparities? In C. Valero-Garcés & A. Martin (Eds.), *Crossing borders in community interpreting: Definitions and dilemnas* (pp. 187–201). Amsterdam/Philadelphia: John Benjamins Publishing Company.

Vlaamse Overheid. (2014). *Inburgering.* Retrieved from http://www.inburgering.be/en

Wets, J., & de Bruyn, T. (2011). La migration: une solution aux pénuries de personnel dans le secteur des soins et de la santé? Brussels: King Baudouin Foundation.

Whitehead, M., & Dahlgren, G. (2006).*Concepts and principles for tackling social inequities in health: Levelling up Part 1.* Copenhagen: WHO Regional Office for Europe.

Legislation Cited

Chancellery of the Prime Minister, Justice FPS, Personnel & Organisation FPS, Federal Agency for the Reception of Asylum-Seekers. Arrêté royal fixant le statut organique du Centre fédéral pour l'analyse des flux migratoires, la protection des droits fondamentaux des étrangers et la lutte contre la traite des êtres humains en exécution de l'article 5 de la loi du 15 février 1993 créant un Centre fédéral pour l'analyse des flux migratoires, la protection des droits fondamentaux des étrangers et la lutte contre la traite des êtres humains [Royal Decree establishing the organic status of the Federal Center for the analysis of the migration flows, the protection of fundamental rights of the foreigners and the fight against human trafficking, executing the article 5 of the law of February 15, 1993, creating a Federal Centre for the analysis of the migration flows, the protection of fundamental rights of the foreigners, and the fight against human trafficking] (2014).

Communauté Francaise de Belgique. (2015). *Circulaire sur le parcours d'accueil des primo-arrivants.* Décret du 27 mars 2014 remplaçant le Livre II du Code wallon de l'Action sociale et de la Santé, relatif à l'intégration des personnes étrangères et d'origine étrangère. —Titre III : Parcours d'accueil 2015027035 C.F.R. Bruxelles: Author.

Council of the European Union. (2003). Council Directive 2003/86/EC of 22 September 2003 on the right to family reunification. *Official Journal of the European Union*, L251, 12–18.

Home Affairs FPS. Arrêté royal du 12 décembre 1996 relatif à l'aide médicale urgente octroyée par les centres publics d'aide sociale aux étrangers qui séjournent illégalement dans le Royaume [Royal Decree of December 12, 1996, related to urgent medical aid delivered by the public centres of social aid to foreigners residing illegally on the territory] (1996).

Home Affairs FPS. Arrêté royal du 13 janvier 2003 modifiant l'arrêté royal du 12 décembre 1996 relatif à l'aide médicale urgente octroyée par les centres publics d'aide sociale aux étrangers qui séjournent illégalement dans le Royaume [Royal Decree of January 13, 2003, modifying the Royal Decree of December 12, 1996, related to urgent medical aid delivered by the public centres of social aid to foreigners residing illegally on the territory] (2003).

Home Affairs FPS. Loi du 15 décembre 1980 sur l'accès au territoire, le séjour, l'établissement et l'éloignement des étrangers [Law of December 15, 1980, on access to territory, short-term and long-term residency, and deportation of foreigners] (1980).

Home Affairs. Loi du 6 juillet 1983 concernant l'obligation scolaire [Law of July 6, 1983, related to school obligation] (1983).

Ministry of the Flemish Community. Decreet betreffende het onderwijs XVI. [Decree related to school system XVI] (2006).

Ministry of the French Community. Décret du 20 décembre 2001 relatif à la promotion de la santé à l'école [Decree of December 20, 2001, related to health promotion at school] (2001).

Ministry of Justice. Code de la Nationalité Belge [Code of the Belgian Nationality], 1984-06-28/35 C.F.R. (1984).

Ministry of Public Health and Social Affairs. Loi du 22 aout 2002 relative aux droits du patient [Law of August 22, 2002, related to patient rights] (2002).

Social Integration, Fight against Poverty and Social Economy PPS. Loi organique des Centres publics d'aide sociale du 8 juillet 1976 [Law of Public Centres of Social Aid of July 8, 1976] (1976).

Social Integration, Fight against Poverty and Social Economy PPS. Loi du 12 janvier 2007 sur l'accueil des demandeurs d'asile et de certaines autres catégories d'étrangers [Law of January 12, 2007, related to the reception of asylum-seekers and other categories of foreigners] (2007).

Public Policy, Immigrant Experiences, and Health Outcomes in Germany[1]

Gudrun Hentges and Heinrich Bollinger

Chapter Objectives

This chapter focuses on the immigration and integration of immigrants into German society. The objectives of this chapter are:

- to realize that migrants as a group are highly heterogeneous and to examine their heterogeneity—with a special focus on the differentiation between so-called ethnic Germans and immigrants without German citizenship;
- to explore the access of different categories of immigrants to the health care system in Germany;
- to review the evidence concerning health outcomes among immigrants in Germany; and
- to analyze the interrelationship between public policy, integration, and health outcomes of immigrants in Germany.

Introduction

Health and migration is a subject area that combines a variety of dimensions and aspects. Migration comprises processes of immigration and emigration, transnational migration, shuttle migration, and also social integration into host societies and the participation of migrants in social life. Dealing with questions of migration also requires a clear definition of terms. In the German debate, which groups of people are called migrants, immigrants, people of migrant background, people with migrant experience, or foreigners? Which status of residence do these respective social groups have?

When focusing on health with respect to migration, it is important to differentiate between the health status of immigrants, their subjective state of health, access to the health care system, outpatient and inpatient health care, and prevention of disease among immigrants. One question to be answered is whether immigrants are equally affected by the widespread diseases—heart and circulatory system diseases, diabetes, cancer—as the majority population, or whether there are differences. Regarding the morbidity of immigrants, studies investigate maternal and infant mortality, suicides, and deaths as a result of drug abuse and infections. Further studies deal with the immigrants' lifestyle with respect to nutrition and exercise, as well as with the consumption of addictive substances such as nicotine and alcohol. However, besides these questions, which essentially concern the total population as much as the minorities, the specific health issues of migrants also play a role. Those are, above all, post-traumatic stress disorders (PTSD) as a result of political persecution, torture and flight, the health status at the moment of immigration, and the life situation of immigrants who are without legal resident status or asylum-seekers under the asylum-seekers benefit act and tolerated refugees. Not least, it is important to identify the specific current health care policy projects and to see how much these projects manage to improve the health status of migrants and decrease barriers to the health care system.

This article further examines immigration and health based on the situation in Germany. This chapter cannot claim to present and assess the wide spectrum of individual studies; rather, it traces the megatrends and gives insight into the health policy and migration policy debates in Germany.

Statistical Questions

People of Migration Background

For many years—since the establishment of the Federal Republic of Germany—the concept of the "foreigner" was the essential social-structural category in questions of interior policy and security as well as in the context of migration and integration policy. The term "foreigner" was and still is clearly defined: A person who lives in the territory of the Federal Republic who does not have a German passport but is a foreign citizen. People who have neither German nor foreign citizenship are regarded as "stateless."[2]

Foreign citizens do not enjoy civic rights (freedom of assembly, freedom of association, freedom of movement, freedom to choose an occupation). The Residence Act lists the circumstances that may lead to the expulsion of foreigners who live on the Federal territory (Act on the Residence, Economic Activity and Integration of Foreigners in the Federal Territory, sections 53–55). People of foreign citizenship are thus considered—implicitly or explicitly—as a risk to the internal security of the Federal Republic of Germany.

Since the beginning of the 1990s—as a result of the collapse of the Soviet Union—Germany experienced an influx of so-called *Russlanddeutsche* (Russian Germans) from the states of the former Soviet Union. As "status Germans" (i.e., people with the legal status of Germans), these late repatriates were naturalized speedily and thus acquired unlimited civic rights. As German citizens, they blended into the general population; it was therefore difficult for many years to examine more closely the effects of immigration and integration with respect to these late repatriates.

When the new citizenship law was reformed in 2000, the children of foreign parents born in Germany not only acquired the citizenship of their parents but were also entitled to a German passport. Hence the territoriality principle (*jus soli*) became part of German citizenship law, where the principle of descent (*jus sanguinis*), stemming from the German empire, had been in force unaltered since 1913. Yet the dual citizenship of children and adolescents was considered only temporary. By the age of 23 the law required young people to choose between the two citizenships, as they could keep only one passport as adults.[3] In 2013, the new governing coalition—a so-called grand coalition consisting of Christian Democrats and Social Democrats—decided in their coalition agreement to abolish this compulsory choice. The draft bill submitted by the federal government was debated and passed in Parliament on July 3, 2014. Thus the legal obligation to choose between citizenships no longer applies to children of foreign parents who were born and raised in Germany; this group of young adults is allowed dual citizenship.

The increase in naturalization of formerly foreign citizens gave rise to the passing of the Micro-Census Act. In accordance with the Act, the statistical census of 2005 contained the category of "people of migrant background" for the first time. Since then, statistics not only recorded whether or not a person had a German passport, but also recorded the citizenship of parents and grandparents, the time of arrival in the host country, etc., so migration background became part of the statistics.[4]

According to the definition of the Federal Statistical Office, people of migrant background are "all those who have immigrated into today's territory of the Federal Republic of Germany as well as all foreigners born in Germany and all Germans born in Germany with at least one parent who is an immigrant or a foreigner born in Germany" (Statistisches Bundesamt, quoted from: Bayerisches Landesamt für Gesundheit und Lebensmittelsicherheit, 2011, p. 7; authors' translation).

In 2012, 80.8 million people lived in Germany—with or without a German passport, of whom 16.3 percent had a **migration background**. Almost 11 million people of migration background immigrated after 1949; another 5.4 million people were born in Germany. Thus, every fifth German resident (20 percent) has a migration background, and 7.6 percent of the migrants living in Germany have only a foreign passport (Website of the Federal Ministry of the Interior, May 15, 2015).

In some of the Federal states more than a quarter of the population has a migration background, for example, in Hamburg (27.5 percent), Baden Württemberg (25.2. percent), and Bremen (25.1 percent), whereas the percentage of people with a migration background is below 4.5 percent in the eastern German states.

More than two-thirds of all people of migration background originate from European countries: 37.7 percent of all people of migration background come from EU member states and another 36 percent from other European states. Almost 18 percent of all people of migration background are Turkish.

Foreigners or Foreign Citizens

Foreign citizens[5] belong to the group of people of migration background. At the end of March 2014, about 7.7 million foreigners lived in Germany. The Central Register of Foreigners, which records "foreigners according to the most frequent nationalities," states that people of Turkish nationality are the biggest group among foreigners (about 20 percent), followed by foreigners born in Germany of Polish (8.1. percent), Italian (7.2 percent), Greek (4.1 percent), Romanian (3.7 percent), Croatian (3.2 percent), and Russian (2.8 percent) nationality, and foreign nationals from other states (50.9 percent) (Bundesministerium für Familie, Senioren, Frauen und Jugend, 2007, p. 25).

It is also worth mentioning that about a third of the Turks and Italians living in Germany were also born in Germany, and one in five Greeks living in Germany (23.4 percent) was born in the Federal territory (Bundesamt für Migration und Flüchtlinge, 2014, p. 105).

In the context of migration and health, the length of stay in Germany is also relevant. Among the Turkish nationals, the majority have lived in Germany for 30 years or more. Over 35 percent of all Turks living in Germany have lived there for more than 30 years. Among the Poles living in Germany, the largest group has lived there for six to eight years (around 17 percent). As for Italians, the largest group has lived in Germany for 30 years or more (around 14 percent).

The average age of the population groups varies depending on the status of migration. People without migration background currently have an average age of almost 45 years, foreigners are 36 years old on average, Germans of migration background have an average age of 29, and non-naturalized migrants are 39 years old on average (Bundesministerium für Familie, Senioren, Frauen und Jugend, 2007, p. 25). Clearly, Germans of migration background constitute the youngest age group. Here, the effects of the citizenship reform of January 1, 2000, become apparent. Also, the group of foreign nationals living in Germany is nine years younger on average than the group of people without migration background.

There are no statistical data on immigrants without valid documents. Depending on the terminology, they are called "sans papiers," "undocumented," "illegalized," or "illegal residents from third countries" (Sinn et al., 2006, pp. 1–13; Straubhaar, 2007).

In May 2006, the Joint Analysis and Strategy Centre Illegal Migration (GASIM), based at the Federal Police Headquarters in Potsdam, was set up to deal with illegal immigration and residence. Obviously, the number of those "sans papiers" can only be estimated. The figures vary between 500,000 and 1 million people staying in Germany without valid documents (Bundesministerium des Innern, 2007, p. 16). The Süddeutsche Zeitung, for instance, reported hundreds of thousands of people living illegally in Germany (Gräf, 2014), and the weekly magazine *Der Spiegel* estimates the number of the so-called illegal at 1 million (Götsch, 2005).

Access to the Health Care System

This section provides both an overview of the different kinds of immigrants living in Germany and describes their access to health care. Not every person living in Germany has health insurance coverage. The Ethics Commission of the German Medical Association estimates that between 200,000 and 600,000 people are without health insurance in Germany—that is, those who have gone underground to avoid deportation, asylum-seekers who have been denied asylum, stateless people, or people without a secured status of residence (Berger & Conrad, 2013).

The law requires that doctors in Germany treat emergency patients—even if they have no health insurance. The costs of the treatment can then be reimbursed by the social services offices. In reality, however, it is more complicated. Numerous immigrants report being turned away by doctors—even when they were in acute pain and needed emergency treatment. Moreover, many patients without papers avoid visiting a doctor. They fear that doctors or medical staff might transfer their data to the authorities and that this might lead to their deportation.[6] By now, there are medical networks in many big German cities that nevertheless treat uninsured patients who do not have residence status. The so-called Medinetze are NGOs that were initiated by voluntary members and have been operating in about 34 cities since 1994.

The charity Malteser Hilfsdienst has been involved since 2001, when the organization Malteser Migranten Medizin (MMM) was founded for uninsured "people without a secured residence status," (Malteser Migranten Medizin, 2016) but also for citizens from the new EU member states Romania (2007), Bulgaria (2007), and Croatia (2013). Now Malteser Migranten Medizin has contacts and branch offices in 13 German cities.

In September 2014, the Federal government submitted a statement to the health committee of the German Bundestag. It reported approximately 80,000 people without health insurance in Germany. This group comprises people who have been unable to pay their contributions to private health insurers or statutory health insurance funds; they are therefore in default with the insurer and excluded from coverage. The uninsured are mostly indebted self-employed people or basic security-benefit recipients—that is, those who receive unemployment benefits. The government statement does not specify, however, the percentage of foreign nationals or migrants among the non-health insured.

There is no overall answer to the question of immigrants and their access to the health care system. Conditions depend on the country of origin and the employment status of the particular groups of people, as well as on the duration of stay (Szent-Ivanyi, 2014; Deutsches Rotes Kreuz, 2013).

Foreign Employees and the German Health Care System

This section describes the different kinds of immigrants in Germany and their access to health care. Foreign employees have compulsory health insurance if they engage in legal employment subject to social security contributions. EU citizens with an EU work permit are members of a statutory health insurance fund, like other employees. The EU work permit is issued by the Employment Agency (Deutsches Rotes Kreuz, 2013, p. 7; Frings, 2012). The situation is more complicated for foreign nationals who are not engaged in gainful or legal employment.

Unemployed EU Citizens

EU citizens who are not gainfully employed (e.g., tourists, students) and are temporarily living in Germany are entitled to free medical treatment, covered by the European Health Insurance Card. Such medical treatment is, however, limited to cases of emergency.

For an extended stay in Germany, the health insurance funds recommend that EU citizens apply for a special form, the European Document S1. In combination with the European Health Insurance Card, it gives access to the standard services in Germany.

EU citizens who have registered as unemployed may join a health insurance fund as well. Since the introduction of labour mobility within the EU (May 2011), EU citizens from the new member states (Estonia, Latvia, Lithuania, Slovakia, Slovenia, Czech Republic, and Hungary) may also register as unemployed.

Romanians and Bulgarians were granted unlimited labour mobility on January 1, 2014. Hence, Romanian and Bulgarian citizens may register as unemployed or seeking work; they may engage in gainful employment and apply, if necessary, for unemployment benefit II (German basic security benefit). As social security recipients they have health insurance coverage. The percentage of uninsured people was particularly high among Romanians and Bulgarians before unlimited labour mobility came into force (Loerzer, 2012).

Furthermore, since 2007 Book V of the Social Code has required compulsory health insurance. Compulsory health insurance applies to "persons with no other claim to coverage in the event of illness and a) those who were previously statutorily health insured or b) have so far not been statutorily or privately health insured" (Section 5, Subsection 1, Number 13).

Unemployed People from Third Countries

The situation is far more difficult for foreign citizens from non-EU states who are not gainfully employed. In exceptional cases, the health insurance funds will give coverage to certain people after a stay of one year. Yet most third-country nationals need to take out private health insurance to obtain coverage (Cf. Website: Krankenkassen. Deutschland, June, 2016).

Asylum-Seekers and the Health Care System

Specific legislation applies to migrants who are asylum-seekers, tolerated refugees, or foreigners who have been ordered to leave the country, i.e., the **Asylum-Seekers' Benefits Act (AsylbLG)**, which has been in force since 1993. With regard to "benefits in case of illness, pregnancy and birth" (Section 4), the Act limits medical treatment to instances of "acute illness and pain" and grants medical help to "pregnant women and women who have recently given birth." This limitation of medical treatment is highly controversial and has often been criticized. From the medical perspective, the legal distinction between acute and non-acute illness and pain is problematic as there are transitional stages that make it difficult to distinguish between the two. This compulsory differentiation, moreover, allows for a variety of possible interpretations; added to that, decisions on whether to offer medical treatment or not are made by administrators in social services offices—not by doctors (Knipper & Bilgin, 2009, p. 69). In view of this, asylum-seekers cannot be said to have regular access to the health care system; they are entitled only to emergency treatment.

The same is true for tolerated refugees. To date, about 86,000 tolerated refugees live in Germany, mostly people who have fled from the former Yugoslavia, Iraq, and Turkey. Another 33,000 people have been ordered to leave the country (UNHCR, 2006; Hentges & Staszczak, 2010, p. 38ff).

Heterogeneity and Recent Immigration Patterns

It should be evident by now that migrants are very heterogeneous; they can be subdivided into the following groups:

- guest workers of the first generation who immigrated during the phase of active foreign worker recruitment

- spouses, children, and now also grandchildren of this first guest worker generation from Turkey, Southern Europe, Southeastern Europe, and Northern Africa
- (late) repatriates and their families from the former Soviet Union, Romania, and Poland
- Jewish quota refugees, also from the former Soviet Union
- civil war refugees from the former Yugoslavian states
- refugees from the crisis regions in Africa and Asia
- EU citizens from the western and southwestern member states
- EU citizens from the Baltic states and the Eastern and Central European states that joined the EU in 2004
- EU citizens from Romania and Bulgaria, which joined in 2007
- EU citizens from Croatia, the twenty-eighth member state (2013)
- people coming to Germany to study at a university
- highly qualified professionals or people with a "shortage occupation" who are employed in Germany on the basis of the Immigration Act (2005) or who have a Blue Card (2007)

Given such a variety, it is quite difficult to make precise and general statements about all immigrants or foreigners. Meaningful and precise conclusions on the connection between migration and health require a focus on more homogeneous subgroups rather than on "migrants," "people of migration background," or people of foreign citizenship.

Current State of Research

Even though the first medical dissertations on "epidemiology and areas of conflict in the health behavior of foreign workers" were published in the 1980s (Mehle, 1981), compared to the international discourse, it took a while for immigration and health to become a subject of importance in the German debate. At the beginning of the 21st century, policy-makers, and institutions showed initiative and started to commission surveys and expert opinions.

The Government Commissioner for Migration, Refugees and Integration, for example, presented a study entitled "Healthy Integration" in 2003 (Beauftragte der Bundesregierung für Migration, Flüchtlinge und Integration, 2003). A few years later, a *Manual for Good-Practice Models* was published, also initiated by the commissioner (Beauftragte der Bundesregierung für Migration, Flüchtlinge und Integration, 2007), followed by an analysis of "migration-sensitive data collection for health and nursing care documentation" (Beauftragte der Bundesregierung für Migration, Flüchtlinge und Integration, 2010) and a practical guide for culture-sensitive hospitals (Beauftragte der Bundesregierung für Migration, Flüchtlinge und Integration, 2013a).

In 2008, the Robert Koch Institute—in co-operation with the Federal Center for Health Education—published a study of child and adolescent health in Germany with extensive material on children and adolescents of migration background (Robert Koch-Institut & Bundeszentrale für gesundheitliche Aufklärung, 2008). In the same year, the comprehensive study *Migration and Health* was published, also commissioned by the Robert Koch Institute and the Federal Center for Health Education (Robert Koch-Institut & Statistisches Bundesamt, 2008). The study *Migration and Health Promotion* was published in 2009, edited by the Federal Center for Health Education (Bundeszentrale für gesundheitliche Aufklärung, 2009).

The Federal Office for Migration and Refugees (BAMF) published a study called *Migrant Morbidity and Mortality* in 2011 (Kohls, 2011). Political foundations, such as the Konrad Adenauer Foundation, began to address the topic as well. Thus, the authors Michael Knipper and Yasan Bilgin presented a study that was co-edited by the Konrad Adenauer Foundation and the Turkish-German Health Foundation (Knipper & Bilgin, 2009). This list is far from complete and should only clarify that the subject of migration and health—after having been neglected by German debate for decades—gained momentum at the beginning of the new millennium.

In recent years, cities or boroughs such as Nuremberg/Gostenhof (1997), Bielefeld (2004) and Berlin/Mitte (2011), or Federal states such as Bavaria initiated regional health reports with a focus on migration; these not only presented and interpreted statistical material, but also contained practical and political recommendations (Gesundheitsamt der Stadt Nürnberg, 1997; Stadt Bielefeld, 2004; Bezirksamt Mitte von Berlin—Abteilung Gesundheit, 2011; Bayerisches Landesamt für Gesundheit und Lebensmittelsicherheit, 2011).

Numerous studies concentrate on specific groups of immigrants, such as children and adolescents (Gesundheitsamt der Stadt Nürnberg, 1997; Robert Koch-Institut & Bundeszentrale für gesundheitliche Aufklärung, 2008), women (Borde, David & Kentenich, 2000), or people with a Turkish migration background (Collatz et al., 1985; Theilen, 1985, pp. 292–322; Yildirim-Fahlbusch, 2003).

The studies mentioned here mostly have a secondary-analysis approach and refer to comprehensive sets of data (e.g., population statistics; cause-of-death statistics; foreigner central register; micro-census; socio-economic panel; Federal Health Survey, 1998; German Dental Health Studies, 1997, 2005; Health Behaviour in School-Aged Children; Child and Adolescent Survey (KiGGs); Foreigner Survey of the German Youth Institute, 1998; etc.) (Robert Koch-Institut & Statistisches Bundesamt, 2008, p. 26ff.).

In research and political counselling, studies using quantitative methods are predominant; only very few studies have a qualitative approach. As a consequence, a great deal can be learned about statistical correlations, but relatively little about causalities and underlying motivations.

Discussion: Healthy Migrant Effect

Numerous studies conclude that migrants' status of health—compared to the non-migrant population (the autochthones)—is not worse but actually better (Razum, 2006, pp. 255–270; Kohls, 2008; Höhne & Schubert, 2010, pp. 103–126; Knipper & Bilgin, 2009, p. 34).

The mortality rate of migrants is even lower, compared to the majority population. Correspondingly, epidemiology refers to a "healthy migrant effect" (HME), which might be explained as follows: Generally, people who are young, healthy, and able-bodied are more likely to decide to emigrate, as only those migrants know they will be able to cope with the physical and mental challenges of emigration.

The Federal Employment Agency conducted health checks and capability tests on behalf of companies that were interested in hiring guest workers. Before a guest worker was allowed to travel to Germany, he or she had to undergo a selection procedure in which the individual's physical condition was tested. The German industry paid a fee of 165 DM for the successful placement of each foreign worker during the first year (later 300 DM were paid; since July 1973 the fee was at 1,000 DM) and, as Seidel-Pielen (1989) points out, demanded "impeccable goods."

A guest worker who had been recruited from Turkey, Filiz Yüreklik, remembers the humiliating procedure: "It was terrible. We had to strip to our drawers and were examined by a German doctor. We were standing in line, and he looked into our mouths—as if we were horses—to check if our teeth were healthy. Then we had to give a sample of blood and urine, so that they could find out if we were pregnant or had diabetes" (Filiz Yüreklik, quoted in Seidel-Pielen, 1998; authors' translation).

A further explanation of the HME is connected with demography and re-emigration. Due to migrants' low average age and lower incidence of age-related diseases (heart and circulatory diseases, diabetes mellitus), the total mortality rate is lower (Knipper & Bilgin, 2009, p. 35). Another tendency that can be observed is the re-emigration of older migrants to their countries of origin. Thus the authors Knipper and Bilgin conclude that "migrants are not 'healthier', but demographic and sociological factors make it relatively more difficult to record cases of illness" (Knipper & Bilgin, 2009, p. 35; authors' translation).

As in other countries, in Germany we observe that this healthy migrant effect decreases during migrants' stay in Germany, and that their health status converges with that of non-migrants. On closer inspection it becomes clear that a "convergence of risk of illness" can be observed for diseases that are associated with age and lifestyle; in part, there is even an increase that surpasses the risk of illness of the population without migration background (Knipper & Bilgin, 2009, p. 35).

For example, there is a significantly higher incidence of diabetes mellitus in the group of Turkish migrants than in the average population in Germany (Knipper & Bilgin, 2009, p. 36). Incidences of cancer diseases increase in the group of Turkish migrants, whereas there is a downward trend in the total population.

Evidence Concerning the Integration of Immigrants into Society

Numerous empirical and theoretical publications have investigated immigrants' integration into society. In the following, some central findings will be presented and then assessed with reference to social and health policy. The relevant sources used here are, among other publications, a report of facts edited by the Government Commissioner for Migration, Refugees and Integration (Beauftragte der Bundesregierung für Migration, Flüchtlinge und Integration, 2013b), as well as the labour market report of the Federal Employment Agency (Bundesagentur für Arbeit, 2004).

Education

Even though the formal education levels of Germans and foreigners have become somewhat less disparate in recent years, it is still evident that foreign children and adolescents tend to graduate from school with lower qualifications. A closer look at the years from 2004/2005 to 2010/2011 makes clear that the number of foreign children and adolescents with graduation diplomas improved gradually. The number of those dropping out of school without a diploma decreased by 44 percent; the number of foreign graduates of lower secondary schools (*Hauptschule*) dropped by 14 percent; at the same time, the rate of foreign students graduating from intermediate secondary school (*Realschule*) rose by 12 percent; and there was also an increase in the number of foreign students achieving the German university entrance qualification *Abitur* on completing higher secondary school.

Nevertheless, there are still considerable disparities: While 40 percent of all German adolescents leave school with the general *Abitur* or at least the *Fachabitur* (a university entrance qualification for a limited number of subjects), the rate of young foreigners graduating from higher secondary schools is only 18 percent (Bundesagentur für Arbeit, 2004, p. 18).

Considering other factors—the parents' educational level and income—it becomes clear that the parents' graduation diploma and the family's household income influence the children's and adolescents' school career in a significant way.

The Federal Employment Agency confirms that the higher the parents' graduation diploma (and the higher the household income), the more likely the children are to attend higher secondary school (Bundesagentur für Arbeit, 2004, p. 20; authors' translation). Correspondingly, as to the 14-year-olds who emigrated from EU states as children and whose parents have the same educational level and income as the parents of children without migration background, there is no correlation between migration background and choice of school (Bundesagentur für Arbeit, 2004, p. 20). By contrast, the "migration background" factor has an "independent effect" on second-generation children of immigrants and young immigrants from third countries. These young people are less likely to attend higher secondary schools (Bundesagentur für Arbeit, 2004, p. 20).

Vocational Training and Higher Education

Similar to secondary education, the number of young adults without any **vocational training** decreased between 2005 and 2011. This group includes young adults with or without migration background and Germans as well as non-Germans (Bundesagentur für Arbeit, 2004, p. 24).

In the total population the rate of 25- to 35-year-olds without vocational or higher education dropped by a proportion 16 percent of the original rate (from 17.6 percent in 2005 to 14.8 percent in 2011). In the group of people without migration background there was a proportional decrease of 14 percent (from 10.8 percent in 2005 to 9.3 percent in 2011), while the group of foreigners saw a proportional decrease of 11 percent (from 42.6 percent in 2005 to 37.8 percent in 2011).

Quite obviously, there is still an enormous gap between the groups. While only 9.3 percent of the 25- to 35-year-olds without migration background were without vocational or higher education in 2011, the rate of people of migration background was at 31.2 percent in the same year and as high as 37.8 percent in the group of foreigners (Bundesagentur für Arbeit, 2004, p. 26).

With respect to university entrance qualification, the education levels show a slight tendency to converge. In the group of 25- to 35-year-olds without migration background, 19.6 percent had a degree; in the same age group with migration background, 17.1 percent held a degree; in the same age group with migration experience, 18.9 percent had completed higher education courses; and 20.6 percent of all foreigners aged 25 to 35 held a degree (Bundesagentur für Arbeit, 2004, p. 29). Hence, one in five foreigners in this age group living in Germany had graduated from university or another institution of higher education. However, the statistics include degrees acquired in the country of origin as well as in Germany, so that conclusions about the accessibility of the German educational system have to be drawn with caution.

Employment Rates

The Federal Employment Agency considers as unemployed all people who "are currently not gainfully employed or are working fewer than 15 hours a week"; they also need to seek work subject to social security contributions and be registered as unemployed (Bundesagentur für Arbeit, 2004).

People who participate in employment policy programs (e.g., further and continuing education, job application training) or who do "one-euro jobs" on work opportunity schemes are excluded from the unemployment statistics of the Federal Employment Agency. The Federal Employment Agency does not consider either foreigners who need a work permit and their family members, or asylum-seekers who do not receive benefits as unemployed if they are excluded from the labour market (Bundesagentur für Arbeit, 2004, p. 3).

Since August 2012, the labour market statistics of the Federal Employment Agency include a category for "people of migration background" in addition to the former differentiation between Germans and foreigners (Beauftragte der Bundesregierung für Migration, Flüchtlinge und Integration, 2013b, p. 33).

Current labour market reports of the Federal Employment Agency indicate that people of migration background and foreigners show an above-average unemployment rate. In December 2013, 36 percent of the unemployed were people of migration background (although they make up 20 percent of the total population).

The far-reaching social and labour policy reform implemented by the "red-green" governing coalition (i.e., the Social Democrats and the Green Party) was introduced as "Agenda 2010"; its purpose was to combine unemployment benefits and social assistance. Unemployment benefit I under Book III of the German Social Code is based on social security contributions, while unemployment benefit II (Book II of the Social Code) is funded by taxation.

Since 2004, unemployment benefit I is granted only to people who have been gainfully employed and subject to social contributions for at least one year. Unemployment benefit I is paid for a maximum of one year (older unemployed people are entitled to a maximum of two years). A person who has worked and paid social contributions for 24 months within two years qualifies for unemployment benefit I for a maximum of 12 months. The amount of the benefit depends on the gross salary (minus social security payments, income tax, and the solidarity supplement—a kind of German reunification tax). After this time, the unemployed are entitled only to basic security benefits called unemployment benefit II, and only if the person does not have any savings nor lives in a joint household with people who could support him or her financially.

Unemployment benefit II is funded by taxation and is means-tested; it is granted to people who do not engage in gainful employment, have no savings, and do not live in a joint household (marriage or common-law marriage, etc.) that might provide for them. In contrast to unemployment benefit I, unemployment benefit II can be granted for an unlimited time.

From the beginning, the reconstruction of the German welfare state has been based on the principle of "support and challenge." Transfer payments are thus granted only if a person signs a so-called integration agreement with the Federal Employment Agency. If recipients of unemployment benefit I or II do not comply with the objectives (e.g., participate in programs such as job application training), they risk potential sanctions such as reduced or stopped benefits (Butterwegge, 2013a, 2013b, 2014).

Statistics show that there is a considerably higher percentage of people of migration background among the recipients of unemployment benefit II (Book II of the Social Code) than among the recipients of unemployment benefit I (Book III of the Social Code). Forty percent of all recipients of unemployment benefit II are migrants, whereas they account for only 26 percent of those entitled to unemployment benefit I (Bundesagentur für Arbeit, 2014, p. 2).

The statistics also show that a lack of vocational education leads to a higher risk of unemployment. More than two-thirds (68 percent) of all unemployed people of migration background have no vocational or professional qualification. On the other hand, vocational training—acquired through in-company training or at school—does not prevent unemployment. One in four unemployed people of migration background have completed vocational training (Bundesagentur für Arbeit, 2014, p. 8).

A closer look at the different age groups makes clear that the elderly are overrepresented among the unemployed without migration background, whereas the unemployed of migration background are significantly younger (27 percent of all unemployed people with a migration background are between 35 and 45) (Bundesagentur für Arbeit, 2014, p. 9).

Poverty Rates

A person is considered at risk of poverty if his or her income is lower than 60 percent of the average income. The National Social Report 2013 states that "people of migration background are still twice as much at risk of poverty as the population without migration background. In eastern Germany, migrants are even more affected by poverty; they represent a much smaller percentage of the population in eastern than in western Germany, though" (Datenreport, 2013, pp. 177, 199 ff.; authors' translation).[7]

Twenty-three percent of all people of migration background are at risk of poverty, but only 15 percent of the population without migration background is at risk (Datenreport, 2013, p. 199). A particularly high risk of poverty can be observed in people with a Turkish migration background (33 percent), with an Eastern European background (28 percent), migrants from former Yugoslavia (26 percent), (late) repatriates (22 percent), and people with a Southwestern European background (17 percent). A person of Turkish origin, for example, has an average income of €1,188 and pays an average rent of €493 (Datenreport, 2013, p. 199).

Evidence Concerning Health Outcomes among Immigrants

The following section focuses on the health status, health behaviour, and health care of people of migration background. Box 8.1 provides an overview of ways of thinking about health inequalities.

Box 8.1: The Phenomenon of Health Inequality

For a number of years, international social science research and social epidemiology have been establishing a new field of research that focuses above all on the analysis of health inequality. This term refers to social differences with respect to the health status of the population as well as health behaviour and health care (Datenreport, 2013, p. 259; Richter & Hurrelmann, 2006a, 2006b, pp. 11–31). According to health inequality research, an individual's health status and behaviour are largely determined by income level, education level, employment status, and, finally, also migration.

Some empirical findings illustrate the phenomenon of health inequality. People with a low income or people living in relative poverty (less than 60 percent of the average income) tend to describe their health status as "fair or poor," unlike people with a medium or high income (Bundesministerium für Arbeit und Soziales, 2014, pp. 45ff., 137ff., 287ff.).

In addition, the life expectancy of men and women correlates with their income. Men in the lowest income group have an average life expectancy of 70.9 years; women in that group have a life expectancy of 76.9 years. Men in the highest income group, by contrast, have a life expectancy of 80.9 years, women of 85.3 years.

In terms of formal educational levels, men and women with a low formal education level have a higher degree of considerable health-related restrictions in daily living. In the past four weeks, people with a low education level had been—by their own account—either "always" or "often" in "bad physical pain" (Datenreport 2013, p. 262).

Income levels also correlate with questions of (mal)nutrition and obesity (BMI ≥ 30). Hence, women as well as men of the lowest income group show a higher obesity rate than people from the medium- or high-income groups.

As to smoking behaviour and sports activities, there are also differences with respect to education level. Men and women with little education—regardless of age—are more likely to smoke than people with a medium or high education level. People with little education—regardless of age—take less exercise than people with a medium or high education level.

→

Approaches to Explaining Health Inequalities

The correlation between health, education, gainful employment or unemployment, and income has been proven internationally. Matthias Richter and Klaus Hurrelmann have discussed different explanatory approaches, which will be presented below.

Selection hypothesis: A classical explanatory approach attributes the phenomenon of health inequality to processes of selection. It is argued that people who are particularly healthy and able-bodied have higher socio-economic status while illness leads to social decline. Correspondingly, health influences social mobility (not vice versa).

Principle of causation: A second explanatory approach argues that low socio-economic status causes greater health hazards, which leads to health inequality.

Material explanatory approach: A third approach attributes health inequality to an "unequal social distribution of material living conditions" (Richter & Hurrelmann, 2006b, p. 19), which affects income as well as housing and work conditions. Accordingly, people who are at a socio-economic disadvantage are also exposed to an unhealthy environment.

Cultural-behavioral explanatory approach: The fourth approach presumes that people with a low education level and a low income share a culture that promotes unhealthy behavioural patterns (tobacco and alcohol consumption), unhealthy nutrition, and physical inactivity.

Inequalities in health care: A fifth explanatory approach argues that people who are at a socio-economic disadvantage have relatively poor access to health care. Richter and Hurrelmann raise the question of whether economic measures in the German health care system (e.g., the introduction of a consultation fee) might still have increased existing health inequalities (Richter & Hurrelmann, 2006b, p. 19).

Psycho-social explanatory approach: A sixth approach questions the explanatory power of the material approach and stresses that it is not enough to consider health hazards in the working and living environment. In explaining health inequalities, it is also important to take into account the "psychological and psychosocial factors (e.g., critical life events, chronic daily hassles or professional gratification crises)" (Richter & Hurrelmann, 2006b, p. 20). The psychosocial explanatory approach refers, for example, to studies proving that not only is there an unequal distribution of stress but also of resources to deal with stress. Thus, people on the lowest rung in the social hierarchy are "affected doubly." They are to a greater extent exposed to health hazards in their environment; at the same time, they have fewer resources to cope with them (Richter & Hurrelmann, 2006b, p. 20).

Mortality

As recently as 2008, the Robert Koch Institute concluded in its study: "It is difficult to say whether migration has an effect on life expectancy. A striking phenomenon in the cause of death statistics—which only record citizenship at the time of death—is the lower mortality of non-Germans as opposed to Germans living in Germany" (Robert Koch-Institut & Statistisches Bundesamt 2008, p. 31; authors' translation).[8] It remains unclear, though, whether the main difficulty is the method of recording the deaths of foreigners living in Germany—and thus merely a statistical problem.

Statistics show that mortality of non-German infants is slightly elevated. Until the age of 15, the death rate of foreign adolescents is slightly higher than that of Germans. From then on, the death rates of non-Germans parallel those of Germans, yet on a considerably *lower* level. In the age group of 80- to 84-year-olds, the German death rate is 2.5 times higher than that of non-Germans. This difference is even clearer in the age group of men over 90. In this group, the death rate of German men of the same age is 6.7 times higher (Richter & Hurrelmann, 2006b, p. 32).

Cause-of-death statistics that also record citizenship exist only for the group of Turkish nationals. There are records for the period from 1980 to 1997. The statistics show a significantly lower mortality rate for heart and circulatory diseases or cancer diseases in the group of Turkish nationals.

Parallels exist with respect to the specific cause of death. The most frequent cause of death by cancer for German and Turkish men was lung cancer; for German and Turkish women it was breast cancer. (Over 65-year-olds were not considered in this study.)

The cause-of-death statistics of 2011 show that the most frequent causes of death for German nationals are heart and circulatory diseases; most deaths of migrants are caused by cancers (Datenreport, 2013, p. 270).

This study refers to other international studies that come to similar conclusions and have already proved the existence of a healthy migrant effect. "In terms of overall mortality and individual causes of death, immigrants often show lower rates than the population of the host country" (Datenreport, 2013, p. 32; authors' translation).[9]

This healthy migrant effect applies above all to migrants from countries with a well-established tradition of transnational migration. Possibly, therefore, the healthy migrant effect is partly due to statistical problems in recording the deaths of foreigners living in Germany. It is assumed that elderly foreign nationals, in the context of transmigration, spend longer periods of their lives in their country of origin. If they die in their country of origin, their death is not recorded in the statistics of the host country. However, as the healthy migrant effect is not only a German but an international phenomenon, the study of the Robert Koch Institute concludes: "It remains a challenge for epidemiological migration research to search for further and more precise explanations accounting for the complexity of correlations between risk factors, selection mechanisms, and mortality" (Datenreport, 2013, p. 33; authors' translation).[10]

Between 1994 and 2001, foreign pensioners had a slightly higher life expectancy than German retirees. This tendency, however, changed gradually from 2001/2002 onward. In 2008 one notices a slightly higher life expectancy for German pensioners than for foreign pensioners (men: 1.5 years longer, women: 1.2 years longer) (Datenreport, 2013, p. 270).

Morbidity

Dealing with health and migration also involves the question of specific health risks and health conditions that might affect migrants more so than the rest of the population. Research has pointed at two health risks of migrants in particular, namely, tuberculosis and *Helicobacter pylori*.

While tuberculosis had almost disappeared until a few years ago, there has been an increase in cases of the disease in the course of immigration processes. The Robert Koch Institute observes a rather high incidence of tuberculosis among foreign nationals. In the group of 25- to 29-year-olds of foreign citizenship, there are approximately 35 cases of tuberculosis in 100,000 people, as opposed to around three or four cases in the group of 25- to 29-year-old Germans (Datenreport, 2013, p. 40).

The infectious disease *Helicobacter pylori* frequently leads to stomach cancer. People from Turkey or Eastern European states and their children are affected to a higher degree by this infectious disease. While migrants show a higher incidence of tuberculosis and *Helicobacter pylori*, all migrant groups are less affected by other diseases—heart and circulatory diseases—than people without migration background.

Subjective State of Health

The following findings refer to the National Social Report 2013, which again is based on the 2009 micro-census. With regard to their subjective state of health, migrants (up to the age of 44 years) indicate slightly less often than the majority of the population that they were ill or had an accident within the past four weeks. The opposite effect can be observed for the older age groups (45–64 years and 65+ years). Over-45-year-olds with a migration background indicated slightly more often than people without migration background that they had been ill in the past four weeks or suffered from an injury as a result of an accident (Datenreport, 2013, p. 266).

Turkish migrants in particular reported that they had ("always" or "often") suffered from bad physical pain in the past four weeks. This applies to both the male (23.4 percent) and female (51.2 percent) Turkish migrants who were questioned. The figures relating to the female Turkish migrants are particularly striking. More than one in two (51.2 percent) women of Turkish background answered in the affirmative when asked about bad physical pain in the past four weeks. (In the same age group (45+ years), every fifth non-migrant (21.5 percent) indicated that they had suffered from bad pain.) The risk of physical pain is evident for Turkish migrants, but not for non-Turkish migrants.

Health Behaviour

Some differences can be observed in health behaviour (nutrition, smoking, etc.). Overweight and obesity (BMI > 30) seem to be a more important issue for migrants than for non-migrants. This is true to a lesser extent for male migrants of all age groups, but to a greater degree for female migrants, especially those 45 to 64 years old (23.1 percent) and the age group of the over-65-year-olds (27.5 percent).[11]

There are also differences in terms of smoking: 37 percent of all male migrants are smokers, whereas only 30 percent of all male non-migrants smoke. In contrast, the rate of smokers among female migrants is lower than among non-migrants: 23 percent of all female migrants and 25 percent of all female non-migrants smoke regularly.

Health Care

There are also differences with respect to the use of the health care system. Male and female migrants, unlike German patients, "use emergency rooms rather than GPs as a first contact point and visit them more often in the late evening or at night as well as on weekends" (Robert Koch-Institut & Statistisches Bundesamt, 2008, p. 110f.; authors' translation).

A study by Theda Borde et al. found a number of reasons for this practice. Migrants often face barriers in the health care system, for example, with respect to language, socio-cultural communication, and access to information. In contrast to GPs and medical specialists, an emergency room seems to present fewer obstacles. This may be because the hospital is located near the place of residence; it may be a place the patient knows as a result of a previous hospital stay or visit or while accompanying other family members or friends to the hospital's emergency room (Borde et al., 2009, p. 149).

Further specifics may be noted briefly:

- Migrants use preventive, health-promoting measures less frequently.
- If family members are in need of care, migrant families make use of nursing services less frequently.
- Medical rehabilitation measures are used less often by people of foreign citizenship.
- In addition, foreign patients have less rehabilitation success.
- Compared to German employees, the rate of early retirement is higher for migrants.

The National Social Report 2013 points out that:

> People of migration background are in a worse state of health in some areas than the rest of the population. In terms of prevention, medical and nursing care, the male and female migrants' situation is to some extent less positive than for the population without migration background. However, a general

> health disadvantage of migrants cannot be confirmed. Current research findings suggest a differentiated assessment that needs to take into account the individual living conditions and chances of participation, but also cultural specifics, migration experiences and the social and health situation in the country of origin. (Datenreport, 2013, p. 271; authors' translation)

The Ethno-Medical Centre (EMZ) in Hanover, founded in 1989, aims to improve the health care of migrants. By its own account, the EMZ wants to facilitate access to existing health care options through culture-sensitive and language-specific concepts and services. Furthermore, it wants to motivate migrants to make better use of the health care system and its services, so that they take more responsibility for their own health. The project, (MiMi mit Migranten—für Migranten (i.e., with migrants, for migrants)) focuses on providing migrants with more information on health questions. As a first step, committed bilingual migrants (mostly women) are trained as mediators. As intercultural health guides, they offer information and educational events on health topics. So far, 1,000 migrants from 40 countries have been trained as intercultural health mediators. A combination of basic training and successive further education enables the migrants to further develop their skills and to update their knowledge and methods continuously. The Government Commissioner for Migration, Refugees and Integration is the patron of the project, which has also been adopted in Austria.[12]

Analysis of the Interrelationship between Public Policy, Living Conditions and Experiences of Immigrants, and Health Outcomes

A comprehensive analysis of the interrelationship between social policy, labour market policy, living conditions, and experiences of migrants with respect to their effects on health would require an extensive research effort; a project of such a scale has not been achieved so far. Therefore, only a few findings based on analysis of secondary sources can be presented here.

The reforms in social and labour market policy of recent years constitute an unparalleled reconstruction of the German welfare state. As a consequence of the combination of unemployment benefit and social assistance, the number of people affected by relative poverty has greatly increased. This includes people who live on unemployment benefit II (or unemployment benefit I), but also those whose work is limited to one-euro jobs or mini-jobs, people who work part-time (involuntarily) or are engaged in precarious employment. Even though these people are not considered unemployed (according to the statistics) because they work more than 14 hours a week, they still do not manage to escape poverty. High costs of living—above all, the increasing rents in areas of high population density—make it more and more difficult to cope with working and living conditions.

Although migrants as a whole are an extraordinarily heterogeneous group, individual groups of migrants are particularly affected by the social and labour market policy reforms of recent years, called Agenda 2010 (Deutscher Bundestag, 2002). This is true for migrants of the first, second, and third generation, and it is particularly true for children and adolescents from migrant families, an increasing number of whom are growing up in poverty (Bundesministerium für Arbeit und Soziales, 2014).

It should have become clear that a low education level and a low income have negative effects on health—this applies to all people, but more so to migrants. Therefore, it can be concluded that a policy of social welfare cuts has far-reaching consequences for migrants' status of health and will continue to do so.

Given the explanatory approaches outlined above, the psychosocial approach seems the most convincing explanation of health inequality, especially with respect to migrants. It is true, on the one hand, that individual groups of migrants are exposed to higher health risks in their working and living environments; it is also true, on the other hand, that they suffer from greater stress caused by psychological and psychosocial factors.

Attitudes in the Population

The longitudinal analysis (2002–2011) entitled "Deutsche Zustände" (German conditions) has proved that, over a period of 10 years, a constantly growing proportion of the German population shows feelings of hostility toward specific groups of people; a high percentage of people agree with xenophobic statements.

Hence, 60 percent of all respondents agreed with the statement that too many foreigners live in Germany. Thirty-five percent believe that foreigners should be sent back to their home countries at times of job scarcity. Homeless people and Muslims also face aggressive forms of rejection, as 30 to 40 percent of the responses confirm. At the same time, more than 40 percent of the respondents demanded more rights for those who have established themselves in Germany (Heitmeyer, 2008).

Wilhelm Heitmeyer and his colleagues are particularly worried about the fact that the observed ideologies of social marginalization are not limited to the fringes of society, but can be found in mainstream society as well. These attitudes are thus setting standards of normality and becoming more and more difficult to challenge and question. In addition, the extreme right, with its political offerings, might also profit from such normalization of marginalization and racism.

There is an obvious interrelationship here between the development of attitudes and the increasing processes of social disintegration. Experiences of insecurity as a result of increased racism and xenophobia lead to increased disorientation and a search for security, which is reflected by values such as nation, home, but also "race" and ethnic affiliation in the general population. This study shows a clear link to the topic of xenophobia (Heitmeyer, 2008, p. 43f.).

The results of the study "Deutsche Zustände" correspond to some extent to the empirical study by Decker et al. (2012), which was commissioned by the Friedrich Ebert Foundation. This study illustrates the widespread racist, xenophobic, and authoritarian attitudes of a majority of the population.

- Around 37 percent of the respondents agreed with the statement "Too many foreigners in the Federal Republic have led to foreign domination" (authors' translation); (14.9 percent agreed strongly, 21.7 percent agreed on the whole).
- Thirty-six percent agreed with the statement that "Foreigners only come here to abuse our welfare state" (authors' translation); (14.3 percent agreed strongly, 21.7 percent agreed on the whole).
- And 31.6 percent believed that "Foreigners should be sent back to their home countries if jobs are scarce" (authors' translation); (13.2 percent agreed strongly, 18.4 percent agreed on the whole).

Hence, the studies show that hostility toward specific groups of people is widespread among Germans. There is resentment against immigrants, open or hidden racism directed against refugees, and also against people of Turkish and Arab origin and, increasingly, against Sinti and Roma (Benz, 2014; Antidiskriminierungsstelle des Bundes, 2014). These groups repeatedly face racist attitudes and actions—in everyday situations, in the housing market, in the education system, with public authorities, or in the health care system.

As employees they are often at the bottom of the job hierarchy, their work offers little recognition, and they face hidden or open hostility. If they are not gainfully employed (unemployment benefit II recipients), they are often accused of living off tax money, and they need to justify their life in the Federal Republic again and again, even if they are second-generation immigrants and were born in the Federal territory.

The recent Ebola epidemic in Western Africa provides an example of how even health catastrophes outside Germany are exploited in the xenophobic debate. Even though only two Ebola patients have been treated in Germany since August 2014 (in the university clinics of Hamburg and Frankfurt/Main), the topic has already entered the right-wing populist discourse. A politician from the Alternative für Deutschland (Alternative for Germany) Party, for instance, took advantage of this epidemic for her political objectives. Alluding to movements of refugees and the epidemic, Petra Federau, AfD politician, wrote on her Facebook page: "Not only do we attract the religious wars into the country but also all the diseases of the world" (authors' translation).[13] This political instrumentalization was replaced by the xenophobic debate regarding the great number of refugees who were allowed to enter Germany. Again the AfD, as a party, used the xenophobic attitude found in segments of the German population to run successful campaigns in several elections.

All these experiences of marginalization, discrimination, and racism have an effect on migrants' daily life and, eventually, also on their well-being and health. The extent of these harmful effects also depends on the migrants' ability to cope with mental and physical stress.

Implications for Immigration and Other Policy

A number of implications for immigration and integration policy can be derived from the findings presented above. Regarding migration and health, it has become clear that people with a low education level and social status face health risks to a greater extent. It should also have become apparent that the subject area must not be "ethnicized." Rather, academic analysis needs to pay attention to the question of social status in the context of migration as well. All studies used here (e.g., the government report on poverty and wealth) (Bundesministerium für Arbeit und Soziales, 2014) point to the interrelationship between the state of health and social status—and this applies to all age groups.

Under the Asylum-Seekers' Benefit Act, certain groups—asylum-seekers, tolerated refugees, or refugees whose deportation has been ordered—are excluded per se from specific medical services. They are entitled only to emergency care and are thus marginalized within the health care system.

Exclusion from the health care system applies even more so to the approximately 500,000 to 1 million people living in Germany who do not have valid documents. Medical networks and charities are crucial for those particularly vulnerable social groups so they can gain access to medical care.

A policy—above all in the context of Agenda 2010—that is geared toward deconstructing social security systems and shows an increasingly neo-liberal orientation contributes to the emergence of poverty, unemployment, and a precarious existence. Even though the Agenda 2010 or the Hartz laws did not focus on migrants, that group of socially vulnerable people (migrants, among others) is particularly affected by the reconstruction of the German welfare state.

Special multilingual educational programs on health and the health care system for migrants, such as the MiMi project—with migrants, for migrants—offered by the Ethno-Medical Centre are certainly a groundbreaking approach.

Conclusion

It is difficult to draw clear and unambiguous conclusions from the existing academic research findings. Migrants as a whole comprise many different subgroups with different migration experiences, heterogeneous educational backgrounds, and correspondingly different life situations and problems. This differentiation is taken into account in very different ways by the predominantly quantitative empirical studies, which makes it nearly impossible to compare the results. Therefore, the academic investigation of the interrelationship between migration and health/illness needs to be intensified and coordinated considerably, and above all must be complemented by group-specific qualitative studies.

Essentially, it is assumed that individual groups of migrants—above all migrants with little formal qualification and, of course, especially those with no secured residence status—are subject to particular health risks. All of them are exposed to relatively hard-working conditions, have low incomes, and often live in unhealthy housing conditions. At the same time, the legal migrants with low qualifications are particularly affected by the socio-political reforms in Germany. The psychosocial strain on illegal migrants and those without a secured residence status is increased by a constant fear of being caught or deported; also, they often lack access to appropriate medical care.

All migrants suffer to a greater or lesser degree from the latent or open xenophobia in German society. It remains unclear, however, whether or not and to what extent this has a pathogenic effect or which personal or social resources are able to help migrants cope with these negative attitudes. To our knowledge, there are no pertinent studies on this topic.

There is also an urgent need for more intensive investigation into the actual existence (and if so, weakening) of the healthy migrant effect; it needs to be clarified whether or not it is merely a methodological artifact or a result of selection processes of transnational migration.

With respect to the medical and nursing care of migrants, the challenge is above all to create easier, low-threshold access to the health care system. In this context, the increasing and state-supported immigration into Germany of international medical and nursing experts might become a highly significant factor. This would imply, however, to orientate the acquisition and immigration policy for such experts more strongly along the structural parameters (language, cultural area) of the migrant population in Germany. This might lead to greater and easier access to health care for the existing migrant population in Germany.

Critical Thinking Questions

1. What are the factors that contribute to the healthy migrant effect in Germany?
2. How can policies in the field of public health contribute to the improvement of immigrant health in Germany?
3. What role do NGOs play in the field of immigrant health?
4. What role does the nation-state play in immigrant health?
5. What are some means of shifting attitudes towards immigrants?

Glossary

Asylum-Seekers' Benefits Act (AsylbLG) regulates the benefits granted to asylum-seekers and tolerated refugees in Germany. For those living in reception facilities, food, heating, clothing, health care, etc., are covered by benefits in kind. Asylum-seekers who are entitled to cash benefits are paid a monthly allowance to cover their personal needs (Section 44 of the Asylum-Seekers' Benefits Act).

In its decision of July 18, 2012, the Federal Constitutional Court criticized the cash benefits for asylum-seekers—which have not been raised since 1993—as "evidently insufficient." An amendment of the Asylum-Seekers' Benefit Act, which came into effect on March 1, 2015, provides for an increase in benefits. Also after the 2015 amendment, medical care is still limited to "treatment of acute illness and pain" as well as "medical and nursing care and support" of pregnant women and women in childbirth (Section 4 of the Asylum-Seekers' Benefit Act).

Migration background of people entering Germany has been recorded in the statistics of the Federal Republic of Germany since 2005. This group comprises the following subgroups: firstly, migrants who have entered Germany after 1949; secondly, all foreigners born in Germany; thirdly, all people born in Germany with at least one parent who has migrated to Germany or was born in Germany as a foreign resident.

Vocational training in Germany is very specific and different from most systems in other countries. There is a formalized educational track for about 350 specialized occupations (*Berufe*) such as locksmith, hairdresser, or mechanic, which usually takes three years of education and combines theoretical knowledge (taught in state schools) and practical experience in companies. To qualify for this kind of vocational training, applicants usually have to be at least 16 years old and have successfully finished a 10-year education in secondary schools. At the end of the training there is a theoretical and practical examination, which is certified. The German labour market and the recruitment strategies of the companies rely on these certificates. More than 50 percent of the German population holds such a certificate. People without any vocational certificate or university degree have fewer opportunities in the labour market. For migrants who did not go through the German school system, it is very hard to enter and complete this vocational education system, and without a vocational certificate, they must concentrate on low-paid jobs with hard-working conditions.

Recommended Readings

Butterwegge, Christoph. (2014). *Hartz IV und die Folgen. Auf dem Weg in eine andere Republik?* Weinheim: Beltz Juventa.

The author argues that the Hartz reforms have turned Germany into a different republic. Besides an ever-growing low-pay sector, the other effects of the Hartz reforms are social tendencies toward "de-solidarization" and increasingly indifferent social attitudes. The Hartz laws not only increased the risk of poverty for the long-term unemployed and their families, but also strongly influenced the political climate in the Federal Republic. Butterwegge thus concludes that "Hartz IV," i.e., the basic security benefit for long-term job-seekers, is now associated all over Europe with social benefit cuts and is seen in Germany itself as the most significant turning point in the history of the German welfare state since 1945.

Knipper, Michael, & Bilgin, Yasar. (2009). *Migration und Gesundheit.* Edited by Konrad Adenauer Stiftung and Türkisch Deutsche Gesundheitsstiftung. Sankt Augustin/Berlin: Konrad-Adenauer-Stiftung.

This study summarizes the current state of knowledge and questions regarding migration and illness. It presents examples of specific findings (migrants' health situation, frequency of diseases in different migrant groups). The authors point out that with regard to medical questions, migration is "a difficult-to-grasp and often insufficient criterion." The study concludes by giving recommendations for action in terms of comprehensive strategies and projects to facilitate intercultural access to the health sector.

Richter, Matthias, & Hurrelmann, Klaus. (Eds.). (2006). *Gesundheitliche Ungleichheit. Grundlagen—Probleme—Perspektiven.* Wiesbaden: VS-Verlag.

Starting from the widespread assumption that "the poor, the lowly educated and occupationally disadvantaged are more often ill and have to die earlier," this volume attempts to explain the connection between social inequality and health. The volume provides an overview on theories and research findings. The authors' contributions also deal with the implications for policy and practice. Moreover, the anthology gives insight into the sociological and health science explanations of health inequality and discusses methodological challenges that the research area is facing at present.

Robert Koch-Institut & Statistisches Bundesamt. (2008). *Migration und Gesundheit. Schwerpunktbericht der Berichterstattung des Bundes.* Berlin: Robert Koch-Institut. Retrieved from http://www.rki.de/DE/Content/Gesundheitsmonitoring/Gesundheitsberichterstattung/GBEDownloadsT/migration.pdf?__blob=publicationFile

The Federal Health Report offers a comprehensive overview of the available data on the health of people with a migration background. The 135-page report concludes that "the spectrum of disease in the group of people with a migration background resembles that of the non-migrant population." At the same time, there are higher health risks in certain areas. These are infant mortality, infectious diseases such as tuberculosis, and illnesses caused by psychosocial stress as a result of separation from family and of political persecution in the country of origin. The health report identifies particularly vulnerable groups such as children, adolescents, and women with a migration background, as well as elderly migrants and people without a legally secured status of residence.

Related Websites

Beauftragte für Migration, Flüchtlinge und Integration—http://www.bundesregierung.de/Webs/Breg/DE/Bundesregierung/BeauftragtefuerIntegration/beauftragte-fuer-integration.html

The website of Minister of State Aydan Özoğuz has information on her political function and personality, and provides various publications focusing on immigration and integration. Since Aydan Özoğuz considered 2015 as the "year of health," this site provides a wide range of information and publications on the topic of health and care.

Ethno Medizinisches Zentrum Hannover—http://www.ethno-medizinisches-zentrum.de/

The site of the Ethno Medical Centre presents various intercultural projects of the centre—among them MiMi (with migrants, for migrants); AIDS and mobility in Europe; and translation services—and provides information on training as "transcultural mediator for the prevention of addiction and AIDS."

Federal Office for Migration and Refugees (BAMF)—http://www.bamf.de/SiteGlobals/Forms/Sprachumschaltung/DE/Sprachumschaltung_Formular.html

The website of the Federal Office for Migration and Refugees provides information about regulations on immigrating to Germany, subsequent entry of families and spouses, working in Germany, studying and education, asylum and refugee protection, reception procedure for Syrian refugees, ethnic German resettlers, and Jewish immigrants.

Federal Statistical Office— https://www.destatis.de/EN/Homepage.html;jsessionid=2C2BF6F05F8D7A3424C29173A5417049.cae4

The Federal Statistical Office provides and disseminates statistical information on a wide range of different topics, among them health and migration and integration. This site also offers a "Common Archive of Online Publications," among them various publications on population and the health care system.

Robert Koch Institute—http://www.rki.de/EN/Home/homepage_node.html

This site, administered by the central federal institution responsible for disease control and prevention, provides data on the health of people with migration backgrounds. The Robert Koch Institute developed methods and standards to encourage immigrants to participate in health surveys.

Notes

1. Many thanks to Sabine Kirschenhofer, Fulda, for assisting us with the translation.
2. Currently, around 14,000 stateless people are living in Germany, according to the Federal Office for Migration and Refugees. Numerous people without citizenship come from the former Soviet Union or the former Yugoslavia and have lost their citizenship in the course of the dissolution of the socialist system of states. In the first eight months of 2014, 807 stateless people applied for asylum in Germany; they described their ethnic origin as Palestinian (377), Arab (216), and Kurdish (133) (Cf. Deutscher Bundestag & Wissenschaftlicher Dienst, 2014, p. 2).
3. Many EU citizens or Swiss citizens are allowed dual citizenship. Bilateral agreements were concluded with other states (the United States, Canada, etc.), allowing dual citizenship under certain conditions.
4. The term "migration background" needs to be differentiated from the term "migration experience." Not every person of migration background has migration experience as well. For example, children and adolescents born and raised in Germany whose parents are foreign citizens have a migration background but no migration experience.
5. In the following we refer to figures from the Central Register of Foreigners (as of March 31, 2014).
6. The residence act stipulates an "obligation to transfer data and inform." Until 2006, doctors were obligated to inform the authorities if they assumed a patient was an illegal resident. Since 2009, doctors are exempt from this obligation and may maintain medical confidentiality. The obligation to inform continues to apply to other professional groups as well as to the public health departments. The obligation to inform is stipulated in the residence act (Section 87): "Transfer of data and information to foreigners authorities": "(1) On request, public bodies with the exception of schools and other educational and care establishments for young people shall notify circumstances of which they obtain knowledge [...], insofar as this is necessary for the purposes stated in said Section. (2) Public bodies within the meaning of sub-section 1 shall notify the competent foreigners authority forthwith, if, in discharging their duties, they obtain knowledge of 1. the whereabouts of a foreigner who does not possess a required residence title and whose deportation has not been suspended, 2. a breach of a geographic restriction, 3. any other grounds for expulsion [...]." (Bundesministerium der Justiz und für Verbraucherschutz, 2008).
7. "Personen mit Migrationshintergrund sind unverändert einem doppelt so hohen Armutsrisiko ausgesetzt wie die Bevölkerung ohne Migrationshintergrund. In Ostdeutschland ist die Armutsbetroffenheit bei Migranten noch höher, allerdings ist ihr Bevölkerungsanteil hier weit geringer als in Westdeutschland" (Datenreport, 2013, p. 177, 199ff.).
8. "Es ist schwer zu beurteilen, ob sich die Migration auf die Lebenserwartung auswirkt. Ein auffälliges Phänomen in der Todesursachenstatistik, die nur eine Differenzierung nach Staatsangehörigkeit zum Zeitpunkt des Todes zulässt, ist die niedrigere

Sterblichkeit von in Deutschland lebenden nichtdeutschen Personen gegenüber Deutschen" (Robert Koch-Institut & Statistisches Bundesamt, 2008, p. 31).

9. "Zugewanderte Personen weisen bei der Gesamtsterblichkeit und auch bei einzelnen Todesursachen häufig niedrigere Raten als die Bevölkerungen des Zuzugslandes auf" (Robert Koch-Institut & Statistisches Bundesamt, 2008, p. 32).
10. "Die Suche nach weitergehenden Erklärungen, die die Komplexität der Zusammenhänge zwischen Risikofaktoren, Auswahlmechanismen und Mortalität genauer fassen, bleibt daher eine Aufgabe für die epidemiologische Migrationsforschung" (Robert Koch-Institut & Statistisches Bundesamt, 2008, p. 33).
11. Robert Koch-Institut & Statistisches Bundesamt, 2008, p. 267. The figures, in comparison, for female non-migrants: 14.8 percent of all women without migration background are obese in the age group between 45 and 64 years; 18 percent of all women without migration background are obese in the age group over 65.
12. EMZ website. The EMZ has developed flyers and brochures in several languages on the following subjects: new flu, psychotherapy, and health guides for different federal states.
13. "Wir holen uns nicht nur die Religionskriege, sondern auch alle Krankheiten der Welt ins Land."

References

Antidiskriminierungsstelle des Bundes. (2014). Zwischen Gleichgültigkeit und Ablehnung. Bevölkerungseinstellungen gegenüber Sinti und Roma. Berlin: Antidiskriminierungsstelle des Bundes.

Bayerisches Landesamt für Gesundheit und Lebensmittelsicherheit. (2011). Gesundheit und Migration. Bayerischer Bericht. Gesundheitsberichterstattung für Bayern 4. Unter Mitarbeit von Josef Kuhn und Dunja Grimmer. Nürnberg.

Beauftragte der Bundesregierung für Migration, Flüchtlinge und Integration. (2003). Gesunde Integration. Berlin, Bonn.

Beauftragte der Bundesregierung für Migration, Flüchtlinge und Integration. (2007). Gesundheit und Integration. Ein Handbuch für Modelle guter Praxis. Berlin.

Beauftragte der Bundesregierung für Migration, Flüchtlinge und Integration. (2010). Migrationssensible Datenerhebung für die Gesundheits- und Pflegeberichterstattung. Berlin.

Beauftragte der Bundesregierung für Migration, Flüchtlinge und Integration. (2013a). Das kultursensible Krankenhaus. Ansätze zur interkulturellen Öffnung. Praxisratgeber. Berlin.

Beauftragte der Bundesregierung für Migration, Flüchtlinge und Integration. (2013b). Faktenbericht 2013. Integration in Bildung und Arbeitsmarkt. Berlin.

Benz, W. (2014). Sinti und Roma: Die unerwünschte Minderheit: Über das Vorurteil Antiziganismus. Berlin: Metropol Verlag.

Berger, Alois & Conrad, Naomi. (2013, May 2). Ohne Krankenversicherung in Deutschland, in: *Deutsche Welle*.

Bezirksamt Mitte von Berlin—Abteilung Gesundheit. (2011). Migration und Gesundheit im Bezirk Berlin Mitte. Gesundheitliche und soziale Lage der Bevölkerung unter Berücksichtigung des Migrationshintergrundes. Beiträge zur Gesundheitsförderung und Gesundheitsberichterstattung. Unter Mitarbeit von Jeffrey Butler. Berlin.

Borde, T., Braun, T., & David, M. (2009). Unterschiede in der Inanspruchnahme klinischer Notfallambulanzen durch deutsche Patient/innen und Migrant/innen. Berlin: Schlussbericht.

Borde, T., David, M., & Kentenich, H. (Hg.). (2000). Migration - Frauen - Gesundheit. Perspektiven im europäischen Kontext. Frankfurt am Main: Mabuse.

Bundesagentur für Arbeit. (2004). Begriff der Arbeitslosigkeit in der Statistik unter SGB II und SGB III. Online verfügbar unter https://statistik.arbeitsagentur.de/Statischer-Content/Grundlagen/Statistik-SGBII-SGBIII/Generische-Publikationen/Arbeitslosenbegriff-unter-SGBII-und-SGBIII.pdf

Bundesagentur für Arbeit. (2014). Arbeitsmarktberichterstattung, Juni 2014. Der Arbeitsmarkt in Deutschland—Menschen mit Migrationshintergrund auf dem deutschen Arbeitsmarkt. Nürnberg. Online verfügbar unter http://statistik.arbeitsagentur.de/Statischer-Content/Arbeitsmarktberichte/Personengruppen/generische-Publikationen/Broschuere-Migranten-2014-07.pdf

Bundesamt für Migration und Flüchtlinge (BAMF). (2014). Das Bundesamt in Zahlen 2013. *Asyl, Migration und Integration*, Nürnberg. July, 2014. Retrieved from www.iaf-bremen.de/files/bundesamt-in-zahlen-2013.pdf

Bundesministerium der Justiz und für Verbraucherschutz. (2008). Residence Act in the version promulgated on 25 February 2008. *Act on the Residence, Economic Activity and Integration of Foreigners in the Federal Territory Residence Act*. Retrieved from http://www.gesetze-im-internet.de/englisch_aufenthg/englisch_aufenthg.html#p1122

Bundesministerium des Innern. (2007). Illegal aufhältige Migranten in Deutschland. Datenlage, Rechtslage, Handlungsoptionen. Bericht des Bundesministeriums des Innern zum Prüfauftrag "Illegalität" aus der Koalitionsvereinbarung. November 11, 2005. Kapitel VIII 1.2. Berlin.

Bundesministerium für Arbeit und Soziales. (2014). Lebenslagen in Deutschland. Armuts- und Reichtumsberichterstattung der Bundesregierung. Der Vierte Armuts- und Reichtumsbericht der Bundesregierung, Berlin.

Bundesministerium für Familie, Senioren, Frauen und Jugend. (2007). Der Mikrozensus im Schnittpunkt von Geschlecht und Migration. Möglichkeiten und Grenzen einer sekundär-analytischen Auswertung des Mikrozensus 2005. Berlin.

Bundeszentrale für gesundheitliche Aufklärung. (2009). Gesundheitsförderung konkret. Band 12: Migration und Gesundheitsförderung. Köln.

Butterwegge, C. (2013a). Krise und Zukunft des Sozialstaats. 5. Aufl. Wiesbaden.

Butterwegge, C. (2013b). 10 Jahre Agenda 2010. Auf dem Weg nach unten. In *Süddeutsche Zeitung*. Online verfügbar unter http://www.sueddeutsche.de/politik/zehn-jahre-agenda-auf-dem-weg-nach-unten-1.1638856.

Butterwegge, C. (2014). *Hartz IV und die Folgen. Auf dem Weg in eine andere Republik?* Weinheim: Beltz Juventa.

Collatz, J., Kürsat-Ahlers, E., & Korporal, I. (Hg.). (1985). Gesundheit für alle. Die medizinische Versorgung türkischer Familien in der Bundesrepublik. Hamburg.

Datenreport. (2013). Ein Sozialbericht für Deutschland (hg. vom Wissenschaftszentrum Berlin für Sozialforschung und vom Statistischen Bundesamt), Berlin.

Decker, O., Kiess, J., & Brähler, E. (2012). Die Mitte im Umbruch. Rechtsextreme Einstellungen in Deutschland 2012. Bonn: Verlag J. H. W. Dietz Nachf. Online verfügbar unter http://www.fes-gegen-rechtsextremismus.de/pdf_12/mitte-im-umbruch_www.pdf

Deutscher Bundestag. (2002, November 5). Gesetzentwurf der Fraktionen der SPD und Bündnis 90 / Die Grünen. Entwurf eines ersten Gesetzes für moderne Dienstleistungen am Arbeitsmarkt. Drucksache 15/25.

Deutsches Rotes Kreuz. (2013). Gesundheitsversorgung für EU-Bürgerinnen und EU-Bürger in Deutschland. Handreichung zu den rechtlichen Grundlagen, Berlin.

Federal Ministry of the Interior. (2016). Migration and integration. Retrieved from http://www.bmi.bund.de/EN/Topics/Migration-Integration/migration-integration_node.html

Frings, Dorothee. (2012). Sozialleistungen für Unionsbürger/innen nach der VO 883/2004.

Gesundheitsamt der Stadt Nürnberg. (1997). Stadtteilgesundheitsbericht Gostenhof. Zur Gesundheit von Kindern und Jugendlichen. Nürnberg.

Götsch, A. (2005, March 8). Illegale Einwanderer: Ohne Papiere—aber immer mit Fahrschein, in: *Spiegel-Online.*

Gräf, C. (2014, February 6). Bloß nicht krank werden. In *Süddeutsche Zeitung.*

Heitmeyer, Wilhelm. (Hg.). (2008). Deutsche Zustände. Folge 7. Frankfurt am Main: Suhrkamp Verlag.

Hentges, G., & Staszczak, J. (2010). Geduldet, nicht erwünscht. Auswirkungen der Bleiberechtsregelung auf die Lebenssituation geduldeter Flüchtlinge in Deutschland, Stuttgart.

Höhne, A., & Schubert, M. (2010). Vom Healthy-Migrant-Effekt zur gesundheitsbedingen Frühberentung. Erwerbsminderungsrenten bei Migranten in Deutschland. *DRV-Schriften* (55), S. 103–126.

Knipper, M. & Bilgin, Y. (2009). *Migration und Gesundheit.* (Ed. Konrad Adenauer Stiftung; Türkisch Deutsche Gesundheitsstiftung). Sankt Augustin/Berlin: Konrad-Adenauer-Stiftung.

Kohls, M. (2008). Erfassungsfehler, Healthy-Migrant-Effect und andere Schwierigkeiten bei der Analyse der Mortalität von Migranten - Eine Bestandsaufnahme. Nürnberg.

Kohls, M. (2011). Morbidität und Mortalität von Migranten in Deutschland. Nürnberg.

Krankenkassen, Deutschland. (2016). Health insurance. Retrieved from https://www.krankenkassen.de/

Loerzer, S. (2012, August 12). Wenn die Armut sichtbar wird. In *Süddeutsche Zeitung.*

Malteser Migranten Medizin. (2016). Malteser Migranten Medizin. Retrieved from http://www.malteser-migranten-medizin.de/startseite.html

Mehle, J. (1981). Evaluation der deutschsprachigen medizinischen Literatur von 1962 bis 1979 über die Epidemiologie und die Konfliktfelder im Gesundheitsverhalten ausländischer Arbeitnehmer in der Bundesrepublik. Dissertation an der Universität Bochum. Bochum.

Razum, O. (2006). Migration, Mortalität und der Healthy-migrant-Effekt. In M. Richter & K. Hurrelmann (Eds.): Gesundheitliche Ungleichheit. Grundlagen—Probleme—Perspektiven (pp.250–270). Wiesbaden: VS-Verlag.

Richter, M., & Hurrelmann, K. (Hg.). (2006a). Gesundheitliche Ungleichheit. Grundlagen—Probleme—Perspektiven. Wiesbaden: VS-Verlag.

Richter, M., & Hurrelmann, K. (2006b). Gesundheitliche Ungleichheit: Ausgangsfragen und Herausforderungen. In M. Richter & K. Hurrelmann (Eds.), Gesundheitliche Ungleichheit. Grundlagen—Probleme—Perspektiven (pp.11–31). Wiesbaden: VS-Verlag.

Robert Koch-Institut & Bundeszentrale für gesundheitliche Aufklärung. (2008). Erkennen—Bewerten—Handeln. Zur Gesundheit von Kindern und Jugendlichen in Deutschland. Berlin.

Robert Koch-Institut & Statistisches Bundesamt. (2008). *Migration und Gesundheit. Schwerpunktbericht der Berichterstattung des Bundes.* Berlin: Robert Koch-Institut. Retrieved from http://www.rki.de/DE/Content/Gesundheitsmonitoring/Gesundheitsberichterstattung/GBEDownloadsT/migration.pdf?__blob=publicationFile

Seidel-Pielen, E. (1998). *Unsere Türken. Annäherungen an ein gespaltenes Verhältnis.* Berlin: Espresso/Elefanten Press.

Sinn, A., Kreienbrink, A., & von Loeffelholz, H. (2006). *Illegal aufhältige Drittstaatsangehörige in Deutschland.* Nürnberg.

Stadt Bielefeld. (2004). *Gesundheitliche Lage & Versorgung von Migrantinnen & Migranten.* Bielefeld.

Straubhaar, Thomas. (2007). Illegale Migration. Eine ökonomische Perspektive. *Politische Essays zu Migration und Integration,* (3). 1–13.

Szent-Ivanyi, T. (2014, September 23). 80.000 Menschen ohne Krankenversicherung. *Berliner Zeitung.*

Theilen, I. (1985). Überwindung der Sprachlosigkeit türkischer Patienten in der Bundesrepublik Deutschland. Versuch einer ganzheitlichen Medizin als Beitrag zur transkulturellen Therapie. In J. Collatz, E. Kürsat-Ahlers, & I. Korporal (Eds.), *Gesundheit für alle. Die medizinische Versorgung türkischer Familien in der Bundesrepublik* (pp.292–322). Hamburg: ebv Rissen.

Yildirim-Fahlbusch, Y. (2003). Kulturelle Missverständnisse (Türkische Migranten). *Deutsches Ärzteblatt* (5); 100 (18): A-1179 / B-993 / C-928.

Legislation Cited

Act on the Residence, Economic Activity and Integration of Foreigners in the Federal Territory (Residence Act in the version promulgated on February 25, 2008) (Federal Law Gazette I p. 162), last amended by Article 3 of the Act of September 6, 2013 (Federal Law Gazette I p. 3556)—Gesetz über den Aufenthalt, die Erwerbstätigkeit und die Integration von Ausländern im Bundesgebiet. Aufenthaltsgesetz.

Asylum-Seekers' Benefits Act (AsylbLG).

UNHCR-Position zur Diskussion um ein Bleiberecht für geduldete Ausländer in Deutschland, November, 2006.

Nordic Nations: Can the State Provide Equity for All?

Public Policy, Immigrant Experiences, and Health Outcomes in Denmark

Romana Careja and Heidi Vad Jønsson

Chapter Objectives

This chapter discusses on Denmark's immigration and integration policies, with a focus on immigrants' health issues. The objectives of this chapter are:

- to introduce immigrant integration outcomes in present-day Denmark;
- to present immigration policies in Denmark, with emphasis on developments since 1990;
- to review evidence concerning key aspects of immigrants' health status; and
- to discuss the relationship between immigrants' integration and access to health care.

Introduction

"Nobody wants to do research on immigrants' health."

—Allan Krasnik[1]

There is little discussion about **immigrants'** health in the Danish public sphere and few health policy measures have been adopted to address immigrant-related problems. This does not mean that Allan Krasnik's provocative statement is true. On the contrary, the health research community has long recognized that immigrants in Denmark face specific challenges when it comes to their health and their interactions with the Danish health system. In the last decade the number of studies focusing on immigrants' health has increased.

Over the last 50 years Denmark has become the home of a relatively large immigrant community. Although resisted by some political groups, these immigrants have become part and parcel of society. Several reforms have been passed to regulate **immigration** as well as **integration** over the last couple of decades. As it will be shown, the reforms have increasingly restricted immigrants' access to welfare benefits, and have attempted to limit opportunities to enter Denmark through a few well-managed channels. In this process, immigrants' health has been less of a concern as compared to issues such as employment, culture, and recently national security (Jønsson, forthcoming). However, immigrants' health is particularly important because they are exposed to significant health risks in the migration process itself, they may differ in their disease profiles as compared to the non-migrant population, and immigrants may also experience barriers to accessing health services in their new country, thereby affecting their overall post-migration health status.

Understanding these issues is of utmost importance for several reasons. First and foremost, integration and health policies can be adjusted to cope better with immigrants' reality. Secondly, improving immigrants' health is crucial since poor health can have a negative impact on immigrants' ability to interact with mainstream society and thus may limit their integration in their new home. Last but not least, improving the access to health and thus increasing health access equity is an important policy objective in itself as a means of reducing inequalities and tackling social exclusion at the European Union (EU) level, a goal recognized and thus promoted by EU member states.

This chapter begins by discussing the context of immigration in Denmark, immigrants' current status and integration outcomes, followed by a brief presentation of immigration and integration policies. Thereafter, a description of the health care system and various health policies are presented. The last part reviews the health status of immigrants and the health-related problems that have been identified. The conclusion will consider how the Danish welfare state is responding to immigrants' health needs.

Patterns of Immigration and Integration

According to Statistics Denmark, at the end of 2014 the immigrant population[2] comprised 653,041 people, of whom 233,484 were immigrants from Western countries and 419,557 from non-Western countries. Currently, the immigrant population makes up 11.5 percent of the total Danish population. Immigrants arrive in Denmark as labour immigrants, asylum-seekers, or as reunited family members. Over the last several years all immigrant categories have registered an increasing trend, as shown in Table 9.1. Of course, illegal immigration and human trafficking also occur, but these figures are difficult to estimate.

Immigrant integration has become an increasing concern for Danish politicians, academics, and public administrators alike, especially as gaps in many important indicators of societal participation have emerged among immigrants, especially between those coming from non-Western Europe and native Danes (Liebig, 2007). In the following, the most important aspects of these gaps are presented.

Table 9.1: Residence Permits Granted, by Region of Origin, Year, and Category of Entry

	2006	2007	2008	2009	2010	2011	2012	2013	2014
Western countries									
Asylum	0	0	0	0	0	4	3	0	0
Family	2,378	3,385	4,936	3,746	3,379	3,244	3,689	3,589	3,969
Education	9,340	9,398	10,571	11,491	12,133	11,635	12,287	13,155	13,488
Work	15,971	20,625	24,194	12,886	12,195	12,915	14,485	16,009	18,489
Other reasons	1,617	1,380	1,385	1,758	2,597	3,427	4,018	4,288	4,704
Non-Western countries									
Asylum	1,095	1,278	1,453	1,376	2,124	2,245	2,580	3,889	6,110
Family	3,140	4,050	3,586	4,557	4,881	3,195	3,420	5,406	6,157
Education	7,380	9,606	11,846	9,471	8,684	7,949	7,569	7,818	8,273
Work	3,129	5,347	6,281	7,301	9,216	8,147	7,702	10,261	10,891
Other reasons	356	422	390	459	399	218	228	147	253

Source: Authors' calculations, data from Statistics Denmark

Labour Market Participation

Immigrants' participation in the labour market is significantly lower than that of Danes.[3] However, the immigrant group is not homogeneous. For example, country of origin plays an important role in explaining labour market performance. As Figure 9.1 illustrates, the gap between the employment rates of immigrants and their descendants and the employment rates of native Danes is higher for non-Western immigrants than for Western immigrants. Gender, too, makes a difference. Women of immigrant background are less educated and have higher unemployment rates than both male immigrants and women with Danish citizenship, both natives and naturalized immigrants (Jønsson, 2014; Bievelander et al., 2013). Figure 9.2 illustrates the worrying situation of young people: among those younger than 24, both male and female immigrants who are neither in school nor in the workforce are much more numerous than their corresponding Danish peers. Numerous immigrants turn to self-employment, but in spite of long hours and hard work, self-employed immigrants usually earn less than Danes in comparable positions, and also compared to Danes in regular employment.

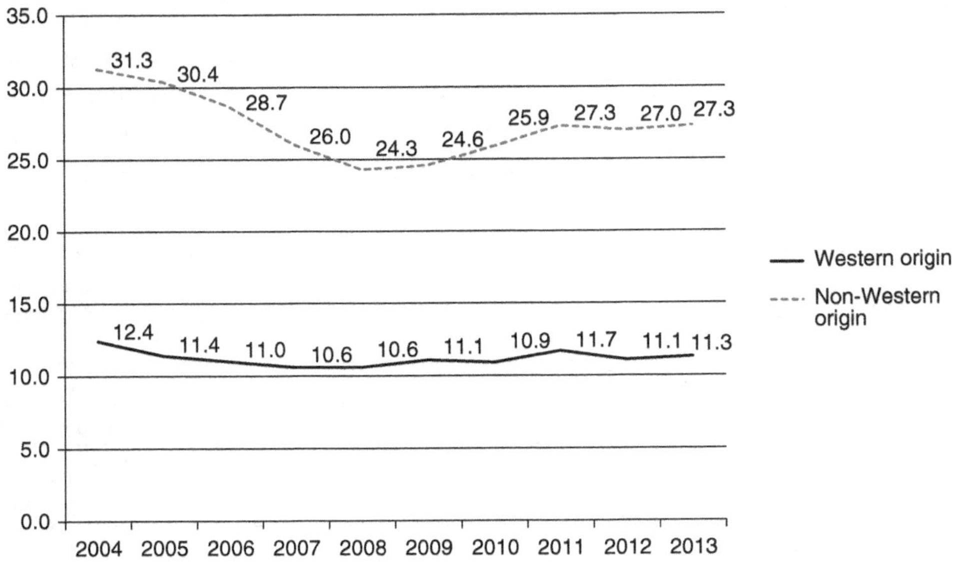

Figure 9.1: Employment Gap between Non-Western Immigrants and Native Danes, Compared to the Employment Gap between Western Immigrants and Native Danes

Note: The *y*-axis indicates the difference between different categories of immigrants and native Danes.

Source: Ministry of Children, Gender Equality, Integration and Social Affairs, *Fact Sheet: Immigrants and Descendants*. Retrieved from http://sm.dk/publikationer/fact-sheet-immigrants-and-descendants

Education

Immigrants also differ from native Danes in their distribution of educational achievement. For example, almost 50 percent of immigrants have only basic education, while only 33 percent of native Danes are so educated. At the other end of the spectrum, rates of tertiary education are similar between migrants and natives. However, good education translates into corresponding jobs only for roughly half of these highly educated migrants, due in particular to absence of language skills and the difficulty in assessing quality of foreign education/diplomas (Pohl Nielsen, 2007). Discrimination might also play a role. The situation is better for immigrants who have arrived at younger ages and for descendants of immigrants who are born in Denmark. This is probably because they enter the Danish education system at earlier ages. Although they are more likely to continue education after the compulsory nine years, their participation rates in the labour force remain below those of native Danes (Roseveare & Jorgensen, 2004).

Discrimination

Although notoriously difficult to measure objectively (T. G. Jensen et al., 2010), there is little doubt that immigrants experience discrimination in the labour market (Liebig, 2007) and in other social interactions such as membership in various associations, school boards, and other activities that are defined under the category "active citizenship" (see Integrationsbarometeret, www.integrations-barometer.dk), as well as in their experiences with the justice system (Holmberg & Kyvsgaard, 2003). As to what effects discrimination may have on immigrants, there are no definitive answers. Some studies find the experience of discrimination does not affect generalized trust (Thysted Dinesen, 2010), while others find it may lead to mental problems and failure in social adaptation (Montgomery & Foldspang, 2007).

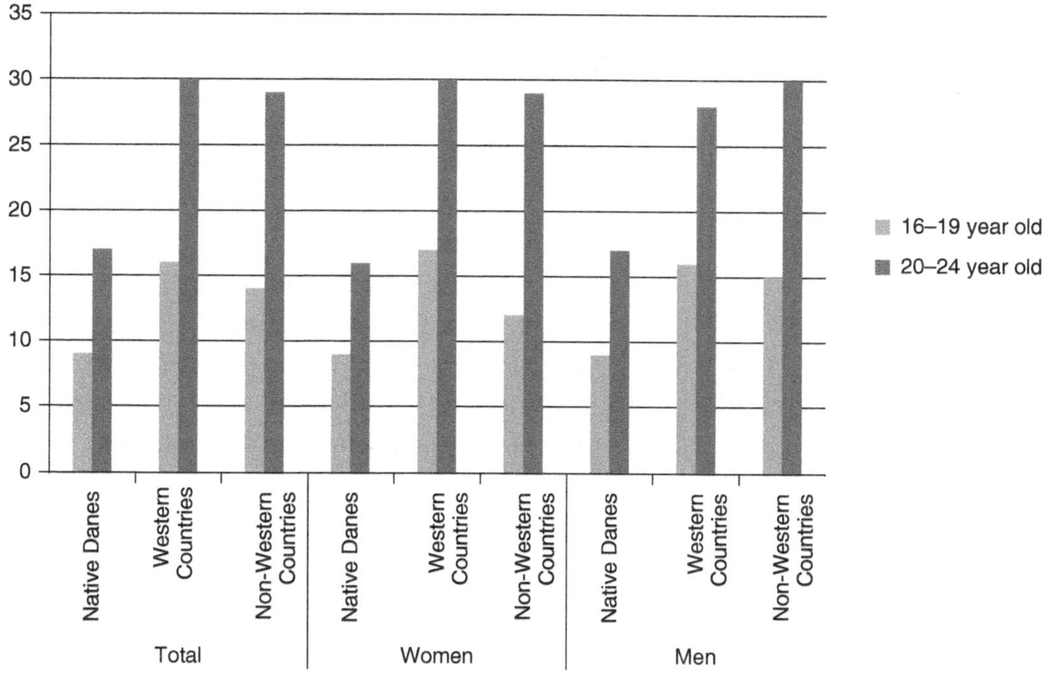

Figure 9.2: Percentage of Young People Not in Education and Not Employed, Comparison between Immigrants and Native Danes

Source: Calculation based on data from Ankestyrelsen (2015) *Integration: Status Og Udvikling 2014*. For further statistical information, see also Ministry of Children, Gender Equality, Integration and Social Affairs, *Fact sheet: Immigrants and descendants*. Retrieved from http://sm.dk/publikationer/fact-sheet-immigrants-and-descendants

Social Mobility and Poverty

Immigrants are likely to experience poverty. A panel study has shown that since the mid-1980s, the poverty rate among non-Western immigrants has increased from about 30 percent to 50 percent and stabilized at this high level from the mid-1990s to the present (Pedersen, 2011). The consequence of this sharp increase has been many immigrants' continued dependence on welfare benefits. Among other things, living in poverty has negatively affected immigrants' social mobility, which has been very limited. A few studies have shown that some immigrants focus on achievement in sports-related activities (Agergaard & Kahr Soerensen, 2009), while others prefer educational achievement (Moldenhawer, 2005) as a means of improving their social and economic status.

Immigrants' weak socio-economic positions in Danish society, coupled with evidence of few opportunities for improvement, have generated calls for more responsive integration policies to address these problems. This has been the case particularly over the last three decades. Therefore, recent reforms have been built around the goal of having immigrants develop skills to facilitate their labour market integration, thereby reducing their dependence of welfare assistance. The next section briefly presents Danish immigration and integration policies in the 1990s and 2000s.

Immigration and Integration Policies in Denmark

Until the 1950s Denmark was a net emigration country with more leaving than entering. However, in the aftermath of the Second World War, labour demand increased, and, over the next two decades, Denmark received a steady flow of labour immigrants, mainly from Turkey and Yugoslavia. The scale of immigration remained, however, much lower than in other European countries. During this period, immigration was regulated by the Aliens Act. Until 1973, this Act left much room for flexibility in interpreting regulations for the institutions managing immigration. As a result, immigrants were able to easily obtain labour permits. Similarly to other Western European countries, Denmark ended labour immigration in 1973 in reaction to the economic crisis prompted by the first oil crisis. However, immigration was allowed to continue for family reunification and asylum-seekers (Liebig, 2007).

The Aliens Act has since remained in effect, but has had numerous changes over time, with major modifications in 1983, 1998, 2002, and 2006. The 1983 reform aimed to improve immigrants' legal status and extended the right to family reunification to parents above the age of 60. It also specified the grounds for expulsion and broadened the category of **refugees** by introducing the de facto refugee concept.[4]

Over time, however, the liberal 1983 Aliens Act became more restrictive. The principle of legal claims and provision of a temporary residence permit for a certain number of years were maintained, but the requirements for gaining a residence permit were changed several times. In 1992 temporary residence permits were extended from two to three years, but the passing of the Integration Act in 1998 required active participation in an individual integration program as a requirement for obtaining a permanent residence permit. Additionally, in 1992 the family reunification right was granted only to immigrants who had resided in Denmark for at least five years.

The first Integration Act institutionalized integration of immigrants as a new pillar in the Danish welfare policy. This move is important in two aspects. First, it officially recognized the need to promote immigrants' integration in Danish society and, second, it specifically identified Denmark's welfare state as a means through which this integration could be achieved.

Denmark's Social Democratic welfare system emphasizes equality between individuals in terms of social rights. An often-referred to example of the Nordic model, the Danish welfare state is funded through taxes and is very generous, especially in comparison with the Liberal and Conservative **welfare state regimes** (Esping-Andersen, 1990). Access to welfare benefits has historically been granted on the basis of legal residency, not of citizenship. This is of particular relevance for immigrants, who, on the basis of their legal right to reside in the territory of Denmark, have had access to a large array of services that include social support as well as child and family benefits. As we will show in the next section, immigrants' access to benefits has been significantly curtailed since 1998.

The 1998 Integration Act included two main aspects. First, a quota-based housing system was designed to limit the formation of clusters of immigrants (mainly refugees) in some municipalities. Second, an integration program was instituted that required lessons in the Danish language, education on various social issues, and labour market participation[5] over a three-year period. Those immigrants who participated in the program received an "Introduction Benefit," which replaced the social assistance benefits. However, the former amounted to only a fraction of the latter.

An important consequence of these reforms was the creation of an entirely new policy area focused on managing immigrants and asylum-seekers. Prior to 1998, responsibility for integrating newcomers had been divided between state-funded private organizations, such as Danish Refugee Aid, and individual municipalities. Since 1998 this policy area has developed its own logic and mechanisms, where the goals and means are defined at the national level and the municipalities are held responsible for implementation (Jønsson, 2014).

The increased concern with the immigrants' situation led to the 2001 national electoral campaign, which was extensively focused on immigrants and their integration. The Danish People's Party argued forcefully that Denmark was not and should not ever be a multicultural society. The liberal and conservative parties espoused the positions that Danish immigration policy should be more restrictive. The election resulted in a change of government. The Social Democratic Party was replaced by a coalition of liberal and conservative parties that received parliamentary support from the Danish People's Party.

In the following decade, immigration issues were frequently debated in Parliament and the Aliens Act was changed several times, with every change leading to imposition of more restrictions (Green-Pedersen, 2012; Jønsson, 2014). The family reunification and family formation as entry channels became more restrictive (Careja, Emmenegger, & Kvist, 2015), and the "temporary protected status" was introduced as a legal category to deal with asylum-seekers whose applications were rejected, but who could not be deported.

The eligibility for social assistance became conditional on a minimum residence period of seven years, which in effect meant that many newly arrived immigrants were denied social assistance. The amount of the Introduction Benefit was reduced greatly in comparison to the social assistance benefits, which previously were available to immigrants. Newly arrived immigrants, who did not qualify for the Introduction Benefit, were granted New Start assistance, which was also significantly lower than social assistance.

Since the mid-2000s, this restrictive immigration policy was complemented with an opening of the Danish labour market for highly skilled immigrants. All subsequent changes were aimed at simultaneously attracting immigrants who, due to education and employment possibilities, were expected to be economic assets, while limiting entry to those immigrants and refugees expected to have high risk of unemployment. It was assumed that this latter group of immigrants were more difficult to integrate in Danish society and therefore would be a burden on its welfare system (Roseveare & Jorgensen, 2004; Liebig, 2007; Kvist, 2004).

The election of a left-leaning government in 2011, formed by the Social Democratic Party, Social Liberal Party, and Socialist People's Party, has led to the reversal of some of the restrictive measures of the previous government; however, many remained in effect. The point system that made family reunification conditional on the acquisition of more than 60 points, virtually limiting family reunification to those who could show good job qualifications and language skills, was changed to a more relaxed system. Other restrictive regulations were maintained and even strengthened, such as the 24-year rule, which means that family reunification is possible only for a married couple when both spouses are over 24 years old, and the attachment rule, which requires the couple to demonstrate a stronger attachment to Denmark than to another country (Jønsson, 2014). For an overview of other measures, see Careja, Emmenegger, and Kvist (2004).

This restrictive trend, which apparently contrasts with the basic tenets of the Danish social democratic welfare state, has been explained in relation to several factors. One key factor is the electoral success of the Danish People's Party, which placed it in a pivotal position, especially after 2001. However, several other larger contextual factors have played a role. First, the number of people entering through asylum and family reunification channels increased at the end of the 1990s. Second, the eastward enlargement of the European Union since the mid-1990s has always been regarded as a potential threat to the viability of the Danish welfare state (Kvist, 2004). Third, numerous studies that have calculated the costs and benefits of immigrants to Danish society often portray immigrants as a strain upon, rather than a contributor to, the welfare system (Nannestad, 2004).

Also important is how the logic of labour market participation and workfare has taken priority in Danish integration approaches. Currently, immigrant integration in Denmark is subordinate to the notion that labour market integration is of foremost importance (Tranæs & Zimmermann, 2004). This integration program offered to all newly arrived immigrants lasts a maximum of three years and includes opportunities and obligations to learn Danish and to enter the education system or labour market training. The intensive introduction program is provided by local municipalities and is tailored to the individual. The aim is to have immigrants find paid work by the end of the three-year period (Liebig, 2007). The efficacy of these measures remains to be conclusively proven. There are concerns that although language skills have a significant impact on immigrants' ability to find work (Clausen et al., 2008), and although immigrants who have taken part in these introduction courses usually find employment (Liebig, 2007), the quality of the jobs is often not enough to lift people over the poverty line or to prevent social exclusion (Brodmann & Polavieja, 2011; Liebig, 2007; Blume et al., 2003).

Health Care System, Outcomes, and Policies

Access to Health Care

Denmark boasts a universal health system financed though taxes. Most health services such as visits to general practitioners, private practice specialists, or hospital treatment are free at point of contact. Dental treatment and medicines, however, require patients to pay part of the costs. Each municipality automatically issues a health insurance card to every person officially registered as the municipality's resident. The card entitles the holder to receive medical services and must be presented at each visit to the doctor (Jensen et al., 2011; Petersen, 2014).

This procedure gives automatic access to the heath system to all legal residents. In the case of immigrants, this includes the categories of accepted asylum-seekers, family reunification, and labour migrants. A recent 2013 amendment to the Integration Act obliges municipalities to offer "an integration plan for newly arrived refugees and persons involving family reunification cases as well as *medical screening for newly arrived refugees and their family members*. Medical screenings, carried out by family doctors, are activated as early as possible to provide adequate health treatment or social measures that would support successful integration of migrants and their family" (EMN, 2013, p. 1; emphasis added). By singling out asylum-seekers, this new procedure indicates that the Danish authorities have identified them as the category most likely to need support on health issues and closer observation. All the other categories are considered well served by the current system.

The asylum-seekers in reception centres are in a category of their own. They have the right to health care and dental care, and health services are provided by health practitioners in the reception centres. The expenses are covered by the Immigration Service "if the treatment is to relieve pain or if the treatment cannot be postponed because there is a risk of permanent injury, development or progression of a condition, or a risk that a condition may become chronic" (Danish Refugee Council, n.d., p. 7).

However, the question of access to health services for people not recognized as legal residents, such as illegal and undocumented migrants, remains open. Denmark is a signatory of several international conventions proclaiming the individual's right to health. This is a basic human right, and therefore it is considered the duty of medical personnel to provide the best possible care for patients, even if they have no documents or provide false identities (Hansen, Krasnik, & Høg, 2007). At the same time, however, the policies that regulate the access of aliens without residence permit to health care are limited and/or contradictory (Hansen, Krasnik, & Høg, 2007). For example, the only explicit reference to this topic is in the Aliens Consolidation Act, whose section § 42a states that undocumented migrants registered with the authorities and residing in an asylum centre will acquire rights to health care on the same terms as asylum-seekers (Jensen et al., 2011). If a person registers with the authorities and lives in an asylum centre, the Danish Immigration Service is obliged to notify the police about where the person is staying. According to Hansen and colleagues, "the Aliens Consolidation Act conditions access to health care for undocumented immigrants upon their immigration status. This means discriminatory practice based on their group identity as undocumented immigrants as opposed to the rest of the population" (Hansen, Krasnik, & Høg, 2007, p. 51). More importantly, however, this regulation indicates that undocumented immigrants not registered at an asylum centre have no "official" access to health care, which thus remains a completely informal process. In this informal process, health care professionals are caught between their professional oath and uncertainties about rules (Hansen, Krasnik, & Høg, 2007; Jensen et al., 2011).

Health Outcomes

It is likely that the explicit concern with asylum-seekers is related to the results from numerous studies indicating that refugees and asylum-seekers are at high risk for health problems. Despite this recognition, policy-makers and medical practitioners in Denmark have only recently become interested in systematically studying the health status of immigrants and assessing its causes, mechanisms, and implications. The health research is limited by the fact that non-Western immigrants are either not included in national health surveys or when they are, the samples include too few immigrants to produce meaningful generalizations (Andersen et al., 2008). However, the availability of registration data on immigration status that can be merged through unique personal registration numbers with health data (Nørredam et al., 2014) has produced useful insights into the differences between different immigrant categories, and between immigrants and native Danes (Sundhedsstyrelsen, 2005; Holmberg et al., 2009).

Use of Health Services

Several studies have mapped the use of health services by ethnic groups and entry categories. They found that, compared to native-born Danes, immigrants from non-Western countries use at least the same or more emergency services (Folmann & Jørgensen, 2006), while immigrants from European countries use them less (Nørredam et al., 2004). Both refugees and labour immigrants have higher health service (hospital and GP) usage than native-born Danes (Dyhr et al., 2007). Some studies have proposed that lower morbidity for certain ages and groups of immigrants (Rutle & Steihaug, 1997, cited in Dyhr et al., 2007) and socio-economic factors are likely determinants of the observed patterns. For example, immigrants may use emergency services more because they lack knowledge about the primary-care opportunities; are concerned that language barriers might limit good communication with the primary-care doctors; are afraid of being discriminated against; or because their previous experiences with primary care have been unpleasant (Nørredam et al., 2004). Unfortunately, due to lack of survey data, these factors currently remain more speculative than empirically proven.

Morbidity and Mortality

Overall, immigrants report poor health more often than native Danes (Dinesen et al., 2011). Immigrants are more at risk when it comes to illnesses as diverse as coronary heart disease (Bo et al., 2014) and vitamin D deficiency (Andersen et al., 2008). With regard to mortality during early ages, Villadsen and colleagues (2009) found stillbirths and infant mortality rates are higher among immigrants than among native Danes. Since socio-economic characteristics did not explain their findings, the authors conclude that ethnicity serves as a marker of risk than as a risk factor per se in the sense that ethnicity is an indicator of other individual characteristics that may play a role in adverse health outcomes.

Sunby and Petersen's (2003) study shows that occurrence of illnesses also depends on health-related attitudes. Among children between three and seven years of age in Copenhagen, children of immigrants had poorer oral hygiene than children of native Danes. Interviews with parents indicated that this was due to both higher consumption of sugary products and parents' attitudes toward oral hygiene.

While many studies find health differences between native Danes and immigrants, the study of Andersen et al. (2008) found no such differences among residents of a deprived neighbourhood. The authors argue that this result only apparently contradicts the previous studies. More precisely, they argue that the previously observed differences are due to the fact that immigrants are compared to average Danes, who are likely to have more economic and social resources than average immigrants. However, because the self-reported health status varies with the amount of economic and social resources individuals and families have, when immigrants are compared to Danes with similar life resources, these differences disappear.

Mental Health

Bancila et al. (2012) and Bancila and Singhamer (2013) have found that stress is higher among immigrants than Danes. The risk of anxiety is two to four times higher among non-Western immigrants than among native Danes (Singhammer, 2008). When mental stress is compared across gender and ethnic groups, women show increased stress risk. The authors argue that the pattern of stress risk indicates that socio-economic characteristics are not enough to explain the differences, but life circumstances may play a role. This is confirmed by research on asylum-seekers and refugees (Masmas et al., 2008), which finds that mental disorders are affected by duration of stay in asylum reception centres (Hallas et al., 2007; Vitus & Smith-Nielsen, 2011) and experiences outside the reception centres (Cantor-Graae et al., 2003; Cantor-Graae & Selten, 2005).

Effects of Policies and Medical Practice on Immigrants' Health

The effects of health care–related policies on immigrants' health have not been directly researched. However, they can be indirectly assessed by exploring health care practitioners' opinions about the existing issues the health system faces when dealing with immigrants, issues that may have an impact on immigrants' health risks and professionals' ability to provide diagnosis and treatment. Several factors have been identified as problematic and in need of improvement.

Cultural Differences and Mutual Knowledge

The health system has difficulties in dealing with cultural differences that affect both patients and medical personnel (Jønsson, forthcoming). On one hand, immigrant patients appear to have different understandings of illnesses and treatment than service providers. Cultural variation in perception of illness has led to late referrals to doctors and/or reluctance to follow recommended treatments (Vinter-Jensen, 2010; Folmann & Jørgensen, 2006). On the other hand, doctors' lack of information about their patients and limited time for consultations led doctors to misunderstand patients' attitudes and behaviours, resulting in risk for misdiagnosis.

In order to deal with these effects of cultural differences, specialized clinics for immigrant patients have been suggested as a solution. There has been such a clinic at Odense University Hospital since 2008, and it was set up as an experiment to investigate whether specialized interaction with immigrant patients improves diagnosis and treatment. The five-year evaluation of the program concluded that the procedures at the clinic had positive results (Sodermann et al., 2013).

Language

Linked to cultural differences, immigrants' limited ability to speak Danish is overwhelmingly seen as a major barrier for access to health care. This has been the case since the 1970s, when communication problems led to the death of three infants of immigrant parents. Due to limited language skills, immigrants avoid going to the doctor, and, when they do, they have problems in effectively communicating their symptoms or in understanding treatment options provided to them (Priebe, 2011; Michaelesen et al., 2004; N. K. Jensen et al., 2010).

Since the 1970s, the practical solution to this problem has been the use of free translation services provided by the state. The cases where professional interpreters have mediated communication between health care professionals and immigrant patients have been unanimously identified as a good practice with significant results. These positive results correlate with provision of translations that are accurate not only linguistically, but also medically. In this context, the November 2010 decision to stop the provision of free interpretation services for immigrants who have lived in Denmark for more than seven years (with exception of very specific circumstances) (N. K. Jensen et al., 2010) raised numerous questions from the medical community. Under the new rule, these immigrants were offered interpretation services, provided they paid a fee. Following the implementation of this measure, immigrants resorted to using relatives as translators. This is considered a suboptimal solution, which presents increased risk of misdiagnosis (N. K. Jensen et al., 2010). Under vocal protests from health care professionals, concerned with its potential negative effects, the rule was reversed.

Limited Information

In addition to these cultural and language barriers, medical care specialists emphasize that often they miss relevant information about their patients and their environment (medical history, living conditions, family-related problems).

Currently, there is only limited co-operation with institutions concerned with immigrants, such as social services that can provide the relevant missing information (Priebe et al., 2011; N. K. Jensen et al., 2010; Sodermann, 2013). Therefore, there is plenty of room for improvement in this respect.

Regulatory Environment

Health care professionals are unanimous that the lack of a clear regulatory environment in relation to health care provision to undocumented immigrants has a negative effect on their ability to provide the best possible treatment (Hansen, Krasnik, & Høg, 2007; Jensen et al., 2011). Currently, no solution has been implemented.

Discussion

At the beginning of the chapter we emphasized three reasons why assessment of the health status of immigrants is important. We now discuss these in light of the presented evidence.

Integration and Health Policies Can Be Adjusted to Cope Better with Immigrants' Realities

Although the extent of immigrants' health-related difficulties is hard to know with precision due to specific challenges associated with investigating immigrants, the evidence reviewed in this chapter indicates that compared to native Danes, immigrants not only have inadequate economic and social resources, but are also in poorer health. Some categories of immigrants, such as asylum-seekers, have significantly more health problems, which are also likely to be of longer duration, such as mental health problems.

Currently there is little evidence that the knowledge accumulated by practitioners is being translated into health policy measures. With exception of the 2013 amendment requiring municipalities to enact health screenings of asylum-seekers' families, which implicitly recognizes the long-term problems of this group, we are not aware of other proactive measures targeting immigrants' health. Moreover, the limited communication between the health system and the relevant components of the welfare system not only deprives doctors of relevant information, but also hampers the ability to tailor integration policies to these target groups. Currently, integration policies in Denmark overwhelmingly focus on building labour market skills. However, in absence of support for coping with the physical and mental stress generated by the migration process, immigrants may not be able to take full advantage of the opportunities offered.

Improving Immigrants' Health Can Be Crucial Since Poor Health Can Have a Negative Impact on Immigrants' Ability to Interact with Mainstream Society and May Limit Their Ability to Integrate

Unlike the United States or Canada (Vineberg, 2015), Denmark has never in its history implemented measures to assess immigrants' and refugees' health status. This suggests that Danish governments have not considered health as a potential impediment to immigrants' integration and ability to contribute to Danish society. The only mention of health in the Aliens Act is a paragraph that allows for the possibility of expelling immigrants who are considered a threat to "national security or public health." However, this reason for expulsion is rarely used, if ever.

There is evidence that links health to important indicators of social cohesion such as trust and social capital. For example, using European Social Survey data, Poortinga (2006) found that trusting and socially active individuals are more likely to report good health. Other studies focus on the formation of vicious circles by which unemployment or low-quality work makes good-quality food unaffordable. This then affects health status, which in turn affects individuals' ability to find and maintain employment (see, for example, Schuring et al., 2013; Wanberg, 2012). Although these studies do not focus on immigrants in particular, it is not difficult to extend their results to these groups, which may exhibit low levels of trust and might find themselves on the fringes of the labour market. Thus, they are likely to fall into a cycle of declining health like the one described earlier.

It is difficult to assess whether the measures in place are able to break such vicious circles, if they occur. However, the fact that responsibility for such measures is often divided among different institutions or services and administrative levels is likely to render their coordination difficult and ultimately limits their efficiency. Moreover, the increased decentralization of immigrant-related measures (including health-related measures) opens the door for discrepancies across municipalities in what concerns their implementation, with direct consequences for the immigrants' integration.

Improving Access to Health and Thus Increasing Health Access Equity Is a Policy Objective Related to Reducing Inequalities and Tackling Social Exclusion at the EU Level, Thus Promoted in All EU Member States

In line with Vallgårda's (2003) argument that the long tradition of high levels of regulation of public health in Denmark has led to a high level of citizens' self-regulation, it could be argued that the efficient functioning of the health system relies on a high degree of knowledge, understanding, and self-regulation on the part of users. Consequently, even though the Danish health care system is designed to provide free and equal access to health care, the system does not cope effectively with patients who are not "educated" in how to understand and navigate it.

How can this system deal with an increasingly culturally diverse population? Two solutions have been proposed. First, it has been suggested that immigrants need to be better informed about their health rights and about the health care system. However, this is strongly dependent on resources available at the municipal level. Some municipalities present newly arrived immigrants with a "welcome package" that contains some information regarding the health system. This is a relatively recent practice. However, it is unclear whether this is a measure directed to all the newly arrived, or only to those who communicate to the authorities that they have special needs—for example, families with small children. Although a great deal of information is online, and therefore in principle freely available, it implies that immigrants are computer literate and speak Danish or English, which is often an unrealistic assumption. Thus, future measures could require a better tailoring to the target group.

Second, it has been argued that health care professionals should be informed on immigrant-related issues. In absence of qualified information programs, a recent study showed that health care personnel take mass-media or peers as their main information sources about immigrants (Michaelsen et al., 2004). Their study shows attitudes toward immigrants differ across categories of medical personnel: doctors and nurses had more positive attitudes, while assistant nurses had more negative attitudes. The authors suggest that lower education, plus a feeling of potential job competition with immigrants, is responsible for the latter's likelihood to express negative prejudices.

In this sense, co-operation with institutions or organizations that focus on cultural aspects might help health care professionals to acquire knowledge about the cultural differences and particularities of different immigrant groups. This is of utmost importance because the immigrant population in Denmark is very diverse as to ethnic background and reasons for migration, which is reflected in their health practices (Kristiansen, Mygind, & Krasnik, 2006; Thomas & Thomas, 2004). For example, it has been shown that compared to nationals, migrants from Eastern Europe exhibit more medication compliance (Hedelmalm et al., 2010), while migrants from non-European countries exhibit less medication compliance (Van Dijk et al., 2007).

Summing up, there is a great deal to be done in Denmark to address immigrants' health issues. However, this discussion cannot conclude without addressing a collateral, but very relevant matter. In spite of health professionals' concerns and an increasing body of evidence, immigrants' health seems to be of limited concern for Danish politicians. This conclusion is supported by the main parties' lack of public positions on health issues, accompanied by the limited measures taken to improve the ability of the health system to deal with a diversified group of patients. Moreover, the above-mentioned case of a user fee for state-provided interpretation services suggests that immigrants' health is framed more in terms of costs for the welfare state than in terms of immigrants' needs and challenges.

It is unclear whether there currently is a process that brings together health care professionals and public authorities to address how the health care system can meet the specific needs of immigrants. At the same time, the existing gaps of the regulatory framework—for example, in cases of undocumented migrants—could be read as a sign of health care specialists' limited input in the formulation of immigration/integration policy. A more negative interpretation would point to a limited political will to address the problem of specific groups of immigrants, who are often perceived as "undesired."

Conclusion

Migrant integration in Denmark has been, to a great extent, evaluated through the lens of employment success. Since the 1990s, successful integration has been equated with high labour market participation. Attachment to the labour market is seen both as a goal as well as a means for immigrants' integration. The Danish integration policy can therefore be conceived as a part of the active labour market policies that were introduced in the 1990s, when welfare services were not only a system of social and economic security, but also increasingly designed to provide access to the labour market through targeted initiatives.

Health care professionals, researchers, and the National Board of Health have identified immigrants as a highly vulnerable group of patients in the health care system. In spite of this recognition, policy-makers regard immigrants' health with somewhat limited interest, and prefer to focus on immigrants' labour market participation. However, in the future, health care concerns might gain more importance because, as we argued at the beginning of this chapter, health and access to health care is interconnected not only to personal well-being, but also to the ability to be an active citizen who can participate in the labour market and thereby contribute to the welfare system. Hence, even though immigrant integration policy is not defined as health policy per se by the authorities, integration policy is de facto health policy. Since integration as defined by Danish authorities is also an important social determinant of health, the integration policy is also health policy. Danish health care policy is divided between treatment policy (e.g., hospital policy) and public health policy (e.g., prophylaxis). In this connection, immigrant integration has been identified as an important aspect in connection to diagnostics, treatment, and preventive health care. Therefore, an integration of the two policy areas—immigrant integration policy and health care policy—would enable authorities to better respond to the difficult circumstances that many immigrants are experiencing not only when they first arrive, but also across generations.

Critical Thinking Questions

1. How can integration policy contribute to improving immigrants' health?
2. Which are the main causes of differences in health outcomes between native-born Danes and immigrants?
3. How can the Danish health care system be improved to respond better to cultural diversity?

Glossary

Discrimination in this chapter is defined as actions and patterns of actions that explicitly or implicitly lead to discriminatory practices targeted at people or groups of people due to their ethnic origin, gender, religion, or sexual orientation. In practice, discrimination is both difficult to identify and prove.

Immigrant is a category that includes both people who have moved temporarily and permanently from one country or region to another. In Denmark, guest workers as well as reunited family are included in the immigrant concept. In public debate, the immigrant concept (*indvandrer*) is often used to describe newcomers as well as second-generation immigrants.

Immigration describes the process of human movement from one place to another. In the second half of the 20th century, immigration debates include both immigration from non-Western countries to Western countries and inter-European immigration.

Integration is a dynamic two-way process of mutual adaptation between immigrants and the receiving society. Integration is a multifaceted process, involving interactions in the economic, social, cultural, and political arenas. Integration can be described as a policy objective, as a means and as a goal. In addition to this, it should be noted that integration is also defined as a special welfare policy, which follows some of the same logic as social policy and active labour market policy, but covers a specific group of people (immigrants and refugees) and also includes special culture and value training programs.

Refugee is a term whose definition has been heavily debated and is a highly contested concept. In this chapter, "refugee" is used to describe a person who has received a residence permit based on asylum.

Welfare state regimes are the institutional arrangements, rules, and understandings that guide and shape concurrent social policy decisions, expenditure developments, problem definitions, and even the respond-and-demand structure of citizens and welfare consumers. The existence of policy regimes reflects the circumstance that short-term policies, reforms, debates, and decision making take place within frameworks of historical institutionalization that differ qualitatively between countries (Esping-Andersen, 1990, p. 80). According to Esping-Andersen, there are three types of welfare regimes: (1) a Social Democratic welfare state with universal benefits and a high level of decommodification (e.g., Denmark); (2) a Liberal welfare state with a low level of decommodification and many social benefits provided through the market (e.g., the United Kingdom); and (3) a Conservative/corporatist welfare state with an intermediate level of decommodification and social benefits based on insurance contributions (e.g., Germany).

Recommended Readings

Brochmann, G., & Hagelund, A. (Eds.). (2012). *Immigration policy and the Scandinavian welfare state, 1945–2010*. Basingstoke, UK: Palgrave Macmillan.

This book includes three country chapters: Sweden, Norway, and Denmark, as well as a comparative chapter. The book explores the historical development of immigration politics in Scandinavia and compares how three similar welfare states have responded to immigration. The authors show how the three countries have reacted differently to similar challenges. Denmark became the most restrictive regime, Sweden the most liberal, and Norway ended up somewhere in between.

Kettunen, P., Michel, S., & Petersen, K. (Eds.). (2015). *Race, ethnicity, and welfare states: An American dilemma?* London: Edward Elgar.

Gunnar Myrdal's *An American Dilemma* persuaded many scholars that the United States failed to develop a robust welfare state because of its ethnic heterogeneity, and, conversely, that homogeneity was a precondition for the creation of strong welfare states in European, especially Nordic, countries. With increasing diversity now challenging these welfare states, the kind of "dilemma" that Myrdal identified no longer appears to be solely an American one. In this interdisciplinary volume, leading and emerging scholars examine the relationship between homogeneity and welfare state development.

Kettunen, P., & Petersen, K. (Eds.). (2011). *Beyond welfare state models: Transnational historical perspectives on social policy*. London: Edward Elgar.

In this book, established researchers of welfare history challenge the existing literature of welfare regimes in two ways. First, the standard typologies have omitted important aspects of welfare state developments. Second, the book develops and underlines the importance of a more fluid transnational conceptualization. The chapters cover a wide range of aspects of welfare policy such as social security, religion, family policy, etc.

Recommended Websites

The Danish National Centre for Social Research—www.sfi.dk

The Danish National Centre for Social Research conducts research and carries out commissioned projects in the area of welfare state policies, and disseminates the results. Publications from SFI are available online at this website, many of which are in English.

Danish Parliament—www.ft.dk

The website from the Danish parliament, Folketinget, includes full text versions of parliamentary debates, hearings, and other policy documents. All documents are in Danish.

The "Integrationsbarometer"—www.integrationsbarometer.dk

The "Integrationsbarometer" was developed as a result of the governmental agreement "Et Danmark, der står sammen" in October 2011. This agreement stated that one of the aims was to improve migrants' integration in Denmark by measuring the successful cases and facilitating intermunicipal diffusion and learning. The "Integrationsbarometer" includes nine targets (in 2015) and gives access to data that enables comparison of all Danish municipalities. Improved or good health is not included as one of the nine integration targets.

Ny i Danmark—https://www.nyidanmark.dk

The website Ny i Danmark provides an overview of existing entry rules and regulations.

Retsinformationen—www.retsinformation.dk

Retsinformationen provides full text versions of laws in force as well as historical legislation. The chronology dates back only one decade, but gives easy access to existing legislation in all areas and links to the relevant parliamentary debates and policy documents.

Statistics Denmark—www.danmarksstatistik.dk

Statistics Denmark collects information on various aspects of Denmark, the Danish economy, population developments, etc. "Statistikbanken" gives access to statistical data provided by Statistics Denmark and has free access.

Notes

1. Ingen gider forske i indvandreres sunhed (Nobody wants to do research on immigrants' health). Retrieved from http://videnskab.dk/krop-sundhed/ingen-gider-forske-i-indvandreres-sundhed

2. The national statistics include both newly arrived immigrants as well as immigrants who arrived as guest workers in the 1960s. Furthermore, descendents are included in the category of immigrants.
3. This is not independent from the structure of the Danish labour market, where marginal low-skilled jobs, which in other countries are usually done by immigrants, are relatively scarce and wage structure is relatively compressed.
4. Individuals who were not defined as refugees according to the UN 1956 refugee convention were granted asylum in Denmark as de facto refugees.
5. Active labour market policies are complex and have, as their main aim, limiting individuals' dependency on welfare and activating them in the labour market. For labour market participation, the policies include limitations on duration and amount of benefits, coupled with more help for the unemployed to look for jobs, making benefits conditional on participation in activation programs, re-qualification schemes, job-searching skills, and individually adjusted job-search plans. For an overview, see Kvist and Pedersen (2007).

References

Agergaard, S., & Kahr Soerensen, J. (2009). The dream of social mobility: Ethnic minority players in Danish football clubs. *Soccer and Society, 10*(6), 766–780.

Andersen, P. T., Bak, C. T, Vangsgaard, S., Dokkedal, U., & Larsen, P. V. (2008). Self-rated health, ethnicity, and social position in a deprived neighbourhood in Denmark. *International Journal for Equity in Health, 10*(5), 5–11.

Andersen, R., Mølgaard, C., Theil Skovgaard, L., Brot, C., Cashman, K. D., Jakobsen, J., ..., & Ovesen, L. (2002). Pakistani immigrant children and adults in Denmark have severely low vitamin D status. *European Journal of Clinical Nutrition, 62*(5), 625–634.

Bancila, D., Kronborg Bak, C., & Tanggaard Andersen, P. (2012). Ethnic differences in stress among residents in a deprived neighbourhood in Denmark. *International Journal of Mental Health Promotion, 14*(2), 61–70.

Bancila, D., & Singhammer, J. (2013). The variation of the stress–mental health relationship by ethnicity and gender. *International Journal of Mental Health Promotion, 15*(3), 178–192.

Bievelander, P., et al. (2013). *Scandinavia's population groups originating from developing countries: Change and integration.* Nordic Council of Ministers. Retrieved from www.mah.se/upload/Forskningscentrum/MIM/CT/CT%2014.pdf

Blume, K., Gustafsson, B., Pedersen, P. J., & Verner, M. (2003). *A tale of two countries: Poverty among immigrants in Denmark and Sweden since 1984.* WIDER Discussion Papers/World Institute for Development Economics (UNU-WIDER), no. 2003/36.

Bo, A., Zinckernagel, L., Krasnik, A., Petersen, J. H., & Norredam, M. (2014). Coronary heart disease incidence among non-Western immigrants compared to Danish-born people: Effect of country of birth, migrant status, and income. *European Journal of Preventive Cardiology.* Published online before print September 26. doi:10.1177/2047487314551538.

Brodmann, S., & Polavieja, J. G. (2011). Immigrants in Denmark: Access to employment, class attainment, and earnings in a high-skilled economy. *International Immigration, 48*(1), 59–90.

Cantor-Graae, E., Pedersen, C. B., McNeil, T. F., & Mortensen, P. B. (2003). Migration as a risk factor for schizophrenia: A Danish population-based cohort study. *British Journal of Psychiatry, 182*(2), 117–122.

Cantor-Graae, E., & Selten, J. P. (2005). Schizophrenia and migration: A meta-analysis and review. *American Journal of Psychiatry, 162*(1), 12–24.

Careja, R., Emmenegger, P., & Kvist, J. (2015). An American dilemma in Europe? Welfare reform and immigration. In P. Kettunen, S. Michel, & K. Petersen (Eds.), *Race, ethnicity, and welfare states: An American dilemma?* (pp. 128–149). London: Edward Elgar.

Clausen, J. R., Heinesen, E., Hummelgaard, H., Husted, L., & Rosholm, M. (2008). *The effect of integration policies on the time until regular employment of newly arrived immigrants: Evidence from Denmark.* IZA Discussion Papers, no. 3849. Retrieved from http://nbn-resolving.de/urn:nbn:de:101:1-2008120289

Danish Refugee Council. (n.d.). *Dublin II national asylum procedure in Denmark.* Retrieved from http://www.google.dk/url?sa=t&rct=j&q=&esrc=s&source=web&cd=1&cad=rja&uact=8&ved=0CCEQFjAA&url=http%3A%2F%2Fwww.dublin-project.eu%2Ffr%2Fcontent%2Fdownload%2F549%2F4443%2Fversion%2F3%2Ffile%2FLong_Brochure_Denmark.pdf&ei=wSJJVZC3G8aeywOYr4HYCA&usg=AFQjCNE_6ERofEBTol-zcklx9EssF-rbhg&bvm=bv.92291466,d.bGQ

Dinesen, C., Smith-Nielsen, S., Hvas Mortensen, L., & Krasnik, A. (2011). Inequality in self-rated health among immigrants, their descendants, and ethnic Danes: Examining the role of socioeconomic position. *International Journal of Public Health, 56*(5), 503–514.

Dyhr, L., Sahl Andersen, J., & Engholm G. (2007). The pattern of contact with general practice and casualty departments of immigrants and non-immigrants in Copenhagen, Denmark. *Danish Medical Bulletin, 54*(3), 226–229.

EMN. (2013). *Country factsheet: Denmark 2013.* European Migration Network, European Commission.

Esping-Andersen, G. (1990). *The three worlds of welfare capitalism.* Princeton, NJ: Princeton University Press.

Folmann, N., & Jørgensen, T. (2006). *Etniske minoriteter—sygdom og brug af sundhedsvæsenet. Et registerstudie.* Sundhedsstyrelsen. Retrieved from *http://sundhedsstyrelsen.dk/~/media/2AEF894D15B343F08BE2D5A381DFFE55.ashx*

Green-Pedersen, C. (2012). *Partier i nye tider.* Århus: Århus University Press.

Hallas, P., Hansen, A. R., Stæhr, M. A., Munk-Andersen, E., & Jorgensen, H. L. (2007). Length of stay in asylum centres and mental health in asylum seekers: A retrospective study from Denmark. *BMC Public Health, 7*(288).

Hansen, A. R., Krasnik, A., & Høg, E. (2007). Access to health care for undocumented immigrants: Rights and practice. *Danish Medical Bulletin, 54*(1), 50–51.

Hedelmalm, A., Schaufelberger, M., & Ekman, I. (2010). Reported adherence and social support among immigrants compared to native Swedes. *Journal of Immigrant Minority Health, 12*, 124–131.

Holmberg, L., & Kyvsgaard, B. (2003). Are immigrants and their descendants discriminated against in the Danish criminal justice system? *Journal of Scandinavian Studies in Criminology and Crime Prevention, 4*(2), 125–142.

Holmberg, T., Ahlmark, N., & Curtis, T. (2009). *"State of the art report" Etniske minoriteters sundhed i Danmark.* Statens Institut for Folkesundhed. Syddansk Universitet. Retrieved from http://www.si-folkesundhed.dk/upload/state_of_the_art__etniske_minoriteters_sundhed_i_danmark__pdf.pdf

Jensen, N. K., Nielsen, S. S., & Krasnik, A. (2010). Expert opinion on "best practices" in the delivery of health care services to immigrants in Denmark. *Danish Medical Bulletin, 57*(8), 1–5.

Jensen, N. K., Norredam, M., Draebel, T., Bogic, M., Priebe, S., & Krasnik, A. (2011). Providing medical care for undocumented migrants in Denmark: What are the challenges for health professionals? *BMC Health Services Research, 11*(154).

Jensen, T. G., et al. (2010). *Måling af diskrimination på baggrund af etnisk oprindelse,* SFI. Available online at http://integrationsbarometer.dk/tal-og-analyser/filer-tal-og-analyser/maling-af-diskrimination.

Jønsson, H. V. (forthcoming). Lægestandens møde med migranter som patienter. Den lægefaglige debat om migranter i sundhedssystemet, 1960' erne til 2000'erne. *Temp.*

Jønsson, H. V. (2014). Immigration og integrationspolitik. In J. H. Petersen et al. (Eds.), *Dansk Velfærdshistorie,* (Vol.6, pp. 861–996). Odense: University Press of Southern Denmark.

Kristiansen, M., Mygind, A., & Krasnik, A. (2006). Sundhedsmæssige konsekvenser af migration. *Ugeskrift for Læger, 166,* 3006–3008.

Kvist, J. (2004). Does EU enlargement start a race to the bottom? Strategic interaction among EU member states in social policy. *Journal of European Social Policy, 14*(3), 301–318.

Kvist, J., & Pedersen, L. (2007). Danish labour market activation policies. *National Institute Economic Review, 202*(1), 99–112.

Liebig, T. (2007). The labour market integration of immigrants in Denmark. *OECD Social, Employment and Migration.* Working Paper no. 50. Paris: OECD Publishing.

Masmas, T. N., et al. (2008). Asylum seekers in Denmark. A study of health status and grade of traumatization of newly arrived asylum seekers. *Torture, 18*(2), 77–86.

Michaelsen, J. J., Krasnik, A., Nielsen, A. S., Norredam, M., & Torres, A. M. (2004). Health professionals' knowledge, attitudes, and experiences in relation to immigrant patients: A questionnaire study at a Danish hospital. *Scandinavian Journal of Public Health, 32*(4), 287–295.

Ministry of Children, Gender Equality, Integration and Social Affairs. *Fact sheet: Immigrants and descendants.* Retrieved from http://sm.dk/publikationer/fact-sheet-immigrants-and-descendants

Moldenhawer, B. (2005). Transnational migrant communities and education strategies among Pakistani youngesters in Denmark. *Journal of Ethnic and Migration Studies, 31*(1), 51–78.

Montgomery, E., & Foldspang, A. (2007). Discrimination, mental problems, and social adaptation in young refugees. *European Journal of Public Health, 18*(2), 156–161.

Nannestad, P. (2004). Immigration as a challenge to the Danish welfare state? *European Journal of Political Economy, 20*, 755–767.

Nørredam, M., Krasnik, A., Moller Sorensen, T., Keiding, N., Joost Michaelsen, J., & Sonne Nielsen, A. (2004). Emergency room utilization in Copenhagen: A comparison of immigrant groups and Danish-born residents. *Scandinavian Journal of Public Health, 32*(1), 53–59.

Nørredam, M., Agyemang, C., Hoejbjerg Hansen, O. K., Petersen, J. H., Byberg, S., Krasnik, A., & Kunst, A. E. (2014). Duration of residence and disease occurrence among refugees and family reunited immigrants: test of the "healthy migrant effect" hypothesis. *Tropical Medicine and International Health, 19*(8), 958–967.

Pedersen, P. J. (2011). *A panel study of immigrant poverty dynamics and income mobility—Denmark, 1984–2007*. Study Paper no. 34. The Rockwool Foundation Research Unit.

Petersen, J. H. (2014). Sygesikring og sundhedsvæsen. In J. H. Petersen, K. Petersen, & N. F. Christiansen (Eds.), *Dansk Velfærdshistorie. Bind 6.1. Hvor glider vi hen?*(pp. 469–552). Odense: University of Southern Denmark.

Pohl Nielsen, C. (2007). *Immigrant overeducation: Evidence from Denmark*. World Bank Policy Research Working Paper no. 4234. Washington, DC: World Bank.

Poortinga, W. (2006). Social capital: An individual or collective resource for health? *Social Science & Medicine, 62*(2), 292–302.

Priebe, S., et al. (2011). Good practice in health care for migrants: Views and experiences of care professionals in 16 European countries. *BMC Public Health, 11*, 187.

Roseveare, D., & Jorgensen, M. (2004). *Migration and integration of immigrants in Denmark*. OECD Economics Department Working Papers, no. 386. Paris: OECD Publishing.

Schuring, M., Robroek, S. J. W., Otten Ferdy, W. J., Arts, C. H., & Burdof, A. (2013). The effect of ill health and socioeconomic status on labour force exit and re-employment: A prospective sturdy with ten years follow-up in the Netherlands. *Scandinavian Journal of Work, Environment & Health, 39*(2), 134–143.

Singhammer, J. (2008). *Etniske minoriteters sundhed*. Århus: Centre for Public Health, Central Denmark Region.

Sodermann, M., et al. (2013). *Tak fordi I lavede en bedre version af mig*. Odense: Odense University Hospital.

Sundby, A., & Petersen, P. E. (2003). Oral health status in relation to ethnicity of children in the municipality of Copenhagen, Denmark. *International Journal of Paediatric Dentistry, 13*(3), 150–157.

Sundhedsstyrelsen. (2005). *Etniske minoriteters sundhed og sygelighed—opgørelse af behandlingsrater (2002) blandt indvandrere*. Center for Forebyggelse. Retrieved from http://sundhedsstyrelsen.dk/publ/publ2005/cff/behandlingsrater/behandlingsrater.pdf

Thomas, S. L., & Thomas, S. D. M. (2004). Displacement and health. *British Medical Bulletin, 69*(1), 115–127.

Thysted Dinesen, P. (2010). Upbringing, early experiences of discrimination and social identity: Explaining generalised trust among immigrants in Denmark. *Scandinavian Political Studies, 33*(1), 93–111.

Tranæs, T., & Zimmermann, K. F. (Eds.) (2004). *Migrants, work, and the welfare state.* Odense: University Press of Southern Denmark and the Rockwool Foundation Research Unit.

Vallgårda, S. (2003). *Folkesundhed som politik.* Århus: Århus University Press.

Van Dijk, L., Heerdink, E., Somai, D., et al. (2007). Patient risk profiles and practice variation in nonadherence to antidepressants, antihypertensives, and oral hypoglycemic. *BMC Health Services Research, 7,* 51.

Villadsen, S.F., Mortensen, L. H., & Andersen, A. M. (2009). Ethnic disparity in stillborn and infant mortality in Denmark 1981–2003. *Journal of Epidemiology and Community Health, 63*(2), 106–112.

Vineberg, R. (2015). Healthy enough to get in: The evolution of Canadian immigration policy related to immigrant health. *Journal of International Migration and Integration, 16*(2), 279–297.

Vinter-Jensen, K. (Ed.). (2010). *Etniske minoriteter i det danske sundhedsvæsen—en antologi.* Sundhedsstyrelsen. Available online at http://www.sst.dk/~/media/9FFE65223C8A47328A51CD7DBAFA7466.ashx

Vitus, K., & Smith-Nielsen, S. (2011). *Asylbørn i Danmark. En barndom i undtagelsestilstand.* Copenhagen: Hans Reitzels Forlag.

Wanberg, C. R. (2012). The individual experience of unemployment. *Annual Review of Psychology, 63,* 369–396.

Public Policy, Immigrant Experiences, and Health Outcomes in Norway

Arild Schou and Elisabeth Fosse

Chapter Objectives

This chapter focuses on the immigration and integration of immigrants into Norwegian society. The objectives of this chapter are:

- to examine the role immigration and multiculturalism play in a Scandinavian country like Norway;
- to explore the role that public policy plays in shaping the lived experiences of immigrants to Norway;
- to review the evidence concerning health outcomes among immigrants in Norway; and
- to analyze the interrelationship between public policy, integration, and health outcomes of immigrants and reflect on the implications for policy and program development in Norway.

Introduction

Norway is one of the so-called **Social Democratic** welfare states, as classified by Esping-Andersen (1990). The Social Democratic regime is characterized by its emphasis on solidarity and universalism and the redistribution of resources among social groups, mainly through a progressive tax system and entitlements for vulnerable groups. This is a system of emancipation, not only from the market, but also from the family. The result is a welfare regime with direct transfers to children and one that takes direct responsibility for care of children and thus enables women to engage in paid work.

Lundberg et al. (2008) show that although all rich nations have welfare programs, there are clear cross-national differences with respect to their design and generosity. These differences are evident in variations in poverty rates, especially among children and the elderly. The ways in which social policies are designed, as well as their generosity, are important for health. Hence, such policies are of major importance for how we can tackle the social determinants of health, and population health is best in the welfare regime with the most redistributive and generous welfare arrangements.

However, in order to analyze the special conditions of immigrants, the Social Democratic welfare regime typology needs to be complemented (Sainsbury, 2006). The notion of an immigration policy regime may contribute to the understanding of how different welfare states deal with immigration. The immigration regime consists of rules and norms that govern immigrants' possibilities to become citizens, to acquire residence and work permits, and to participate in economic, cultural, and political life. Sainsbury chooses to utilize an underlying dimension in states' immigration policies, namely, that of inclusion versus exclusion.

The most relevant immigrant category when it comes to issues of both social exclusion and health challenges is that of non-Western immigrants (NWIs). In Norwegian statistics this category refers to people with parents from Asia, Africa, Latin America, Oceania (except Australia and New Zealand), and Europe (except the European Union/European Economic Area [EU/EEA]). In 2014 this group comprised 325,993 people in Norway. However, it has been a common practice to count both immigrants and their descendants as part of the immigrant population. Thus, if we add this latter category of 101,673 people, it amounts to 427,595 NWIs in Norway. This group comprises 8.4 percent of the Norwegian population as a whole.

NWIs in Norway consist of labour, family, and asylum immigrants. The primary immigration to Norway began as Turkish and Morocco labour migrants arrived in the early 1960s. However, because immigration ended for labour immigrants in 1975, most of the immigration from non-Western countries thereafter consists of family and asylum immigrants. Because the arrival of NWIs is a relatively recent historical phenomenon in Norway, this immigrant group is fairly young: 57 percent are between 20 and 44 years of age. The corresponding figure for the majority population is 15 percent. This has implications for the government's overall health promotion policy because an aging immigrant population has different health needs (Baldwin-Edwards, 2004) than a younger one. As one example, older populations have a statistically higher prevalence of non-communicable chronic diseases.

Principles of the Norwegian Incorporation Regime: A Combined Socialist and Individualist Integration Approach

The Norwegian response to its ethnic diversity can, to some extent, be termed multicultural because it preserves and promotes minorities' cultural heritages. But this feature is far more marked in the government's policy toward the **indigenous** Sami people than in its policy toward the immigrant population.

On the Multiculturalism Policy Index (MPI) Norway's score is "Modest," between 3 and 5.5 points on a rank from 0 to 10.[1] The policy toward the Sami people is ranked closer to "Average" than "Modest," whereas its policy toward immigrants is ranked close to "Weak" (Queen's University, 2014). The reason for the ranking of the policy toward the Sami is that Norway recognizes the group's collective rights—not only in terms of control of natural resources but also their rights in the political and cultural realms. The establishment of the Sami Parliament in 1989 provided the Sami population with the right to consultation on issues that might affect Sami interests, and since 1992 the Sami language is recognized as an equal language to Norwegian.

The policy toward the immigrant population, however, has rather few elements of **multiculturalism**. Indeed, the government does support ethnic group organizations and bilingual mother-tongue instruction, and there is a moderate quota for immigrant employees in some public sector agencies. However, there is no system for **affirmative action**. Neither does the constitution recognize dual citizenship, non-Christian holidays, religious schools, or languages other than Norwegian and Sami (Bø, 2013). Thus, all in all, the policy is geared toward the integration of immigrants into the majority culture.

Instead of labelling the policy toward immigrant multiculturalism, it can be classified as an "individualist-integration" type of policy—according to Modood's typology of integration models (Modood, 2013). In this model, the object of the policy is not primarily groups—as in the multiculturalism model—but individuals. The object is the "individuals marked by *difference*" and not the group per se. This policy has a focus on ensuring that individuals are treated equally to the majority population. They are free to cultivate their identity in private, but discouraged from thinking of themselves as a minority. This implies an integration policy that embraces equal citizenship rights and ethnically blind policy instruments.

Moreover, as the Labour Party has to a large extent governed Norway since the Second World War, the Norwegian integration regime has strong socialist elements. Such a policy can be classified as a "socialist integrationalist response," according to Choudhry's typology of integration models (Choudhry, 2008). Socialist integrationalists regard conflicts between minorities and the majority as an expression of different class interests. Thus, their preferred integration policy is the promotion of distributive justice. Social democrats regard substantive social citizenship for all as the best means to the realization of distributive justice (Choudhry, 2008). In Norway such citizenship is promoted by working to actively "integrate new arrivals—especially in working life and also in society" (Brochmann & Grødem, 2013, p. 60).

Norway's Integration Policy in Practice

Integration policies and health promotion policies are closely related because integration policy has bearings on the provision of the prerequisites for good health. A policy that enhances immigrant participation in the labour market and education systems paves the way for healthy lives for those concerned. This mechanism is empirically confirmed in the Norwegian context as a multivariate analysis of NWIs and demonstrates that immigrants with a strong socio-economic position (good education, employment, economic standing, housing, and work conditions) have better health than immigrants without these characteristics (Blom, 2008, 2010).

Mainstream Interventions

The policy implications of the combined "individualist" and "socialist integration" approach is a policy that provides mainstreaming measures and only occasionally establishes targeted measures toward NWIs. Thus, in three of the major areas for integration—the labour market, education, and the housing market—the government's objective is to give immigrants the same access to benefits as those enjoyed by the majority population and to stimulate full labour market participation of all groups, regardless of ethnic characteristics. However, in all these arenas there have been reports of discrimination against immigrants. As a response, the government passed a law against discrimination in 2005, and in 2009 passed the Second Action Plan for Prevention of Ethnic Discrimination (Government of Norway, 2009).

Labour Market

The main foundation for the labour market policy was laid down in a parliamentary report on migration and integration policy in 1987. It emphasizes that immigrants have the same rights and obligations as the native population. This was translated into the goal of "equal status for all." It also underscored the principle of *mainstreaming*, which means that the needs of migrants should, as far as possible, be provided for within the general labour market and social policy measures as part of the general welfare policy (Brochmann & Grødem, 2013).

Labour market programs in Norway traditionally differentiated between "ordinary unemployed" and "vocationally disabled." For both groups, three main sets of active labour market policy instruments can be broadly distinguished—training, work practice measures, and wage subsidies. Since 2008, all measures may in principle be offered to both groups, but this depends on an individual assessment of work capability.

Compared with their share in the working-age population, NWIs are strongly over-represented among the ordinary unemployed, but only slightly represented among the vocationally disabled. Active labour market programs (ALMPs) have been introduced for training and work practice measures for both categories of labour market marginalization—i.e., the unemployed and the vocationally disabled. Evaluations of the ALMPs show that participation in the training programs increases the likelihood of NWIs entering the labour market (Røed & Raaum, 2003). There is also a positive correlation between public work practice measures for NWIs and labour market outcomes (Kavli et al., 2007). The same goes for wage subsidies. In a 2008 evaluation of Nordic countries, evaluations show that wage subsidy programs targeted at immigrants and other disfavoured groups in the labour market consistently yield improved labour market outcomes (Nekby, 2008).

Education

In the education arena the Norwegian government also puts high value on mainstreaming policy measures, combined with some targeted initiatives. As pointed out by the OECD, the key challenge for Norway is to design universal measures that are sufficiently effective so that few targeted measures would be necessary (OECD, 2011).

Norway has a highly inclusive education system. The overall objective of the education policy is to ensure equal education opportunities for all students regardless of gender, ethnicity, geographic location, and socio-economic background. In line with this objective, the public school system is free of charge and higher education is almost free of charge. Moreover, since 1947 both university students and students in upper secondary education have been eligible for loans from the Educational Loan Fund (Lånekassen). It should be noted, however, that early childhood education and care is not free, but the fee is highly subsidized and affordable for most parents. In addition, child care is of high quality and available for all children from one to five years of age. In line with the Social Democratic welfare model, government offers full-time daycare to allow parents to participate in the workforce.

The share of minority-language children attending preschool has more than doubled from 2005 to 2011, from about 13,700 children in 2005 to about 30,000 children in 2011, and this increase is well beyond the corresponding growth of this population over this period (Government of Norway, 2011a). Moreover, there is a state-funded program for language training for minority-language children. As for primary school, in 2010 the government introduced eight hours of free coaching of home lessons per week for first- to fourth-grade pupils. Figures from Statistics Norway show that those who most frequently take advantage of the program are children from low-income and low-education families and first-generation immigrants (Moafi, 2012).

Despite the favourable conditions for entering the education system, there are challenges (low attendance, dropout, low marks) for part of the immigrant population at all levels of education. OECD has pointed out that there is a rather large performance gap between students with and without an immigrant background, which has remained stable since 2000. First-generation immigrant students are twice as likely to perform among the bottom quarter of students when compared to students without an immigrant background (OECD, 2009).

Right to Social Welfare?

Everyone on Norwegian soil has the right to emergency health care. As for care beyond this level, there are variations between different categories of immigrants. Asylum-seekers have the same right to all kinds of health care as the population as a whole. The same goes for refugees—i.e., people who meet the conditions for being recognized as refugees by the UN Refugee Convention or Norwegian law (Government of Norway, 2013). As for illegal (undocumented) immigrants, the situation is different, and has deteriorated since 2012. Prior to 2012, illegal immigrants were entitled to both immediate and necessary medical care from the municipality in which they resided. Since 2012, a new regulation states that emergency health care can be offered only in situations of utmost urgency that cannot be delayed without risk of death, permanently impaired health functionality, severe injury, or severe pain. Critics claim that this regulation is a violation of the United Nations International Covenant on Economic, Social, and Cultural Rights because it implies that people with back pain, bleeding, wounds, and anxiety will no longer be entitled to care from the Norwegian public health system (Sinding Larsen & Kjellevold, 2012).

Targeted Interventions

In the 2000s the government introduced several targeted interventions for the inclusion of the immigrant population—an introductory program for newly arrived refugees, a specific language training course, support to voluntary organizations, and an arrangement for free entrance in preschools.

The introductory program was introduced in 2004 and targets newly arrived refugees and their family members from outside of the EEA who do not master Norwegian or Sami. The program, which is compulsory, provides an introduction to Norwegian society and language in addition to a qualifying course for paid employment. Participants receive an individual salary, which is usually at a higher level than social assistance. In 2005, the right and obligation to participate in 250 hours of Norwegian language training and 50 hours of "social studies" was introduced. There is an obligation to participate in the 300 hours of language and social studies training for all new arrivals from non-EEA countries who do not speak Norwegian. For people in need of training, the actual number of hours of language training can be much higher—up to 3,000 hours.

The program for support to voluntary immigrant organizations was established in 2001 with the aim of strengthening the participation of the immigrant population locally and to providing access to social networks. More than 600 organizations received support in 2009. The local governments are responsible for the implementation of both programs and courses.

In 2006 a program was established offering five-year-old children free preschool for four hours a day. The program is geographically limited to certain areas in Drammen, Oslo, and Bergen, which have a high share of immigrants from non-Western countries. However, all children in these areas—regardless of ethnicity—are eligible for the program. A recent evaluation found that the program had a positive effect on marks in lower secondary school, particularly for girls (Drange, 2013).

The Municipal Level: The Public Health Act of 2012 and New Health Promotion Policies

Norwegian municipalities have a dual role in many of these initiatives. On the one hand they are agents for the welfare state through their responsibility for implementing national policy goals. On the other hand, they form self-standing local democratic arenas that decide how to use national funding in accordance with local preferences and needs (Baldersheim & Ståhlberg, 2002). These needs vary to a great extent as Norwegian municipalities vary in many aspects, among them the number of immigrants.

The Public Health Act of 2012 (Government of Norway, 2011b) represents a new direction in the development of health care services and public health work in Norway. It builds on a broad determinants of health perspective to public health work, and the main aim of the Act is to reduce inequalities in health by levelling the social gradient. The Act states that "a fair distribution of societal resources is good public health policy."

The Act assigns more responsibility for preventive work and health promotion to the municipalities. The Act, which was introduced as part of the Coordination Reform (Government of Norway, 2011c) (coordination between central and local government), includes a statutory provision for the local governments to provide an overview of the health situation, to identify positive and negative prerequisites for health, and, on this basis, to design local adapted public health strategies that are integrated into the municipal plan.

The 428 municipalities in Norway play a significant part in the integration of immigrants at the local level, notably through their responsibilities in the area of social assistance and housing. Within the broad framework defined at the national level, municipalities are also responsible for primary and lower secondary schools and the introductory program for immigrants. Since the 1990s some of the most immigrant-rich municipalities in the city of Drammen, the Fjell areas, and the Groruddalen area in Oslo have introduced area-specific intervention to promote the social determinants of health for immigrants (Drammen Municipality, 2012; Oslo Municipality, 2013).

The findings from a 2014 national survey of all municipalities show that public health work has been given more attention since the reform, not only with regard to more health-related planning, but also to universal and targeted interventions at this level, which are on the rise. The survey shows that more than 15 percent of the most immigrant-rich local governments in Norway have established an overview both of the health situation and the positive and negative health determinants as prescribed in the Public Health Act. Around 39 percent of these have a special focus on public health work for this particular group, and report implementation of a wide variety of measures designed to advance this group in society. Two-thirds of them report introduction of general measures and language training for immigrants, while more than half have introduced interpretation service for immigrants and targeted interventions in schools or preschools (Schou, Helgesen, & Hofstad, 2014; Fosse & Helgesen, 2015).

Evidence Concerning the Integration of Immigrants into Society

NWIs are relatively well integrated into Norwegian society. Nevertheless, there are large variations between this group and the majority population with regard to scores on health determinants such as education, work, and income. A large proportion of NWIs have completed ordinary education at different levels, but there are large gender and country-background variations. As for the group as a whole (in 2008), 26 percent had completed higher education, 41 percent upper-secondary education, 19 percent primary and lower secondary education, and 14 percent have not completed any education (Blom & Henriksen, 2009). The share of women who in 2006 had not completed any education is twice that of men (18 percent versus 9 percent) and the share among Somali women (one of the most recent immigrant groups that has arrived in Norway) was as high as 45 percent.

Young immigrants also have a three times higher risk of being school dropouts (see OECD, 2008). This is particularly worrying since at the outset of schooling, children of immigrants do not have unfavourable school grades. Hægeland et al. (2004) find that after controlling for socio-economic background characteristics, children of immigrants from non-OECD countries achieve roughly the same grade-point averages as children of native Norwegians.

Labour market participation rates are generally high in Norway when compared to other European countries, but are lower among NWIs that the non-immigrant population—59.6 percent against 78.8 percent. Moreover, those who have arrived as refugees tend to have the lowest employment rates, while labour migrants—not surprisingly—have the highest rate. Family migrants are somewhere in between in terms of employment rates. Employment also varies according to length of stay in Norway. It is not surprising that one of the recent refugee populations, the Somalis, has a particular low employment rate (32 percent). The unemployment rate among the NWIs has for years been approximately three times higher than the rate for the rest of the population. From 2002 to 2006 the rate varied between 8 percent and 4 percent while it varied between 2.5 percent and 1 percent for the rest of the population (Government of Norway, 2011a).

The Norwegian labour market reflects the Social Democratic welfare model as it has a compressed wage structure such that low-skilled work is relatively well paid. At the same time there are relative few jobs of this category in Norway as compared to other European countries (OECD, 2009). Nevertheless, NWIs in Norway are strongly over-represented among people with low income, compared to the population as a whole. Figures from 2009 reveal that the share of non-European immigrants with income (after tax) below 60 percent of the median was 33.6 percent in 2006, while the corresponding figure for the general population was 10 percent (Blom & Henriksen, 2009).

The OECD scale defines those who have an income below 50 percent of the median income in the population as poor. The definition set by the EU is 60 percent of the median income. From 2004 to 2006, more than 20 percent of children under 18 years in this group lived in poverty (OECD scale). On the EU scale this number was 37 percent. This group constitutes approximately 40 percent of all children living in poverty. Research found that NWIs in general are at greater risk of living in poverty than the population in general (Bhuller & Aaberge, 2010). There are, however, very few poor among the full-time employed non-immigrants. Still, among full-time employed immigrants, the researchers also find poor groups, including families with children in which both parents are employed. People who receive long-term social benefits are also among the groups at risk of long-term poverty.

In his analyses, Mogstad (2005) found that poverty in Norway is a particular problem in the larger cities. This is because the cost of living is much higher in urban as compared to rural areas. A majority of immigrants live in the cities. At the same time, immigrants are reported to have received more social transfers than the rest of the population. This applies, for example, to social assistance, housing allowance, and cash for care. However, although immigrants reported greater problems with expenses, there were few differences between the two groups (rural and urban) in possession of ordinary capital goods.

Evidence Concerning Health Outcomes among Immigrants

There are variations in health conditions between the majority population and NWIs with regard to non-communicable chronic diseases (NCDs). The most significant difference is for psychological distress among NWIs.[2] In a 2006 survey based on self-reported outcomes, 15 percent of the immigrant respondents reported distress while the corresponding figure for the population as a whole was 5 percent.

However, the profile of the diseases varies considerably. The immigrant population reported more lifestyle-related diseases. There was a high prevalence of type 2 diabetes, thyroid disease, stomach ulcer, angina (heart cramps), osteoporosis, and arthritis. The population as a whole reported greater prevalence of other diseases such as eczema, asthma, allergies, COPD, incontinence, hypertension, and cancer (Blom, 2010). The survey also revealed differences related to gender and country of origin. More women than men reported having psychosomatic ailments and psychological distress. Moreover, type 2 diabetes was most widespread among the population from Pakistan and Sri Lanka (8 percent and 10 percent respectively, twice the average of the entire population). Thyroid disease was most widespread among those from Turkey and Iraq (16 percent and 11 percent—about three times the average), whereas ulcer was most widespread among those from Turkey, Somalia, and Chile (16 percent, 11 percent, and 13 percent respectively, also about three times higher).

There are also variations between the majority population and NWIs with regard to risks that affect the above diseases. The body mass index is, on average, higher among NWIs. Here the share of overweight people is 4 percent higher than in the population as a whole (11 percent versus 7 percent). This difference has to do with the large share of overweight women in this category (12 percent as against 6 percent). However, the immigrant population smokes less than the population as a whole (30 percent as against 39 percent). The difference is mainly because the share of immigrant woman who smoke is less than half the share of immigrant men (17 percent as against 41 percent).

Conclusion

Norwegian immigration policy is geared toward the integration of immigrants into the majority culture. In general, the policy is not geared toward recognizing several cultures, and thus is not multicultural in its nature. It may be characterized as an "individualist-integration" type of policy. In this model, the object of the policy is not primarily groups—as in the multiculturalism model—but individuals. This implies an integration policy that embraces equal citizenship rights and ethnically blind policy instruments.

The Norwegian integration regime includes strong socialist elements. In this perspective, conflicts between minorities and the majority may be viewed as an expression of different class interests. Thus, the preferred integration policy is the promotion of distributive justice. Social democrats regard substantive social citizenship for all as the best means to its realization. This implies active integration of new arrivals, especially in working life and also in society.

The policy implications of the combined "individualist" and "socialist integration" approach are that it is oriented toward mainstreaming measures and only occasionally establishes targeted measures toward NWIs. Thus, in three of the major areas for integration—the labour market, education, and income—the government's objective is to give immigrants equal access to benefits as the majority population and to stimulate full labour market participation of all groups, regardless of ethnic characteristics.

Marmot (2010) states that the principle of "proportionate universalism" is important in levelling the social gradient. The main principle of service delivery should be based on universalism, but some groups may need extra attention and support. The Norwegian policy thus reflects the ideology of the Social Democratic welfare state regime, with an emphasis on universal measures. However, the universal measures are not sufficient to include non-Western immigrants in society. Compared with their share in the working-age population, NWIs are strongly overrepresented among the unemployed, and active labour market programs (ALMPs) have been introduced for training and work practice measure for groups subject to market marginalization.

In the education arena, the Norwegian government also puts a high value on mainstreaming policy measures, combined with some targeted initiatives. Despite the favourable conditions that facilitate entering the education system, there are challenges (low attendance, dropout, low marks) on the part of the immigrant population at all levels.

Although many of the targeted measures are funded by the national government, the municipalities are vital in developing and administrating the measures. This has been further underlined since the Public Health Act was implemented in 2012. The overall aim of the Act is to reduce social inequalities by addressing the social determinants of health. Among the most important determinants are employment and education. Many NWIs are disadvantaged, and should thus be subject to both universal and targeted measures.

Dahl and colleagues state that it is easier to redistribute money than health, and that the Nordic model is definitely more successful than other countries in redistributing money (Dahl et al., 2006). At the core of these arrangements is the political aim of redistribution among social groups (Marmot, 2009). Countries in the social-democratic model have well-developed welfare arrangements, many with universal coverage. In the Norwegian system, NWIs benefit from this system, which may be characterized as "proportionate universalistic" regarding policies aimed at NWIs. As for the overall picture, NWIs are relatively well integrated in Norwegian society. Nevertheless, there are still large variations between this group and the majority population with regard to their scores on positive health determinants such as education, work, and income.

There are several scenarios that might be outlined for the future. Immigration, particularly of NWIs, is a relatively new phenomenon in Norway. Even though there are inequalities regarding education and work life, we also see that the numbers of children and grandchildren of first-generation immigrants in higher education are increasing. The positive scenario is that given the system of easy access to higher education, there is an avenue for social mobility that might level the inequalities. However, in order for more NWIs to enter education, the Norwegian policy needs to address the particular challenges met by young people who experience discrepancy between social expectations about success and the opportunities that society offers.

Acknowledgements

The research presented in this chapter is funded by the Norwegian Research Council projects "Addressing the Social Determinants of Health: Multilevel Governance of Policies Aimed at Families with Children" (Project no. 213841/H10) and "Evaluation of the Coordination Reform: Impact of the Reform on Health Promotion and Disease Prevention in Municipalities" (Project no. 229628).

Critical Thinking Questions

1. What are the factors that contribute to the health of immigrants in Norway?
2. How can policies of multiculturalism contribute to the improvement of immigrant health in Norway?
3. How can health policies change in order to more adequately reflect the cultural diversity of the population of Norway?
4. What strategies can be adopted to improve cultural responsiveness of health systems and professionals?
5. What role does the nation-state play in immigrant health?

Glossary

Affirmative action is positive discrimination (e.g., in the labour market) where a policy favours members of a disadvantaged group who suffer from discrimination within a culture.

Indigenous peoples are those who, having a historical continuity with pre-invasion and pre-colonial societies that developed on their territories, consider themselves distinct from other sectors of the societies now prevailing in those territories, or parts of them.

Multiculturalism is an accommodating policy approach to diversity, including the widespread adoption of accommodation policies for immigrant groups, the acceptance of territorial autonomy and language rights for national minorities, and the recognition of land claims and self-government rights for indigenous peoples.

Social democracy is the idea that the state needs to provide security and equality for its people and should, by democratic means, actively reorder society in a way that is conducive to such developments.

Recommended Readings

Blom, S., & Henriksen, K. (2009). *Living condition amongst immigrants in Norway 2005/2006*. Oslo: Statistics Norway.

A little over half of the NWIs participating in this study have been granted residence in Norway as refugees, most of them on humanitarian grounds. Median length of residence in Norway is 12 years, but this figure varies considerably among the national groups, with shortest residence among Iraqis and Somalis, and longest residence among Pakistanis. A little fewer than one in 10 are born in Norway to immigrant parents. The largest percentages of these national groups are Pakistanis, Vietnamese, and Turks.

Brochmann, G., & Grødem, A. S. (2013). Migration and welfare sustainability, the case of Norway. In E. Jurada & G. Brochmann (Eds.), *Europe's immigration challenge* (pp. 59–76). London: I. B Tauris.

One of the themes running through this book is that governments overestimate the control they have over the movement of people. In fact, the great majority of immigrants crossing EU borders, including EU citizens, are people seeking international protection and irregular migrants that fall outside of, or manage to avoid, immigration controls. However, the book's main underlying concern is that current efforts to select immigrants according to their potential value to the economy underestimate the complexity of the relationship between migrant flows, labour markets, and welfare systems.

Lundberg, O., Yngwe, M. Å., Stjärne, M. K., Elstad, J. I., Ferrarini, T., Kangas, O., et al. for the NEWS Nordic Expert group. (2008). The role of welfare state principles and generosity in social policy programmes for public health: An international comparative study. *Lancet, 372*(9650), 1633–1640.

Welfare states contribute to the resources available for their citizens through cash transfer programs and subsidized services. Although all rich nations have welfare programs, there are clear cross-national differences with respect to their design and generosity. These differences are evident in national variations in poverty rates, especially among children and elderly people. Increased generosity in family policies is linked with lower infant mortality rates.

Marmot, M. (2010). The Marmot Review: *Fair society, healthy lives: Strategic review of health inequalities in England post-2010*. London: UCL Institute of Health Equity.

The key messages of this review is that reducing health inequalities is a matter of fairness and social justice. Focusing solely on the most disadvantaged will not reduce health inequalities sufficiently. There is a social gradient in health—the lower a person's social position, the worse his or her health. Action should focus on reducing the gradient in health. To reduce the steepness of the social gradient in health, actions must be universal, but with a scale and intensity that are proportionate to the level of disadvantage. This is called proportionate universalism.

Sainsbury, D. (2006). Immigrants' social rights in comparative perspective: Welfare regimes, forms in immigration, and immigration policy regimes. *Journal of European Social Policy, 16*(3), 229–244.

In analyzing the social rights of immigrants, this paper draws on insights from comparative welfare state research and international migration studies. The paper examines the social rights of immigrants in three countries generally regarded as exemplars of the welfare regime types. It maps out immigrants' formal incorporation into the welfare systems of the three countries in order to understand the interplay between welfare regimes, the forms of immigration, and the immigration policy regimes in shaping immigrants' social rights.

Related Websites

Ministry of Children, Equality and Social Inclusion—www.regjeringen.no/en/dep/bld/id298/

The ministry has the overall responsibility for children welfare services, family affairs, childhood development, integration and diversity, anti-discrimination, equality, and consumer affairs.

Ministry of Health and Care Services—www.regjeringen.no/en/dep/hod/id421/
The Ministry of Health and Care Services is responsible for providing good and equal health and care services for the population of Norway. The ministry directs these services by means of comprehensive legislation, annual budgetary allocations, and through various governmental institutions.

The Norwegian Centre for Minority Health Research (NAKMI)—http://www.nakmi.no/
The Norwegian Centre for Minority Health Research is a national research, development, and policy centre promoting research-based knowledge about health and care for immigrants and their descendants in Norway.

Notes

1. The index also covers policies toward national minorities. In Norway they comprise Kvens/Norwegian Finns (people of Finnish descent in Northern Norway), Jews, Forest Finns, Roma, and Romani people/Taters. However, numerically speaking these groups are very small, which is probably why Norway is not ranked on this dimension.
2. In this survey the groups of NWI includes people between 16 and 70 years from Bosnia- Herzegovina, Serbia-Montenegro, Turkey, Iraq, Iran, Pakistan, Vietnam, Pakistan, Sri Lanka, Somalia, and Chile.

References

Baldersheim, H., & Ståhlberg, K. (2002). Guided democracy or multi-level governance? New trends in regulatory regimes in central-local relations in the Nordic countries. *Local Government Studies, 28*, 74–90.

Baldwin-Edwards, M. (2004). Immigrants and the welfare state in Europe. In J. Massey & E. Taylor (Eds.), *2004 international migration: Prospects and policies in a global market* (pp. 319–334). Oxford: Oxford University Press.

Bhuller, M., & Aaberge, R. (2010). *Persistent economic poverty among immigrants. An empirical analysis for the period 1993–2007.* [Vedvarende økonomisk fattigdom blant innvandrere, En empirisk analyse for perioden 1993–2007.] Report 32/2010. Oslo: Statistics Norway.

Blom, S. (2008). *Immigrants' health* [Innvandreres Helse]. Statistics Norway, 2005/2006, Report 2. Retrieved from http://www.ssb.no/sosiale-forhold-og-kriminalitet/artikler-og-publikasjoner/innvandreres-helse-2005-2006

Blom, S. (2010). *Social differences in immigrants' health.* [Sosiale forskjeller i innvandres helse.] Report 47. SSB. Retrieved from https://www.ssb.no/a/publikasjoner/pdf/rapp_201047/rapp_201047.pdf

Blom, S., & Henriksen, K. (2009). *Living conditions amongst immigrants in Norway 2005/2006.* Statistics Norway, Report 2. Retrieved from http://brage.bibsys.no/xmlui/bitstream/handle/11250/181005/rapp_200902_en.pdf?sequence=1

Bø, B. P. (Ed.). (2013). *Multicultural theory and practices.* [Multikulturell teori og flerkulturelle praksiser.] Trondheim: Abstract Forlag.

Brochmann, G., & Grødem, A. S. (2013). Migration and welfare sustainability: The case of Norway. In E. Jurada & G. Brochmann (Eds.), *Europe's immigration challenge* (pp. 59–76). London: I. B. Tauris.

Choudhry, S. (2008). *Constitutional design for divided societies: Integration or accommodation?* Oxford: Oxford University Press.

Dahl, E., Fritzell, J., Lahelma, E., Martikainen, P., Kunst, A., & Mackenbach, J. (2006). Welfare state regimes and health inequalities. In J. Siegrist, M. Marmot, & J. Mackenbach (Eds.), *Social inequalities in health* (pp. 193–222). Oxford: Oxford University Press.

Drammen Municipality [Drammen Kommune]. (2012). *Fjell 2010.* Retrieved from www.drammen.kommune.no/no/Budsjettportal-Drammen-kommune/Tertialrapporter-Drammen-kommune/2012-1/Organisasjon-og-prosjekter/Fjell-2020/

Drange, N. (2013). *Evaluation of a program providing free time in day care.* [Evaluering av forsøk med gratis kjernetid i barnehage.] Statistics Norway Report 56. Retrieved from www.ssb.no/utdanning/artikler-og-publikasjoner/evaluering-av-forsok-med-gratis-kjernetid-i-barnehage#content

Esping-Andersen, G. (1990). *The three worlds of welfare capitalism.* Cambridge: Polity Press.

Fosse, E., & Helgesen, M. K. (2015). How can local governments level the social gradient in health among families with children? The case of Norway. *International Journal of Child, Youth and Family Studies, 6*(2), 328–346.

Government of Norway. (2009). *Plan against ethnic discrimination.* [Plan mot etnisk diskriminering.] Retrieved from www.regjeringen.no/upload/BLD/Planer/2009/hpl_etnisk_diskriminering.pdf

Government of Norway. (2011a). *Welfare and migration: The future of the Norwegian model.* [Velferd og Migrasjon. Den Norske modellens fremtid.] Retrieved from www.regjeringen.no/nb/dep/bld/dok/nouer/2011/nou-2011-07.html?id=642496

Government of Norway. (2011b). The Norwegian public health act. [Folkehelseloven.] Retrieved from https://lovdata.no/dokument/NL/lov/2011-06-24-29

Government of Norway. (2011c). *The coordination reform.* [Samhandlingsreformen.] Retrieved from www.regjeringen.no/nb/dokumenter/prop-91-l-20102011/id638731/

Government of Norway. (2013). *Equal health and care services—good health for all.* [Likeverdige helse- og omsorgstjenester—god helse for alle.] Oslo: Ministry of Health and Care Services. Retrieved from www.regjeringen.no/pages/38431748/Likeverdige_tjenester.pdf

Hægeland, T., Kirkebøn, L., Raaum, O., & Salvanes, K. (2004). *Marks across lower secondary schools in Norway.* Statistics Norway Report 2004/11. Oslo/Kongsvinger: Statistics Norway.

Kavli, H., Hagelund, A., & Bråthen, M (2007). *With the right to learn and the duty to participate.* [Med rett til å lære og plikt til å delta.] Fafo-report 2007/34. Oslo: Fafo.

Lundberg, O., Yngwe, M. Å., Stjärne, M. K., Elstad, J. I., Ferrarini, T., Kangas, O., et al. for the NEWS Nordic Expert Group. (2008). The role of welfare state principles and generosity in social policy programmes for public health: An international comparative study. *Lancet, 372*(9650), 1633–1640.

Marmot, M. (2009). Closing the health gap in a generation: The work of the Commission on Social Determinants of Health and its recommendations. *Global Health Promotion, 16*(1), 23–27.

Marmot, M. (2010). *The Marmot review. Fair society, healthy lives. Strategic review of health inequalities in England post-2010.* London: UCL Institute of Health Equity.

Moafi, H. (2012). *First year with legal free homework assistance.* [Første år med lovfestet gratis leksehjelp.] Samfunnspeilet 2012/1. Oslo: Statistics Norway. Retrieved from www.ssb.no/utdanning/artikler-og-publikasjoner/forste-aar-med-lovfestet-gratis-leksehjelp

Modood, T. (2013). *Multiculturalism* (2nd ed.). London: John Wiley & Sons.

Mogstad, M. (2005) *Poverty in Norway: A problem for the capital?* [Fattigdom i Norge: Et hovedstadsproblem?] Economic Analyses 3/2005. Oslo: Statistics Norway.

Nekby, L. (2008). *Active labor market programs for the integration of youths and immigrants into the labor market—The Nordic experience.* Report for the UN Economic Commission for Latin America and the Caribbean (ECLAC). Santiago, Chile: ECLAC. Retrieved from http://labordoc.ilo.org/record/413695

OECD. (2008). *Jobs for immigrants—labour marked integration in Norway.* Paris: Author. Retrieved from http://www.oecd.org/migration/mig/43247521.pdf

OECD. (2009). *OECD employment outlook: Tackling the jobs crisis.* Paris: Author.

OECD. (2011). *OECD reviews of evaluation and assessment in education. Norway.* Paris: Author. Retrieved from www.oecd.org/norway/48632032.pdf

Oslo Municipality. [Oslo Kommune.] (2013). *The Groruddal program.* [Groruddalsatsningen.] Retrieved from www.prosjekt-groruddalen.oslo.kommune.no/programomrade_4/

Queen's University. (2014). *Multicultural policies in contemporary democracies.* Kingston, ON: Author. Retrieved from http://www.queensu.ca/mcp/home

Røed, K., & Raaum, O. (2003). *The effect of programme participation on the transition rate from unemployment to employment.* Department of Economics Memorandum no. 13/2003. Oslo: University of Oslo.

Sainsbury, D. (2006). Immigrants' social rights in comparative perspective: Welfare regimes, forms in immigration and immigration policy regimes. *Journal of European Social Policy, 16*(3), 229–244.

Schou, A., Helgesen, M. K., & Hofstad, H. (2014). [*The effect of the coordination reform on health promotion and disease prevention activities in municipalities.*] *Samhandlingsreformens effekt på kommunen som helsefremmende og sykdomsforebyggende aktør.* NIBR-report 2014:21. Oslo: Norwegian Institute for Urban and Rural Research.

Sinding Larsen, Å., & Kjellevold, A. (2012). Illegal immigration as a basis of rejecting health-care and social services? ["Ulovlig opphold" som grunnlag for å avskjære helse- og sosialhjelp?] *Tidsskrift for velferdsforskning, 2*, 93–108.

Public Policy, Immigrant Experiences, and Health Outcomes in Sweden

Hannah Bradby and Sandra Torres

Chapter Objectives

This chapter focuses on the immigration and integration of immigrants into Swedish society. The objectives of this chapter are:

- to evaluate the development of immigration policy in Sweden in the context of this welfare state's conceptualization of the "people's home" or *folkhemmet*;
- to examine the implications that this development has had for the homogenizing tendencies that characterize Swedish immigration policy and public debate on immigrants;
- to consider the implications that these tendencies have on the ways in which older immigrants are constructed as a category in Swedish policy and public debate;
- to review research on older immigrants' health, appreciate its limitations, and suggest how it can be regarded as an example of the aforementioned homogenizing tendencies; and
- on the basis of the above, to critically assess the Swedish version of multiculturalism.

Introduction

Can welfare benefits persist at current levels in the face of a significant level of immigration that is diversifying the Swedish population, which is one of the oldest in Europe? Sweden represents an interesting test case for how homogeneity, solidarity, and welfare are linked, given that 20 percent of its aging population is of **"foreign background"** and given the high level of public support for the welfare state, both in terms of public opinion and income taxes.

This chapter offers a portrait of the development of immigration and welfare policies in Sweden as a contribution to the wider debate on how the changing nature of immigration and diversity is affecting expectations and configurations of, and aspirations for, the welfare state. Exploring how immigrants have been constructed as a category in Swedish policy allows consideration of the tensions between "integration" and "assimilation" that lie at the core of Sweden's welfare state's approach to immigrants.

A description of Nordic welfare models offers context for characterizing the Swedish model and, in particular, the ways that cultural pluralism arising from immigration challenges the integrative, standardizing logic of the universal welfare state. An account of the relationship between diversity and migration in Sweden precedes a critical discussion of immigration-relevant policy that is divided into four time periods from the 1930s to the present (see Table 11.1). The development of immigration policy, focused on labour immigration from the 1950s and on refugees and family reunification after the 1970s, is described. In the development of policy, immigrants have been constructed as citizens with special vulnerabilities, placing particular demands on the welfare state. The assumptions concerning the status and needs of immigrants encapsulated in policy, which have tended to focus on a presumed lack of integration leading to particular vulnerability, are examined with regard to how policy has played out in practice for older migrants, a group that is seldom considered when migrant policies are discussed. Thus, the way in which the elder care debate on older migrants has evolved in Sweden and the scant evidence that exists about older migrants' situation in this country are discussed to illustrate the homogenizing tendencies that have been characteristic of Swedish policy and the public debate on immigrants. The limited research on older immigrants' health is presented as an example of how the homogenizing tendencies in question limit the insightfulness of such research. By describing the development of immigration policy linked with the response of the welfare state to this particular group of immigrants, the chapter illustrates how Sweden's version of a multicultural society emphasizes positive rights as a result of residence, but offers few exemptions from governance on the grounds of culture or religion, in line with the constraints of the universal welfare system.

Nordic Welfare Models

In international comparative work, Nordic countries exemplify welfare systems that prioritize equity and employ robust redistributive policies through statutory and municipal taxes, benefits, and services in order to mitigate the damaging effects of poverty structured through class and gender inequality. Such welfare states are characterized as comprehensive, institutionalized, solidaristic, and universal (Esping-Andersen, 1990).

Table 11.1: Swedish Migration and Migration Policy

Time Period	Key Events Policy	Key Events Practice	Characteristic Migration
Pre-1964	• No specific immigration policy	Net in-migration, language support, and integration practices developed	Labour migrants from neighbouring Nordic and Baltic countries
1964–1975	• Eventual adoption of multicultural policy • Principles of equality, freedom of choice, and co-operation asserted	Mixed-culture vs. multi-culture debated	Non-Nordic workers begin to arrive from Turkey, the former Yugoslavia, and Southern Europe
1975–1989	• Foreign citizens' right to vote in municipal elections • Consolidation of rights to language support • Refugee dispersal policy • Assertion of "Swedish" values	Restriction of immigration, including for refugees	Labour migrants give way to refugees and asylum-seekers
1990s	• Distinction between migrant and minority group established	• Welfare state accused of creating dependency • Economic crisis	Further entry restrictions, including for family reunification
1999–Present	• EU entry	• Integration emphasized • Election of Sverigedemokraterna (the Sweden Democrats)	Accession migration adding to existing diversity

Source: Adapted from J. Widgren. (1982). *Svensk invandrarpolitik*. Lund: Liber Läromedel; J. Widgren (1988). *Svensk invandrar och flyktingpolitik*. Stockholm: Arbetsmarknadsdepartamentet; C. Dahlström (2004). Rhetoric, practice, and the dynamics of institutional change: Immigrant policy in Sweden, 1964–2000. *Scandinavian Political Studies, 27*(3), 287–310.

This characterization implies that welfare is available to the whole population, not just the most vulnerable, which for immigrants usually means those with legal rights to extended domicile. Nordic welfare systems have, in large measure, alleviated the family of its obligations to care for its vulnerable members and puts great emphasis on the provision of services at a local level, which in turn implies high levels of employment in the production of welfare (Brochmann & Hagelund, 2012) and, particularly for an aging population, the need for immigrant labour.

The Swedish welfare system enjoys popular support and employs fiscal and non-fiscal universal benefits with relatively little means-testing. It is supported by high levels of taxation and social security contributions, as well as extensive public sector employment in health and social care sectors (Thakur, Keen, Horváth, & Cerra, 2003). In understanding the development of this comprehensive approach to welfare, the period from 1932 to 1976 during which the Social Democratic Party governed continuously is important for the set of radical reforms that were enacted. In persuading voters to support these major social reforms, the concept of *folkhem*, which had been developed from the late 1920s, emphasized democracy, citizenship, and modernity, which, together with ideas of solidarity, was central. ***Folkhemmet*** or **"the people's home"** was a model of national co-operation justified by familial models of contribution, rather than **communitarian** or **redistributive political ideology**. Conceptualizing the Swedish population in familial terms rendered the communitarian aspects of solidarity less threatening and allowed a "third way" between socialism and capitalism to develop (Borevi, 2012).[1]

The central ideal of equality within the *folkhem* was predicated on cultural conformity, such that everyone had access to a similarly good standard of living. Borevi (2012, p. 27) refers to a "homogenizing zeal" directed against those thought to deviate from the strong norm of seeking to put "life in order" through social engineering. Without the narrow consensus and paternalistic aspects of the *folkhem*, the emancipation of the individual (and especially women) from the constraints of family life may never have been achieved. A system predicated on conformity to culturally acceptable equality holds within it the possibility of the exclusion of those who do not or cannot conform—high levels of co-operation reliant on strong in-group identification. Thus, from the outset, the Swedish welfare system contained a potential paradox in that the ability of the state to take on what had previously been the familial task of supporting the young, sick, and needy relies on a high level of employment (Andersson, Magnusson Turner, & Holmqvist, 2010; Freeman, 1986). With high levels of public employment comes the potential need for labour migrants, and so the conformity underpinning a communitarian egalitarian redistribution can potentially be disrupted by migration-driven diversity. The identification of new arrivals as part of the in-group—as part of "us" and so belonging to the co-operative, mutually supportive group—would allow the perpetuation of the *folkhem* ideology in the face of migration.

The interaction between employment and immigration is an important feature in understanding the development of the welfare system, especially given the key role that labour organizations have played in negotiating the blocking or promotion of immigration (Borevi, 2012).

Diversity, Equality, and Immigration

Sweden belongs to a group of OECD countries with very low income disparities, which has been linked with elevated life expectancy as compared with other European countries (Marmot, 2005). However, since the economic crisis of the 1990s, these disparities have been growing, even if they remain lower than the OECD average (Andersson et al., 2010). Evidence regarding the health penalty of immigrant status (Lindström, Sundquist, & Östergren, 2001) and a reassessment of how equity in health outcomes should be measured (Popham, Dibben, & Bambra, 2013) has called into question a simplified view of Sweden as a multicultural welfare system success story (Bambra, 2011).

Twenty percent of the population of Sweden is of foreign background[2] and this population is concentrated in the big cities—Stockholm, Gothenburg, and Malmö—where some neighbourhoods have a majority of immigrant residents. Until the 1960s the Swedish population was fairly homogeneous in terms of religion and ethnicity. Long-standing trade and labour-migration with neighbouring Scandinavian and Baltic countries involved immigration, but the Christian and Northern European origins of these immigrants meant that they were absorbed into the national ideal of Swedishness. Since the 1960s labour immigrants have given way to refugee and family reunification, which characterizes the Swedish immigration of the late 20th and early 21st centuries (Andersson et al., 2010).

The political emphasis on integration (which critics might term "assimilation"), explored in more detail below, has led to introductory programs designed to assist newcomers to achieve integration by providing information and employment training. These programs are seen as the key to successful integration. While this worked reasonably well for the labour immigrants of the 1960s, since large-scale refugee immigration began, there has been intermittent debate about the excessive length of time taken for immigrants to become established in the labour market and the difficulty of reducing this time period. Despite the largely successful integration of immigrants into Swedish society, there are significant problems, especially for people arriving from non-European countries, who, in the last 25 years have tended to be subordinated in both labour and housing markets (Andersson et al., 2010). The urban civil unrest from 2009 onward has been interpreted as a strong expression of the frustration of young people of immigrant background at being excluded from the social benefits of a successful society (Schierup & Alund, 2011).

The strong nationalistic sense of having built a good and inclusive society, underpinned by the ideal of *folkhemmet*, is in tension with the sense among visible-minority immigrants that they are excluded from this ideal of solidarity and equality (Pred, 2000). As in many Western European countries, anti-immigration parties have sprung up in Sweden from the 1970s onward, but until recently, Sweden could claim exceptional status in terms of anti-immigration parties having failed electorally (Dahlström & Esaiasson, 2011). In 2014 the explicitly anti-immigration party Sverigedemokraterna (Sweden Democrats, not to be confused with the Social Democrats—Socialdemokraterna) doubled its previous level of voter support to gain a 14 percent stake in the Swedish Parliament, and exceptionalism could no longer be claimed. The election of a party that deems Sweden's immigrant policy a failure and that emphasizes the assimilation or repatriation of existing immigrants, alongside a restriction of further immigration, shows a significant disenchantment with existing immigrant policy. The difficulty of supplying adequate welfare services to the existing Swedish residents is used as an argument to restrict migration and promote **welfare chauvinism** whereby welfare benefits are available only to those who "belong" to Sweden.

Dahlström (2004) has shown that although the rhetoric of immigrant policy in Sweden has changed over past decades, the practice of immigrant policy has remained largely constant. While Sweden's Social Democratic political regime accords rights on the basis of citizenship, the immigration policy regime is actually far more inclusive since it accords rights on the basis of residence (*ius domicilii*) (Sainsbury, 2006). In surveying the development of immigrant policy over time, Widgren (1982, 1988) classified modern Swedish policy regarding immigration and minorities into three distinct phases that could be differentially characterized and that we have drawn on in Table 11.1. From 1930 to 1963 no specific immigration policy had been formulated, although immigration to Sweden exceeded emigration out of Sweden. The integration of immigrants into the workforce was a requirement stipulated by the labour organizations, which were powerful players in Swedish politics (Lundqvist, 2006). By the mid-1960s early policies to aid immigrants' adjustment to Swedish society were being formulated to "incorporate immigrants in a civil community where they could claim individual rights" (Dahlström, 2004, p. 301). These policies consisted of free language training in Swedish and information about Swedish society and political institutions directed to adult immigrants in their native language, together with "home-language" training for immigrant children. So despite the lack of immigration policy, Sweden had de facto policies aimed at the integration of immigrants who could be characterized as labour migrants.

1964 to 1975: Multicultural Policy and the Principle of Equality

Intense public debate but few overtly political stands (Widgren, 1988) characterized the period during which the foundations of an active Swedish immigration and immigrant policy were established. This debate was conducted in a relatively apolitical way (Hammar, 1999) between politically independent commentators rather than between political parties, with Swedish immigrant policy never having been tested through inter-party debate or voter opinion (Dahlström, 2004). The debate in the daily press turned on the pros and cons of a "mixed culture society" (*blandkultursamhälle*) or a "multicultural society" (*flerkultursamhälle*). The advocates of the mixed culture approach argued that the state should neither support the cultural activities of immigrants nor should it force immigrants to assimilate culturally. Rather, immigrants and Swedes should influence one another reciprocally such that the adjustments that were needed as Sweden became an ethnically and culturally diverse society would happen voluntarily.

The advocates of the multicultural approach argued that the mixed cultural approach was actually an assimilationist approach in disguise. Rather than the state effectively forcing immigrants to abandon their cultural identities, it was argued that statutory resources should be made available for the support of minority cultures. Asserting a principle of self-determination for labour immigrants to choose their cultural identity and supporting that choice actively had the potential advantage of facilitating their eventual return to their sending society. Labour immigrants were being drawn into Sweden from further afield than previously, including from Turkey, the former Yugoslavia, and Southern Europe.

Dahlström (2004) argues that even while the public debate on "multiculturalism" versus "mixed culture" was underway, the government sent a bill to Parliament, which included the basic design of Sweden's immigrant policy passed in 1975. The minister of interior who formulated the policies at the time was an advocate of mixed cultural society, and so a Swedish version of assimilationist practices was adopted, even though the public debate never reached an explicit resolution. These policies took equality between immigrants and natives as an official guiding principle. So, for example, immigrants' rights to interpreter and translator services when dealing with Swedish municipalities (if they lacked a decent command of Swedish) were established. At the same time, regulation of immigration was introduced, being regarded as a prerequisite for upholding the principle of equality: levels of immigration had to be matched with the country's capacity to provide immigrants with employment, housing, social care, and education on the same terms as the rest of the population (Borevi, 2012).

The multicultural policy that had been established implied a set of reforms, including the home-language policy based on principles of equality, freedom of choice, and co-operation (Andersson et al., 2010). Future immigrant and minority policy-making would aim for "equality," "freedom of choice," and "co-operation" (sometimes interpreted as "partnership") (Soininen, 1999). By "equality" the Swedish government meant that immigrants were to be guaranteed the same rights, opportunities, and obligations enjoyed by native Swedes—an inclusive multicultural conception based on residence, not birth (Schierup & Alund, 2011). "Freedom of choice" implied that immigrants should have the freedom to determine the degree to which they assimilate, meaning that they could choose between preserving a non-Swedish identity and culture and acquiring Swedish values and traditions. The goal of "co-operation" referred to the expectation and commitment to solidarity and tolerance between Swedes and immigrants. These choices have an "either-or" reasoning that characterize ethnic relations that dichotomize between "us" and "them." The idea launched here was not that immigrants could create hybrid identities but rather that they could choose between the identity they came with (the basis for the assumption that they are different from "us") and the identity that integration into Swedish society could offer (the basis for the "us"—i.e., native Swedes—from which people with foreign backgrounds are excluded).

The newly formulated policies were criticized heavily both by trade unions and the daily press (Román, 1994), but nonetheless concrete immigrant policies had been established in law. Language support and acquisition were adopted as key issues by the labour organizations, since learning Swedish and how society worked was thought to be key in maintaining union influence (Lundqvist, 2006).

1975 to late 1980s: Consequences of Multi-ethnic Declaration

Having voted to declare itself a multi-ethnic country in 1975, the Swedish Parliament had an explicit immigrant policy rather than just a practice. Swedish immigrant policy defined "migrant groups as ethnic minority communities" and aimed "at equality between ethnic groups, while emphasizing separate existences and collective identities" (Soysal, 1994, p. 80). Equality was promoted with the establishment of the right of foreign citizens to vote in local elections in 1976. Services that started in the early 1970s were consolidated by the "native language reform" of 1977, obliging Swedish municipalities to offer training in native languages to immigrant children from preschool to secondary school, confirming immigrants as having "special" rather than "universal" needs.

This multicultural reform was a distancing from the assimilationist character of earlier immigration practice by offering equal access to formal rights of citizenship, including health and welfare benefits, and bolstering the cultural and social resources of immigrants to facilitate involvement in civil society (Schierup & Alund, 2011, p. 48). But the formal access and support of immigrants' participation in civil society was not enough to prevent discrimination and exclusionary labour market practices from systematically limiting immigrants' opportunities (Schierup & Alund, 2011).

Borevi (2012) refers to the multicultural retreat of the mid-1980s as both the character of immigration and its conceptualization shifted. At this time labour immigration gave way to refugees and family reunification, and with the beginning of high unemployment rates among new immigrants came economic motivations for restricting immigration (Lundqvist, 2006). In the early 1980s the immigration board was established and took over responsibility for immigrants from the labour organizations, while changes to the legal regulation of immigration meant that after 1984, refugees could not automatically expect to have their cases approved (Borevi, 2012). The refugee dispersal policy launched in 1984 put great emphasis on municipal authorities organizing the integration of immigrants, directing them away from metropolitan areas (Andersson et al., 2010). Municipalities had to make an agreement to take migrants in return for statutory financial support, which meant that the municipal availability of housing came to dictate where refugees in particular were allocated, rather than the availability of work, as had been the case earlier.

A parliamentary decision of 1986 moderated the "freedom of choice" aspect of the 1975 multicultural declaration, in that primacy was awarded to certain key "Swedish values," in particular gender equality and the rights of children, which could not be compromised with reference to religious or cultural belief systems (SOU, 1997). In the 1960s, when labour migration from neighbouring countries had dominated immigration, the active integration of immigrants to Swedish society through employment was a route to the social benefits of full participatory citizenship, which seemed to work relatively well. With the upturn of refugee migration from the late 1970s, which coincided with the deregulation of the labour marketplace, the merits of diversity and heterogeneity for their own sake came to be vaunted (Lundqvist, 2006). But the promotion of heterogeneity as a social good coincided with the moment when voters in at least one municipality refused to embrace refugees as neighbours. Since local authorities could choose whether or not to make an agreement to accept refugees, a referendum was organized in Sjöbo in 1988. Voters refused to condone accepting refugees, which was interpreted as discontent over immigrant policy and the political establishment (Borevi, 2012).

With the arrival of 28,000 asylum-seekers over six months in 1989/1990, the Swedish reception of refugees had expended the resources allocated for the whole year. During the consequent crisis, the government's need to be seen to limit migration was more pressing than the need to be seen as generous and humanitarian on the world stage (Borevi, 2012). The crisis gave rise to the "All Sweden Strategy" to distribute immigrants to all agreeable municipalities up to the level 2.9 per 1,000 of their population per year (Soininen, 1992). The dispersal policy led to subsequent significant secondary migration from small to larger municipalities during the period

1980 to 1995, but despite refugees choosing to relocate to bigger towns and cities, all municipalities became more diverse (Andersson et al., 2010).

Overall authority for refugee reception moved from the Swedish National Labour Market Board (Arbetsmarknadsverket AMV) to social work with implications for the role of the immigrant in Sweden. Refugees tended to be treated along the same lines as social work's other clients, that is, as people in need of a combination of care and discipline (Soininen, 1999). Thus, problems with refugee reception in the 1980s, such as the long delay to employment in the labour market, were treated as individual problems of immigrant clients' inadequacies. Immigrants came to be seen as a "weak" category, having particular problems to overcome, and this idea perhaps "took root in the population at large—not least the new arrivals themselves" (Borevi, 2012, p. 53).

1990s: Immigration Restrictions

The 1990s brought criticism of the welfare state for having turned people into weak clients who were unable to realize their own innate capacity (Hirdman, 1989) and intensified the need for new solutions. A new period of intensive committee and survey work started with new experts from cultural anthropology traditions specializing in "immigrant research" getting involved in this process. Anthropological critique of welfare providers' homogenizing view of culture led to the suggestion that immigrants should be seen as individuals (Borevi, 2012).

A distinction, which had not been made up until now, between immigrant policy and minority policy was established. These and other adjustments meant that the culture-preserving ambitions of immigrant policies were considerably lowered during this period. Despite the lowering of expectations in terms of the rhetoric of Sweden's immigrant policy, the practices of immigrant policy described earlier remained largely consistent. Dahlström (2004) argues that although most immigrant policies have been criticized on various occasions, the debates surrounding them have never actually addressed whether or not they make sense, but rather the efficiency of the policies has been at the core of debates through the years.

The early 1990s saw a dramatic increase in Swedish unemployment to levels that had not been seen since the 1930s, which together with a declining **gross domestic product** and a budget crisis constituted a serious economic recession. This recession coincided with Sweden's increasing dependency on policies enforced elsewhere due to membership in the EU from 1995; the rise of an immigrant-critical party called New Democracy; and an increase in instances of racialized violence. Over this period refugee policy shifted from liberal to more restrictive in terms of curbing entry, including for reasons of family reunification (Borevi, 2012), while more generally there was a shift from corporatist to individualist approaches to integration.

Late 1990s: New Tensions

The most recent phase of Sweden's immigrant policy can be dated from the late 1990s, when new objectives were formulated. Criticism had grown of the stigmatizing effects of the practice of immigrant policy that creates and maintains a division between "us and them," despite the breadth of diversity represented in Swedish society. As a result, in 1997 Sweden's immigrant policy was reconfigured as an integration policy, meaning that immigrants were not to be singled out as beneficiaries of selective programs but rather should be incorporated in the system of universalist welfare policies. The neo-liberal turn in the wake of the economic crisis saw the stimulation of business being promoted as a means to ensure both economic growth and social inclusion across the population (Schierup & Alund, 2011). This means that, rhetorically at least, the typical 1970s set-up, with statutory support for a system of ethnic groups participating on equal terms, was officially abandoned.

Despite such rhetorical transformations in the immigrant policy over the past four decades, practice implied by Swedish immigrant policy has been fairly stable over time in aiming at integration (Dahlström, 2004). While pluralist policies have appeared on the immigrant policy landscape, Sweden has not become a multicultural society in that it has followed a policy of civic integration without active recognition of ethnic groups, rather than a multicultural policy where a civic notion of the nation coexists with active recognition of minority ethnic groups (Borevi, 2012). The Swedish approach has been to define immigrants' positive rights to obtain resources and uphold their own culture, but to confer very few, if any, negative rights in terms of exemptions from particular practices or regulation on religious or cultural grounds.

Sweden has awarded its immigrants numerous social rights, including the right to vote at the municipal level, since access to rights is based not on one's country of birth but on one's residence or domicile. Moreover, Sweden has an encompassing definition of refugees and a convention for equal treatment of refugees and people granted asylum for humanitarian reasons; it has had generous rules for family reunification; it has offered foreign workers equal access to unemployment and occupational injury benefits at an early date; and it has offered its immigrants national health insurance, child and housing allowances, and social assistance after a short period of residence (Sainsbury, 2006). The Swedish system can be characterized as showing a strong commitment to the integrative logic of the Social Democratic welfare state by its standardizing institutional arrangements and rules that apply to all who enjoy solidarity within the "people's home." The importance of solidarity informs the skepticism toward the formation of special institutions for ethnic groups as disruptive of the solidaristic familial ideal. Mother-tongue teaching is emblematic as a means of recognizing diversity while simultaneously emphasizing institutional integration, educating children so they will eventually become fully assimilated Swedish citizens. Thus cultural pluralism is recognized, but strongly subjected to the constraints of welfare policy with its comprehensive and universal aims (Borevi, 2012).

Any social or cultural features that might attract the label "multiculturalism" are so intertwined with structures of the national welfare state that a culturally pluralist vision can only really be seen in the private spheres of life. Alongside the formal, official generosity, with its integrationist logic, there is palpable segregation between Sweden's native population and its immigrant population (Andersson, 1999; Edin, Fredriksson, & Åslund, 2004; Pred, 1997; Rydgren, 2004). Despite evidence of segregation, the European Social Survey 2010 suggests that Swedes are the most pro-immigrant country in Europe and, furthermore, Sweden has so far resisted the European practice of introducing tests as a condition for obtaining residence or achieving citizenship, despite various proposals (Borevi, 2012).

Integration has been the thoroughgoing practice of Swedish immigrant policy, further strengthened by the standardizing effect of the welfare state's institutional arrangements and the value placed on solidarity. This combination has militated against research developing on the well-being or experience of distinct social groups defined by a dimension of diversity. Not until 2005 was the topic of structural discrimination addressed by an official government report (SOU, 2005), which represented a novel admission of how religious and ethnic difference might be a dimension of discrimination. This report drew on research evidence from outside Sweden by necessity, given the lack of statutory or municipal data on ethnic or religious groups, and was shortly followed by another on health care and discrimination (Groglopo & Ahlberg, 2006), which drew on a very slim Swedish evidence base.

With the possibility of discrimination affecting health care and health outcomes so recently acknowledged by official sources, and the political emphasis on Swedish values rather than supporting distinct groups, there is little material that offers a systematic appraisal of the experience of immigrants or minorities within the welfare system. Furthermore, the welfare system is rationed on the basis of individual identity numbers, such that undocumented or irregular migrants are formally debarred and their experience is even more difficult to document (Médecins Sans Frontières, 2005). While acknowledging this lack of evidence, we focus below on older immigrants to explore what can be said about their health and welfare in Sweden today.

Older Immigrants: A Neglected Group in Migration Policy Discussions

The complexities and paradoxes of how those classified as "immigrants" or of "immigrant background" have encountered the welfare state and how this is reflected in the uptake and experience of elder care and health services is briefly described below with respect to older immigrants. Attending to this particular group is instructive because older people are likely to be out of the workforce and therefore regarded as a particularly vulnerable group within the Swedish immigrant population, where employment has been regarded as such a key mechanism of integration. Moreover, within the feminist debate on "ethics of care," it has long been established that how a welfare state organizes elder care services gives us important insights into a society's moral and political life (cf. Tronto, 1995, 2010) as well as its relationship with "particular Others" (cf. Narayan, 1995). The treatment of older immigrants who are no longer economically active offers insight into the moral and political categorizations to which immigrants are more generally subject in Sweden.

Older immigrants are a heterogeneous group, including "people who are among the most deprived and excluded in our societies ... and others who are in the vanguard of innovative, developmental and positive approaches to later life" (Warnes et al., 2004, pp. 310–311). Two distinct subgroups within the category of older immigrants should be recognized: those who immigrate early in life and age as immigrants, and those who immigrate in old age. The former are often assumed to have immigrated for reasons of either political and/or religious persecution (as in the case of refugees) or for work-related opportunities (as in the case of labour migrants), while the latter are assumed to be motivated by either amenity-seeking reasons (such as better retirement conditions) or family-reunification purposes. The number of older people with foreign backgrounds in Sweden has grown steadily in the two decades such that 12 percent of the population aged 65 and older had a foreign-born background at the end of 2012 (SCB, 2013). The largest increase of older people with this background has occurred among 75–84-year-olds, an "age category where the need for help and support increases" (Socialstyrelsen, 2009, p. 20).

Older immigrants are heterogeneous in terms of ethnic and cultural background, as demonstrated by the 165 countries of birth represented among a group that is largely made up of people who arrived in Sweden as young adult labour immigrants. As workers, they were actively engaged in helping to build up the familial model of egalitarian national co-operation underpinning the Swedish model of welfare or *folkhem*. A small minority of older immigrants came to Sweden late in life for family reunification purposes, and yet this latter group's perceived needs dominate the elder care sector debate (Ronström, 2002; Torres, 2006, 2013; Machat, 2010; Torres, Lindblom, & Nordberg, 2014). The tendency to assume that older immigrants are by definition (and irrespective of when they migrated and of their present situation) vulnerable due to a lack of integration is one means whereby a focus on aspects of immigrants differentiates them from ethnic Swedes, thereby maintaining the "us" and "them" division that permeates the migrant policies discussed earlier.

Older Immigrants: A Policy Category under Construction

It has been established that the debate about elder care tends to homogenize the category of older immigrants, disregarding the range of migration motives, socio-economic backgrounds, and the variety of ethnocultural and religious backgrounds represented, which could have important bearing not only on the way in which they are regarded but also on the way in which we design care services to cater to their needs (Torres, Lindblom, & Nordberg, 2014; Torres, 2006). The public debate about care for older immigrants was instigated at the beginning of the 1980s (Torres, 2006) with the publication of two reports by the National Board of Health and Welfare (i.e., Sachs, 1980; Zetzell, 1980). Neither of these reports included any empirical data on older immigrants in Sweden, but were instead based on reviews of literature gathered in other parts of the world about what it is like to grow old in a foreign country. At that time, the vast majority of people with an immigrant background approaching old age had come to Sweden primarily from other Nordic or European countries as labour immigrants, raising questions as to whether it was relevant or even appropriate to speak of this group as people who were "aging in a foreign country." Reports published since have continued to take for granted that older immigrants are alienated from Swedish society, regardless of when they arrived, how long they have been established, whether or not they are citizens, and how well they have adapted to Swedish society.

Reports on elder care through the years also tend to regard older immigrants as fundamentally different from their Swedish counterparts, while policy documents refer to them as a "specific group" of older people to which the sector needs to respond (Ronström, 2002). Older immigrants are, in other words, often assumed to be vulnerable because they are believed to be socially isolated and ill adapted to Swedish society, even though a study of income mobility among the elderly in Sweden during the 1990s has shown that there are "only small differences between Sweden-born and foreign-born people" (Zaidi & Gustafsson, 2007, p. 90). Despite assumptions of homogeneous vulnerability, there are, in fact, no studies that have looked into older immigrants' actual backgrounds in terms of ethnicity, class, and education level and neither has there been enough inquiry into the present situation of this group. With the exception of the work that has been done on health-related outcomes (described below), most studies of older immigrants in Sweden have been ethnic-specific (but not ethnically representative) qualitative studies with convenience samples. Older immigrants are thus established as an elder-care policy category rather than a group of older people per se. As such, the category hides more than it reveals (e.g., Ronström, 2002; Machat, 2010; Torres, 2006). At the core of the construction of the policy category of older immigrants in Sweden is the idea that they have "special needs" requiring culturally appropriate care, thereby posing particular challenges to the elder-care sector.

The social construction of this vulnerable, needy category of older immigrants in Sweden means that the group is seen as constituting, in and of itself, a welfare challenge (Torres, 2015). As such, the social construction of older immigrants in Sweden is an example of the kind of discussion about immigrants that Borevi (2012) describes as betraying the "homogenizing zeal" to reform heterogeneity to a culturally agreed equality. The construction of the policy category of older immigrants is redolent of the Swedish welfare policies' goals of putting "life in order." The debate on older immigrants in Sweden has not been about who these older people are (i.e., where they come from, their current conditions, and what they need), but rather about what Sweden (and specifically Swedish elder care) can do for them. Designing policies and services to cater to older immigrants requires a move beyond stereotypical ideas of who "they" are and what "they" need, to invest instead in designing studies that build evidence-based policy and practice to cater to the variety of potential needs that may exist. Worth noting is that we write "potential needs" since we do not, in fact, know whether older immigrants have the "special needs" they have been assumed to have, nor do we know how many of them place particular demands on the welfare state.

In the following section we discuss some limited research evidence on the health of older immigrants, aware that we risk reinscribing the problematic homogenizing and dichotomizing effects of the construction of the category "older migrants."

Research on Older Immigrants' Health: The Implications of the "Us" and "Them" Division

Studies drawing on data from national registers enable comparisons between older immigrants and their Swedish counterparts, and contribute to Sweden's long tradition of conducting longitudinal population studies. Swedish research on health disparities that primarily focuses on the adult population up to 65 shows that immigrants have poorer self-reported health than native-born individuals (Lindström et al., 2001; Sungurova et al., 2006; Taloyan et al., 2008; Wiking et al., 2004), as well as higher risks of the following conditions: long-term illness and acute illness (Sundqvist & Johansson, 1997), diabetes (Wändell et al., 2008), cardiovascular or coronary heart disease (Gadd et al., 2003, 2006), acute myocardial infarction (Hedlund et al., 2007), schizophrenia, and psychoses (Hjern et al., 2004).

A European comparative study, the "Survey of Health, Aging and Retirement in Europe" (SHARE), studied health differences between older immigrants and non-migrants by looking at the 50+ age group in 11 European countries and contextualizing the Swedish findings.[3] Solé-Auró and Crimmins (2008) note that older immigrants in Switzerland, Denmark, the Netherlands, and Sweden are "more likely to have functioning difficulties than the native population in each of these countries," and that "in no other country is there a significant difference between immigrants and the native-born in ADL-problems" (Solé-Auró & Crimmins, 2008, p. 871). Notably, these same countries had the best overall levels of functioning and the lowest levels of ADL (activities of daily living) problems, suggesting that any differences in health between migrants and non-migrants must be understood against the backdrop of the very good health of the native population. According to SHARE data, Sweden is part of a group of countries where immigrants have the poorest levels of self-reported health and have had the most disability or disease (the other countries being Switzerland, Netherlands, Germany, and France). When compared to non-migrants, older immigrants were also found to be more likely to be overweight in Germany and Sweden. Moreover, levels of chronic diseases among immigrants in Sweden and Spain were significantly higher than other countries even after controlling for education.

This study indicates that the health of older immigrants in Sweden is not only poorer than the health of their non-migrant Swedish counterparts, but also the poorest among European countries. As such, this suggests that there is reason to question whether or not the Swedish welfare state has the capacity to address the needs of its immigrant population. This conclusion seems quite straightforward at first glance. However, a disaggregation of the category "older immigrant" according to place of birth, reason for migration, level of education, occupational background, and gender might problematize the evidence of immigrant vulnerability. Such disaggregation is not done in this particular study nor has it been done in the various studies that have been conducted over the years.

We can speculate that the centrality of the "us" and "them" parameters that have been at the core of migration policies may have informed the lack of interrogation of the construction of the variable "older immigrant" in the research on health that has been conducted in Sweden. The focus we have had so far directs research interest in the older immigrant population toward between-group differences (i.e., How do they fare compared to their Swedish counterparts?) as opposed to within-group differences (i.e., How do different kinds of older immigrants fare against each other?). In doing so, the category of older immigrants becomes homogenized and the differences between them remain occluded. We suggest therefore that the homogenizing tendencies that characterize Sweden's migration policy have implications not only for the social construction of who immigrants are and what they need in terms of health and welfare, but also for the ways in which research is conducted. In addition, we suggest that researchers' ability to point toward the areas where interventions could be geared is diminished when the "us" and "them" division impedes them from designing inquiries that can help us address the inequalities that immigrants may face.

Conclusion

The electoral success of Sverigedemokraterna (Sweden Democrats) in Parliament, a party with neo-Nazi roots and an anti-immigration stance, has been attributed to the reluctance of established politicians to address the challenges that Sweden's relatively generous immigrant policies have posed over the decades. Immigrant policy hitherto has been shaped apolitically, avoiding debate between political parties through a consensus about the importance of integrating immigrants (Hammar, 1999). The integration of labour migrants from neighbouring countries as contributors to and beneficiaries of the *folkhemmet* worked during an era of full employment. With the shift toward the arrival of refugees and asylum-seekers and the withdrawal of support for ethnic and migrant organizations, the ideal of assimilating immigrants to a (lost and lamented) state of cultural homogeneity is no longer (if it ever was) a realistic strategy (Lundqvist, 2006, p. 197). Solidarity around a set of universal welfare entitlements has served an integrationist immigrant policy but falters in the absence of full employment. The centrality of the rhetoric of caring for the people in the *folkhem* remains politically compelling, as shown by its use in justifying the anti-immigrant and welfare chauvinist politics of Sverigedemokraterna (Mulinari & Neergaard, 2014).

During the era of continuous governance by the Social Democratic Party (1930–1976), Sweden's self-image was determinedly modern, having progressed beyond the limitations of "the national" to embrace rational, scientifically led modernity to be a pioneering country in terms of technology, design, social planning, aiding developing countries, environmental policies, equality, and especially gender equality. Early policy responses to immigration were in line with the self-image of Sweden as a pioneering country, a "moral superpower," and a "leading actor" on the world stage in international refugee work (Borevi, 2012, p. 65). As such, the 1975 multicultural policy that initially emphasized the preservation of cultural diversity went against the narrow cultural consensus implied by the national icon of the *folkhem*, underpinning reform for equality between citizens. The 1975 multicultural policy was inevitably in a state of tension with the prevailing Swedish welfare state ideology (Borevi, 2012, p. 28). The late 1990s emphasis on individualized integration through economic expansion, coinciding with the neo-liberal contraction of welfare support, marks the end of Swedish exceptionalism as a generous welfare state that combines a high tolerance of immigration with unproblematic assimilation (Schierup & Alund, 2011).

A civic nation that actively recognizes ethnic minority groups is inevitably in tension with a universalist and robustly redistributive welfare state that emphasizes equality. In holding equality and solidarity as key values of the welfare system, the inequality of newcomers has come to be viewed as something that must be equalized "up" toward a norm. This conception of "different" as "more needy," "less equal," and "inadequate" rather than "equally valued" has made the provision of welfare in a way that does not stigmatize immigrants as "culturally different" and therefore marginal almost impossible. The example of older immigrants' assumed requirement for welfare services suggests that a presumption of vulnerable neediness has prevented evidence of alternative experience from being gathered, let alone from influencing policy. The reluctance to investigate and measure diversity as a variable means that there is little research evidence on health outcomes by ethnicity or racialized group, nor regarding the experience of health service use.

Critical Thinking Questions

1. What is the Nordic welfare model?
2. How can immigration to Sweden during 1960s be characterized?
3. How did the character of immigration change during the 1980s?
4. Describe the tensions between a multicultural policy and a universal welfare system.
5. Critics have characterized the Swedish welfare system as assimilationist. Drawing on the evidence on older immigrants presented and the evidence there is from other countries, is this a fair critique?

Glossary

Communitarian political ideology is a commitment to understanding people as a product of their relations with their community—usually beyond family—in a particular locality.

Folkhemmet **or "the people's home"** is the ideology associated with the Swedish Social Democratic Party of the mid-20th century. *Folkhemmet* is a metaphor whereby society and the state are compared to a family home, characterized by co-operation, where no one enjoys special privilege and no one seeks advantage at another's expense, and furthermore, where the benefits of productive capacity are shared equally.

Foreign background refers to both foreign-born and Swedish-born citizens with two foreign-born parents.

Gross domestic product is the total value of goods produced and services provided in a country in one year, and is used as an indicator of overall economic activity.

Redistributive political ideology refers to a belief in ensuring that resources—financial, material, social—are shared in society according to people's needs.

Welfare chauvinism or welfarism occurs where resident populations view immigrants as less deserving than themselves of employment opportunities and statutory benefits.

Recommended Readings

Ålund, A., & Schierup, C.-U. (1991). *Paradoxes of multiculturalism: Essays on Swedish society*. Aldershot, UK: Avebury. Retrieved from http://www.diva-portal.org/smash/get/diva2:213706/FULLTEXT02.pdf

A book that addresses different angles that render Sweden's multiculturalism as problematic.

Brochmann, G., & Hagelund, A. (Eds.). (2012). *Immigration policy and the Scandinavian welfare state 1945–2010*. Basingstoke, UK: Palgrave Macmillan.

An edited collection that offers a full and accessible account of post–Second World War developments in welfare states across the Scandinavian region.

Forssell, E., & Torres, S. (2012). Social work, older people, and migration: An overview of the situation in Sweden. *European Journal of Social Work, 15*(1), 115–130.

The care of older people in Sweden is described, with special reference to migrant families and their experience of "otherness."

Kivisto, P., & Östen, W. (2013). *Debating multiculturalism in the Nordic welfare states*. Basingstoke, UK: Palgrave Macmillan.

Investigates how the politics of identity and recognition play out in Nordic countries with a strongly redistributive politics of welfare.

Schierup, C.-U., & Ålund, A. (2011). The end of Swedish exceptionalism? Citizenship, neoliberalism, and the politics of exclusion. *Race & Class, 53*(1), 45–64.

Describes changes in Swedish multicultural politics over three decades, which are seen as culminating in civil disturbances in 2008/2009, marking the end of Swedish exceptionalism.

Related Websites

A Brief History of Immigration in Sweden—http://www.theguardian.com/news/datablog/2014/dec/11/a-brief-history-of-immigration-in-sweden-democrats-election

A British newspaper's brief analysis of Swedish immigration and integration statistics for the last three decades.

Centre of Health Equity Studies—www.chess.su.se/
The institutional website for the Centre of Health Equity Studies, which mostly offers quantitative analysis using immigrant background and country of birth as variables.

Institute for Research on Migration, Ethnicity and Society—www.isv.liu.se/remeso?l=en
The institutional website for the Institute for Research on Migration, Ethnicity and Society (REMESO), Linköping University, with links to publications and project descriptions.

Social Benefits—http://work.sweden.se/living-in-sweden/social-benefits/
The official explanation, in English and aimed at immigrants, of how the benefit system works in Sweden.

Statistics Sweden (Statistika centralbyrån)—http://www.scb.se/en_/Finding-statistics/Statistics-by-subject-area/Population/Population-composition/Population-statistics/Aktuell-Pong/25795/Yearly-statistics--The-whole-country/26040/
This website provides a summary of population statistics from 1960 to 2014, including numbers and proportions of foreign-born residents.

Notes

1. The good-quality employment and welfare provision informed by *folkhemmet* is said to have provoked American President Eisenhower to describe the "sin, nudity, drunkenness and suicide" induced by the generous welfare system in a 1960s speech aimed at discrediting Sweden's Social Democratic system. The speech may be the root of myths about Sweden's excessive suicide rate, and it suggests the radical success that the Swedish model presented compared to other models of welfare development in the capitalist context was seen as a threat.
2. Within the Swedish debate (academically, politically, and in terms of public opinion) the term used to discuss the situation of non-natives in Sweden is not "foreign background" but rather "immigrant background." The term "foreign background" is often used when referring to statistics since this is the wording used in that context. However, both the academic debate and the public debate in Sweden uses the terms "immigrant" and "immigrant background" in order to express the dichotomy between "us" (i.e., Swedes) and "them" (i.e., non- Swedes or people with immigrant backgrounds) that is at the core of these debates. Migration scholars in Sweden have even made a noun out of the term "immigrant" (*invandrare*)—i.e., *invandrarskap* (which could be translated as "migrancy")—in order to describe the social position that migrants tend to be accorded because of their non-Swedishness.
3. Austria, Belgium, Denmark, France, Germany, Greece, Italy, Netherlands, Spain, Switzerland, and Sweden.

References

Andersson, R. (1999). "Divided cities" as a policy-based notion in Sweden. *Housing Studies, 14*(5), 601–624.

Andersson, R., Magnusson Turner, L., & Holmqvist, E. (2010). *Contextualising ethnic residential segregation in Sweden: Welfare, housing, and migration-related policies.* Country Report for Sweden. Uppsula: Uppsala University.

Bambra, C. (2011). Health inequalities and welfare state regimes: Theoretical insights on a public health "puzzle." *Journal of Epidemiology & Community Health, 65*(9), 740–745.

Borevi, K. (2012). Sweden: The flagship of multiculturalism. In G. Brochmann & A. Hagelund (Eds.), *Immigration policy and the Scandinavian welfare state 1945–2010* (pp. 25–96). Basingstoke, UK: Palgrave Macmillan.

Brochmann, G., & Hagelund, A. (2012). Welfare state, nation, and immigration. In G. Brochmann & A. Hagelund (Eds.), *Immigration policy and the Scandinavian welfare state 1945–2010* (pp. 1–24). Basingstoke, UK: Palgrave Macmillan.

Dahlström, C. (2004). Rhetoric, practice, and the dynamics of institutional change: Immigrant policy in Sweden, 1964–2000. *Scandinavian Political Studies, 27*(3), 287–310.

Dahlström, C., & Esaiasson, P. (2011). The immigration issue and anti-immigrant party success in Sweden 1970–2006: A deviant case analysis. *Party Politics, 19*(2), 343–364.

Edin, P.-A, Fredriksson, P., & Åslund, O. (2004). Settlement policies and the economic success of immigrants. *Journal of Population Economics, 17*(1), 133–155.

Esping-Andersen, G. (1990). *The three worlds of welfare capitalism.* Cambridge: Polity.

Freeman, G. P. (1986). Migration and the political economy of the welfare state. *Annals of the American Academy of Political and Social Science, 485*(1), 51–63.

Gadd, M., Johansson, S.-E., Sundqvist, J., & Wändell, P. (2003). Morbidity in cardiovascular disease in immigrants in Sweden. *Journal of Internal Medicine, 254*(3), 236–243.

Gadd, M., Johansson, S.-E, Sundqvist, J., & Wändell, P. (2006) Are there differences in all-cause and coronary heart disease mortality between immigrants in Sweden and in their country of birth? A follow-up study of total populations. *BMC Public Health, 6*, 102.

Groglopo, A., & Ahlberg, B. M. (2006). Hälsa, vård och strukturell diskriminiering (Health, care and structural discrimination; SOU 2006:78). Stockholm: Kulturdepartementet.

Hammar, T. (1999). Closing the doors to the Swedish welfare state. In G. Brochmann & T. Hammar (Eds.), *Mechanisms of immigration control: A comparative analysis of European regulation policies.* Oxford: Berg.

Hedlund, E., Lange, A., & Hammar, N. (2007). Acute myocardial infarction incidence in immigrants in Sweden: Country of birth, time since immigration, and time trends over 20 years. *European Journal of Epidemiology, 22*(8), 493–503.

Hirdman, Y. (1989). *Att lägga livet tillrätta: Studier i svensk folkhemspolitik.* Stockholm: Carlsson.

Hjern, A., Wicks, S., & Dalman, C. (2004). Social adversity contributes to high morbidity in psychoses in immigrants—a national cohort study in two generations of Swedish residents. *Psychological Medicine, 34*(6), 1025–1033.

Lindström, M., Sundquist, J., & Östergren, P.-O. (2001). Ethnic differences in self reported health in Malmö in southern Sweden. *Journal of Epidemiology and Community Health, 55*(2), 97–103.

Lundqvist, T. (2006). Labour migration and organized interests: The Swedish model. In K. Tamas & J. Palme (Eds.), *Globalizing migration regimes: New challenges to transnational cooperation* (pp. 185–199). Aldershot, UK: Ashgate.

Machat, L. (2010). Bilden av "äldre invandrare" i äldrepolitiken. In S. Torres & F. Magnússon (Eds.), *Invandrarskap, äldrevård och omsorg* (pp. 55–68). Malmö: Gleerups.

Marmot, M. (2005, March 19). Social determinants of health inequalities. *The Lancet, 365*, 1099–1104.

Médecins Sans Frontières. (2005). *Experiences of Gömda in Sweden: Exclusion from health care for immigrants living without legal status. Results from a survey by Médecins Sans Frontières.* Retrieved from https://lakareutangranser.se/sites/default/files/reportgomdaswedenen.pdf

Mulinari, D., & Neergaard, A. (2014). We are Sweden Democrats because we care for others: Exploring racisms in the Swedish extreme right. *European Journal of Women's Studies, 21*(1), 43–56.

Narayan, U. (1995). Colonialism and its others: Considerations on rights and care discourses. *Hypatia, 10*(2), 133–140.

Popham, J., Dibben, C., & Bambra, C. (2013). Are inequalities in mortality really not the smallest in the Scandinavian welfare states? A comparative total inequality analysis of life expectancy in 37 countries. *Journal of Epidemiology & Community Health, 67*(5), 412–418.

Pred, A. (1997). Somebody else, somewhere else: Racisms, racialized spaces, and the popular geographical imagination in Sweden. *Antipode, 29*(4), 383–416.

Pred, A. (2000). *Even in Sweden: Racisms, racialized spaces, and the popular geographical imagination.* Berkeley: University of California Press.

Román, H. (1994). *En invandrarpolitisk oppositionell: Debattören David Schwarz syn på svensk invandrarpolitik åren 1964–1993.* Uppsala: Uppsala Multiethnic Papers.

Ronström, O. (2002). The making of older immigrants in Sweden: Identification, categorization, and discrimination. In L. Andersson (Ed.), *Cultural gerontology* (pp. 129–138). Westport, CT: Auburn House.

Rydgren, J. (2004). Mechanisms of exclusion: Ethnic discrimination in the Swedish labour market. *Journal of Ethnic and Migration Studies, 30*(4), 697–716.

Sachs, L. (1980) *Gamla invandrare i Sverige: En probleminventering.* Stockholm: Socialstyrelsens Äldreomsorgsprogrammet, rapport 6.

Sainsbury, D. (2006). Immigrants' social rights in comparative perspective: Welfare regimes, forms of immigration, and immigration policy regimes. *Journal of European Social Policy, 16*(3), 229–244.

SCB. (2013). *Population statistics.* Stockholm: Statistics Sweden.

Schierup, C.-U., & Alund, A. (2011). The end of Swedish exceptionalism? Citizenship, neoliberalism, and the politics of exclusion. *Race & Class, 53*(1), 45–64.

Socialstyrelsen. (2009). *Vård och omsorg om äldre.* Socialstyrelsens Lägesrapport 2008. Stockholm: Socialstyrelsen.

Soininen, M. (1992). *Den kommunala flyktingmottagandet: Genomförande och organisation.* Stockholm: CEIFO.

Soininen, M. (1999). The "Swedish model" as an institutional framework for immigrant membership rights. *Journal of Ethnic and Migration Studies, 25*(4), 685–702.

Solé-Auró, A., & Crimmins, E. M. (2008). Health of immigrants in European countries. *International Migration Review, 42*(4), 861–876.

SOU. (1997). Lika möjligheter. Betänkande av Utredningen om introduktion för nyanlända invandrare samt en ny myndighetsstruktur för det integrationspolitiska området, Pub. L. No. SOU 1997/82. Stockholm: Statens Offentliga Utredningar.

SOU. (2005). *Det blågula glashuset—strukturell diskriminering i Sverige*, SOU 2005/56. Stockholm: Statens Offentliga Utredningar. Retrieved from http://www.regeringen.se/content/1/c6/04/61/88/bcbc2913.pdf

Soysal, Y. N. (1994). *Limits of citizenship: Migrants and postnational membership in Europe.* Chicago: University of Chicago Press.

Sundqvist, J., & Johansson, S.-E. (1997). Long-term illness among indigenous and foreign-born people in Sweden. *Social Science and Medicine, 44*(2), 189–198.

Sungurova, Y., Johansson, S.-E., & Sundqvist, J. (2006). East-west health divide and east-west migration: Self-reported health of immigrants from Eastern Europe and the former Soviet Union in Sweden. *Scandinavian Journal of Public Health, 34*(2), 217–221.

Taloyan, M., Sundqvist, J.. & Al-Windi, A. (2008). The impact of ethnicity and self-reported health and psychological well-being: A comparative study of Kurdish-born and Swedish-born people. *Nordic Journal of Psychiatry, 62*(5), 392–398.

Thakur, S., Keen, Mi., Horváth, B., & Cerra, V. (2003). Sweden's welfare state: Can the bumblebee keep flying? *International Monetary Fund.* Retrieved from https://www.imf.org/external/pubs/nft/2003/sweden/index.htm

Torres, S. (2006). Elderly immigrants in Sweden: Otherness under construction. *Journal of Ethnic and Migration Studies, 32*(8), 1341–1358.

Torres, S. (2013). Healthy aging among migrants in Sweden: What we know and need to find out. In A. Scharlach & K. Hoshino (Eds.), *Healthy aging in sociocultural context* (pp. 42–50). New York: Routledge Press.

Torres, S. (2015). Äldre invandrare: den äldreomsorgspolitiska konstruktionen av ett välfärdproblem. In M. Darvishpour & C. Westin (Eds.), *Migration och etnicitet: perspektiv på ett mångkulturellt Sverige* (2nd ed.) (pp. 423–440). Lund: Studentlitteratur.

Torres, S., Lindblom, J., & Nordberg, C. (2014). Daily newspaper reporting on elderly care in Sweden and Finland: A quantitative content analysis of ethnicity and migration-related issues. *Vulnerable Groups & Inclusion,* November, 2014.

Tronto, J. C. (1995). Care as a basis for radical political judgements. *Hypatia, 10*(2), 141–149.

Tronto, J. C. (2010). Creating caring institutions: Politics, plurality, and purpose. *Ethics and Social Welfare, 4*(2), 158–171.

Wändell, P. E., Johansson, S.-E., Gåfvels, C., Hellénius, M. L., de Faire, U., & Sundqvist, J. (2008). Estimation of diabetes prevalence among immigrants from the Middle East in Sweden using three different data sources. *Diabetes & Metabolism, 34*(4.1), 328–333.

Warnes, A. M., Friedrich, K., Kellaher, L., & Torres, S. (2004). The diversity and welfare of older migrants in Europe. *Ageing & Society, 24*(3), 307–326.

Widgren, J. (1982). *Svensk invandrarpolitik.* Lund: Liber Läromedel.

Widgren, J. (1988). *Svensk invandrar och flyktingpolitik.* Stockholm: Arbetsmarknadsdepartamentet.

Wiking, E., Johansson, S.-E., & Sundqvist, J. (2004). Ethnicity, acculturation, and self-reported health: A population based study among immigrants from Poland, Turkey, and Iran in Sweden. *Journal of Epidemiological Community Health, 58*(7), 574–582.

Zaidi, A., & Gustafsson, B. (2007). Income mobility among the elderly in Sweden during the 1990s. *International Journal of Social Welfare, 16*(1), 84–93.

Zetzell, I. (1980). Äldre invandrare: en bakgrund. Stockholm: Socialstyrelsen Äldreomsorgsprogrammet rapport 5.

PART 3

Analysis and Public Policy Implications

Part 3 presents key themes related to the immigration experience and their implications for research and public policy. In Chapter 12, Dennis Raphael identifies key issues that emerge from the case studies in Section 2. These are wide-ranging and include issues of defining and measuring different forms of immigration, documenting the lived experiences of immigrants, and evaluating health outcomes. Intertwined with these issues are the roles played by public policy and how such public policy is responding to issues of discrimination and racism. Also of importance is how political parties are responding to potentially negative attitudes toward immigrants spurred on by increasing social inequalities resulting from economic globalization.

In Chapter 13, Toba Bryant identifies the public policy implications of the key issues identified by Raphael. She suggests measures that can be taken to promote the integration of immigrants by reducing their social exclusion. These include adopting multiculturalism, reducing discrimination and racism, promoting labour market integration, and increasing democratic participation. Since developed nations are increasingly dependent on immigration to maintain their welfare states, they are therefore compelled to address these issues. Critical to these efforts will be confronting the challenges posed by rising support of anti-immigration political parties.

CHAPTER 12

Key Immigration Issues in Developed Nations

Dennis Raphael

Chapter Objectives

This chapter analyzes some of the key issues that emerged in the case studies. The objectives of this chapter are:

- to identify common themes that emerged across the nine national case studies of immigration;
- to identify systematic variations in immigration approaches across the nine nations;
- to examine the comparative living circumstances of immigrants across the nine nations examined in this volume; and
- to examine the relationship between the form of the welfare state and immigration policy.

Introduction

This chapter explores some of the issues identified in the case studies. It provides an overview of the complexities involved in examining how the lived experiences and health outcomes of immigrants in a jurisdiction are shaped by numerous forms of public policies. By doing so it provides a roadmap for further inquiry into these issues and related public policy debates. It then explores some of the hypotheses identified at the beginning of the volume through analysis of recent data from the OECD on the employment and income situations of immigrants in the nine nations examined in this volume. It attempts to answer the question: How does the form of the welfare state interact with immigration policy and local conditions to shape the lived experiences and health outcomes of immigrants?

Different Forms of Immigration

The case studies illustrate the complexity of the immigration experience and how it takes different forms across jurisdictions. One clear aspect of the immigration story is that Canada and Australia have a longer and deeper history of immigration. This has led to a greater proportion of their population being immigrants or offspring of immigrants and of greater diversity. Austria, Belgium, and Germany also have long experiences of immigration, but in these cases the process was historically connected to immigrants being taken in as temporary workers of which many then came to stay. In these nations, immigrants were usually of European (e.g., Italian, Yugoslavian, or Greek) or European/Asian (e.g., Turkish) descent.

Denmark, Norway, and Sweden initially took in labour immigrants from culturally similar nations, but more recently shifted immigration policies toward family reunification and acceptance of **asylum-seekers**. For all nations, taking in asylum-seekers from non-European nations is creating a situation similar to the settler nations where all forms of immigration have come to consist of immigrants from developing nations. Figure 12.1 provides information on the percentages of national population identified as native- versus foreign-born. These figures do not distinguish between immigrants from European versus non-European sources.

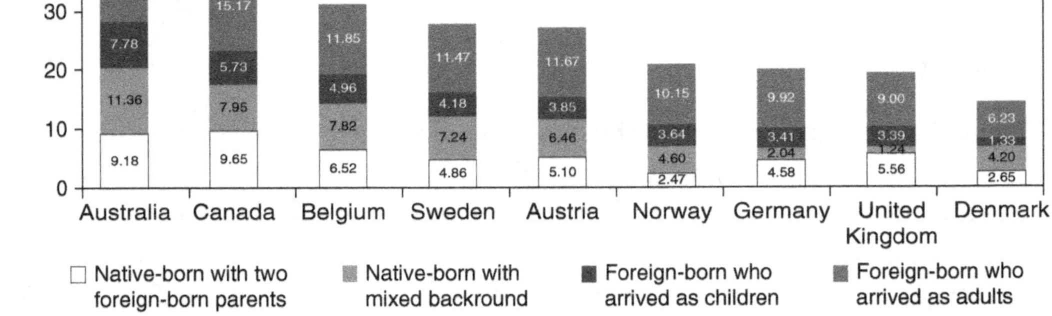

Figure 12.1: Percentage of Population That Are Immigrants and Native-Born Offspring of Immigrants, 2013 or Most Recent Year

Source: Organisation for Economic Co-operation and Development. (2015). *Settling in: OECD indicators of immigrant integration 2015*, Figure 1.1 (p. 17). Paris: Author.

Not surprisingly, Australia (46 percent) and Canada (39 percent) show the greatest proportions of foreign- and native-born with at least one foreign-born parent, while Denmark shows the smallest (14 percent). Belgium (31 percent), Sweden (28 percent), and Austria (27 percent) also have significant proportions of immigrant-related residents. Norway (21 percent), Germany (20 percent), and the United Kingdom (19 percent) have somewhat smaller proportions. We do not know exactly what percentages of these immigrant households consist of people of colour or of differing backgrounds and ethnicities from the dominant cultures, but the case studies suggest that probably a significant proportion of them can be so designated. It is interesting that the nation with the smallest percentage of immigrant households, Denmark, is one of the nations providing the most restrictive immigration policies.

For all nations examined in this volume, immigration was historically restricted to those sharing cultural backgrounds similar to those in the receiving nations. In Canada and Australia there was restriction of immigration to those from the United Kingdom, expanding to those of European background. In Scandinavia, immigration primarily involved those from other Nordic nations. The Continental nations allowed immigrant workers from Turkey, Greece, Yugoslavia, and Italy, and those of similar background from neighbouring nations (e.g., ethnic Germans from Russia). The United Kingdom received immigrants from the Commonwealth in the wake of labour shortages following the Second World War. All nations are now accepting asylum-seekers from the developing world, and European nations must respond to challenges associated with the right of EU residents to work in any EU nation.

The recent shift to accepting immigrants from the developing world—usually involving people of colour and diverse ethnic and cultural backgrounds—takes different forms. For nations such as Australia, Canada, and the United Kingdom, a primary form of such immigration is filling labour shortages and meeting economic goals. Most entrants are considered candidates for citizenship and score high on indicators of economic well-being and education, as well as English language proficiency.

The second form of immigration from the developing world is associated with refugee and asylum claims resulting from political and economic turmoil. These **refugee claimants** are often people of colour with differing traditions and present special challenges to the Scandinavian and Continental nations that do not have the long-term experiences common to the Anglo-Saxon nations of taking in diverse immigrants.

All nations are undergoing policy debates on how to manage these asylum claims, and in all jurisdictions there has been a tightening of eligibility. Also of note, compounding this complexity have been recent changes within the **European Union** that opens borders to employment-related immigration from EU member states. The result of all this is that immigration and its management has become more complex and public policy approaches toward immigration more contested. The following sections identify several issues emerging from the case studies.

Availability of Data Concerning the Immigrant Experience

The case studies identify the importance of having available data on the lived experiences of immigrants and their interactions with the health system that can inform these policy debates. Also of importance is the availability of health outcomes data that can identify the health situations of different groups by nation of origin, residency status and length of residency, and cultural tradition or ethnicity and race, in relation to these lived experiences. Nations differ in their ability to capture and therefore act upon such information.

In Germany, data collection can identify the birthplace of individuals as well as the birthplace of both their parents and grandparents. This does not in itself collect data on ethnicity and race, but does provide the ability to identify various indicators important to specifying the situations of immigrants. In contrast, data collection in Belgium is limited by historical concerns about identification of vulnerable minority groups. Every jurisdiction is attempting to manage these aspects of data collection, and the different experiences provided in the case studies provide much food for thought. The downside to such data collection efforts is the potential for stigmatizing such groups and creating barriers to acceptance and **integration** into the receiving nations.

Nevertheless, from a public policy perspective, it appears essential to detail how race and ethnicity, in addition to birthplace, shape the immigration experience. In cases where such data are available, discrimination has been identified as affecting the living circumstances and health outcomes of immigrants.[1] Across all nations, the data available show that those not of the dominant mainstream culture experience adverse living circumstances and health outcomes that can be traced to these experiences.

Consistent Social Exclusion and Less Positive Profile of Social Determinants of Health

The case studies are consistent in identifying how many immigrants, especially those of colour and differing ethno-racial backgrounds, do not fare as well as the native-born of the dominant culture. In some instances, studies have identified the specific aspects of income, employment, housing, and other social determinants of health associated with these circumstances. Most case studies identify how difficulty with the native tongue, potentially compounded by discrimination, plays a role in producing these adverse living circumstances.

In response, some of the jurisdictions have enacted anti-discrimination laws. It is unclear how effectively these laws are being enforced. In some instances governmental agencies manage these complaints, but in others the individual must initiate action through the courts. A key issue, therefore, is the role that racism and discrimination play in the living circumstances and health outcomes of immigrants and what role the state as well as civil society can play in managing it and its effects. The case studies indicate that issues of racism and discrimination are being researched—and addressed through public policy action—in some, but not all nations.

Evidence Concerning Health Outcomes of Immigrants

Evidence indicates that the health outcomes of immigrants usually fall behind those of the native-born, although these findings may not be able to examine differences between the native-born of the dominant culture and the native-born who may be of colour or ethnically diverse from the dominant culture. In the Anglo-Saxon nations attention has been directed to the healthy immigrant effect whereby immigrants are initially healthier than the native-born population, but over time come to more closely resemble or compare unfavourably with these native populations. The cases studies identify the mental and physical health outcomes associated with these adverse immigrant health profiles.

Mental health seems to be a particularly important dimension upon which immigrants—especially those of colour and differing ethnicities from the dominant culture—differ from the native-born population. This phenomenon has been associated with the experience of lower socio-economic position with its attendant greater unemployment, and lower quality of life with lower pay employment. In other cases it has been associated with the day-to-day experience of racism and discrimination. Particularly noteworthy is the finding that adult-onset diabetes appears to be an affliction to which immigrants of non-dominant nationalities and ethnicities are especially susceptible. In Canada the increased prevalence of adult-onset diabetes among immigrants has been associated with the adverse living circumstances they experience in Canada (Dinca-Panaitescua et al., 2011).

The case studies present additional examples of adverse health outcomes experienced by immigrants. Importance is also placed on the difficulties immigrants may face in accessing the health care system. This issue is especially important when the immigrants may have difficulties with language. In many of the case studies special attention is directed toward the role translators can play in facilitating immigrants' interactions with the health care system.

Differences in State Recognition of the Special Situation of Immigrants

Considering these difficult circumstances to which many immigrants—especially those of divergent ethnicities and race—experience, it is important to consider whether there is state recognition of their special situation and the provisions by which these difficulties can be managed. In some nations this takes the form of increasing research into these issues with the purpose of identifying public policies that can address these situations.

One form of state recognition of these kinds of immigration issues is the acceptance of a public policy of multiculturalism. This is an explicit statement to immigrants of different ethnicities and races of the willingness of the nation to recognize their core identities and not submerge them in the dominant culture. As noted in Chapter 1, nations differ in the extent to which they have embraced this concept. Australia, Canada, and Sweden are distinguished by strong implementation of such an approach, Denmark and Austria rather less so. The question of whether the embrace of multiculturalism has been associated with discrimination toward immigrants is unclear. Figure 12.2 shows OECD data that provide more questions than answers on this issue.

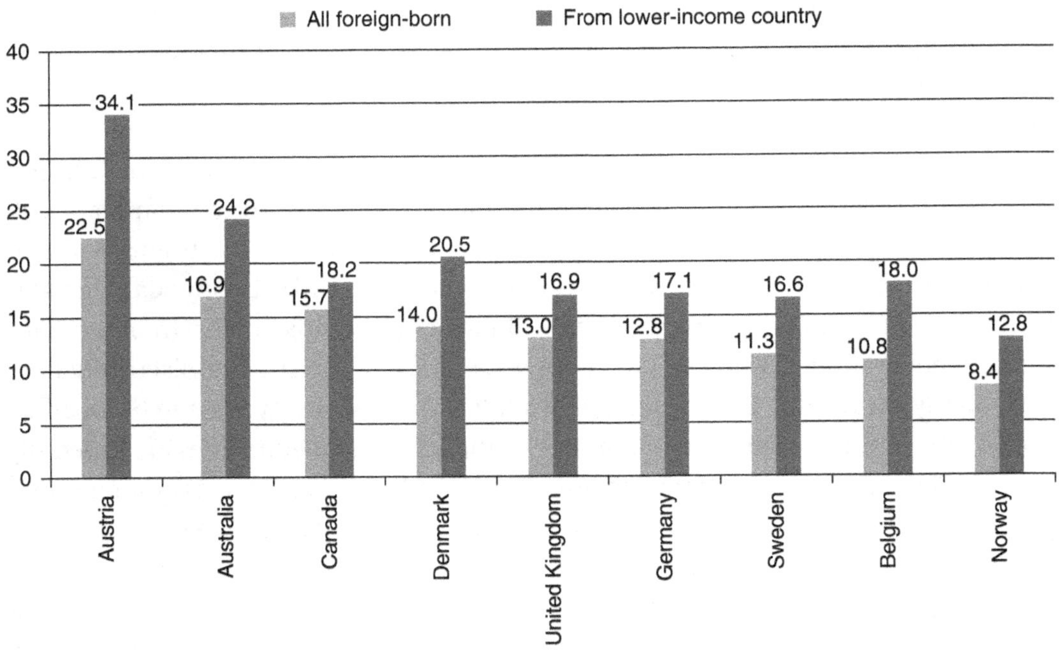

Figure 12.2: Share of 15- to 64-Year-Old Immigrants Who Consider Themselves Members of a Group That Is Discriminated/Has Been Discriminated Against on Grounds of Ethnicity, Nationality, or Race, by Place of Origin, 2002–2012

Source: Organisation for Economic Co-operation and Development. (2015). *Settling in: OECD indicators of immigrant integration 2015*, Figure 1.5 (p. 25). Paris: Author.

In every nation a minority of foreign-born residents believes they belong to a group that has been discriminated against and figures are higher for those coming from low-income nations—a very rough proxy for coming from the developing world. Yet the nations with the two highest discrimination figures, Austria and Australia, differ profoundly in their embrace of multiculturalism, with Australia receiving the highest multiculturalism score of 8 and Austria receiving a low 1.5. The especially well-performing nation regarding discrimination toward immigrants from lower-income nations is Norway, while Austria, Australia, and Denmark provide less favourable profiles. The correlation between these discrimination scores for those coming from a low-income nation and scores on the Multiculturalism Policy Index is -0.26 and the correlation for the larger foreign-born group and the Index is -0.17. *Both coefficients are not close to being either statistically or practically significant.*

Role of Anti-immigration Parties and Sentiments in Setting the Public Policy Agenda

This issue was specifically explored in the case studies of Australia, Belgium, Denmark, and Sweden and provides numerous areas for inquiry. Anti-immigration parties benefit from economic uncertainty to fan racist attitudes that create difficult circumstances for immigrants, especially those of non-dominant races and ethnicities. This has been most obvious in Denmark, where anti-immigration parties have influenced the making of public policy since the 1970s. It was also a focus of attention in the Belgian case study in which regional governments' ministers of immigration have come from nationalistic anti-immigration parties. Sweden has recently experienced a surge in strength of an anti-immigration party. In other nations such as Australia, Canada, and the United Kingdom, anti-immigration sentiment shapes public policy across the mainstream parties and comes to restrict immigration.

Geographical Dispersion

In three nations—Australia, Sweden, and the United Kingdom—immigrants are directed to specific locations within a nation in which they must reside. This raises issues of cultural isolation, social exclusion, and availability of needed programs and services. This issue is highlighted in the United Kingdom case study, but has implications for other nations as well who may be considering such approaches.

Immigrants versus Refugees

The distinction between immigrants and refugees is becoming increasingly associated with receiving nations' differing approaches toward them. Across all the case studies, evidence was presented that the health situation of refugees is especially problematic. This is related both to their experiences in their home nations, as well as the difficulties associated with integration in the destination nations.

In addition, refugees may not possess the kind of social resources that buffer life changes such as higher education and greater wealth that immigrants may possess. The contrast between refugees and these other immigrants' living conditions and health outcomes may be especially great in nations where immigration policy has increasingly come to assess the educational and financial assets of potential immigrants. The significant military conflicts in North Africa and the Middle East will only increase the number of potential refugees to the nations examined in this volume. This phenomenon presents public policy challenges not only for managing the intake process but also integration into the daily life of these nations. There is no shortage of potential areas of inquiry presented by these new developments.

Multiculturalism

Multiculturalism is an attempt to manage the potentially problematic issues identified in the preceding sections. Australia, Canada, and Sweden, and, to a lesser extent, the United Kingdom and Belgium, have adopted policies supportive of the concept. And it is Australia, Canada, and Sweden that score highest in integrating immigrants according to the MIPEX. The nations scoring lowest on adopting multiculturalism, Denmark and Austria, also score the lowest in immigrant integration. Whether the association is a causative one or a reflection of other societal processes that shape both multiculturalism and integration indicators remains unclear.

Citizenship Situations of Immigrants

The OECD also provides information as to the citizenship status of the foreign-born population residing in each nation. In Canada, over 70 percent of these individuals become naturalized while about 30 percent are either landed immigrants or those seeking refugee status. Sweden and Australia provide a similar situation with close to 70 percent of foreign-born individuals in Sweden and about 65 percent of those in Australia having attained citizenship through naturalization.

On the other end, Norway has about 40 percent of foreign-born nationals attaining citizenship through naturalization with another 15 percent apparently having been born abroad to Norwegians. The United Kingdom has about 15 percent of foreign-born individuals having been designated British at birth and another 30 percent having acquired citizenship. However, a full 60 percent of immigrants in the United Kingdom are considered foreign nationals. Finally, in Austria 60 percent of immigrants continue to be considered foreigners with 35 percent having acquired citizenship naturalization and an additional 5 percent having attained citizenship at birth. Creating barriers to attaining citizenship may make it difficult for immigrants to feel attached to their new nation.

Educational Backgrounds of Immigrants

A rather striking pattern is seen in terms of the educational credentials of immigrants across nations. In Canada a full 60 percent of immigrants (versus 46 percent of natives) are considered highly educated (with tertiary education) and only 10 percent (versus 13 percent of natives) are designated as low educated (less than secondary education) (OECD, 2015). A similar situation is seen in the United Kingdom with 47 percent of immigrants (versus 35 percent of natives) being well educated and about 20 percent (versus 23 percent of natives) low educated, and in Australia where 47 percent (versus 29 percent of natives) are well educated and only 19 percent (versus 30 percent of natives) less educated.

The opposite situation is seen in Belgium, Germany, and Austria. In Belgium only 29 percent of immigrants (versus 35 percent of natives); Germany 21 percent of immigrants (versus 28 percent of natives); and in Austria 19 percent of immigrants (versus 18 percent of natives) are considered highly educated with rather more immigrants being low educated; Belgium 41 percent (versus 26 percent for natives); Germany 35 percent (versus 10 percent of natives); and Austria 34 percent (versus 14 percent of natives). In Scandinavia there are fewer differences between immigrants and natives in the proportion highly educated: Denmark (34 percent versus 32 percent); Norway (37 percent versus 35 percent); and Sweden (35 percent versus 32 percent), or low educated: Denmark (28 percent versus 22 percent); Norway (23 percent versus 22 percent); with the exception of Sweden for percentage of low education (31 percent versus 15 percent). These data would suggest that immigrants in Canada, the United Kingdom, and Australia should be doing rather well in terms of poverty rates and unemployment rates.

Comparative Living Circumstances—Social Determinants of Health—of Immigrants across Nations

The OECD provides sets of indicators concerning the living circumstances of immigrants in OECD nations (OECD, 2015). These data do not differentiate between immigrants of similar or dissimilar races and ethnicities to the dominant culture so they need to be interpreted with caution. Four sets of indicators provide some perspective as to issues related to living conditions, the social determinants of health, and health outcomes among immigrants. These provide an overview of circumstances while the case studies provide closer examination of these issues.

These numbers and analyses of labour and other outcomes (see below) contributed to the OECD identifying eight groups of nations of which three groups are of primary interest here (OECD, 2015). One group is that of *settler nations*, which includes *Australia* and *Canada*—as well as Israel and New Zealand. For these nations immigration is seen as part of its heritage of nation building. On average, one in four people is foreign-born and another one in four, while being native-born, has at least one immigrant parent. The OECD sees their integration outcomes as being generally positive. Interestingly, according to the 2015 MIPEX, Australia ranks eighth and Canada ranks sixth of 20 nations in integration.

Another group of nations are identified as *long-standing destinations with many settled low-educated migrants*. This group includes *Austria, Belgium*, and *Germany*—as well as France and the Netherlands. These nations have had flows of less-educated immigrants arriving for employment-related purposes during the boom years of the post-Second World War period. Family members joined them through reunification measures. About 10–15 percent of their populations are foreign-born, and an additional 7–15 percent are native-born with at least one foreign-born parent. These nations are seen by the OECD as facing greater immigration challenges due to the generally lower educational backgrounds of these immigrants. The ranks on overall integration according to the MIPEX of these nations are Austria (twentieth), Belgium (seventh), and Germany (tenth), such that there is little difference between Belgium and Germany with Canada and Australia questioning the generality of the OECD conclusion.

A third group of nations are identified as *destination countries with significant recent and humanitarian migration* and include *Denmark, Norway, Sweden*—and Finland. About 8–15 percent of their populations are foreign-born with an additional 7–12 percent natives with at least one foreign-born parent. However, almost half of the immigrant population have arrived within the past 10 years and include both EU-EFTA free-mobility immigrants and asylum-seekers. The asylum immigrants are seen as struggling to integrate, with labour outcomes less favourable. However, a high share attains citizenship, and these immigrants have similar levels of access to employment training as the native-born. In contrast to the OECD concerns, the ranks on the MIPEX for Sweden (first) and Norway (fourth) are rather favourable, while Denmark compares rather poorly (thirteenth) but still better than the United Kingdom (fifteenth).

Finally, the *United Kingdom* is identified as a *long-standing destination with many recent and highly educated migrants*, many of whom are EU-EFTA free-zone migrants. Other such nations are Luxembourg, Switzerland, and the United States. Many are well educated and their integration is generally seen as positive, although as noted, the United Kingdom ranks fifteenth on the MIPEX.

Labour Outcomes and Relative Poverty

Figure 12.3 provides a quick look at some of the unemployment data that led the OECD to these conclusions. Of particular note is the rather small gap in unemployment rates between the foreign- and native-born of the Anglo-Saxon Liberal welfare states. Double-digit gaps between these groups are seen in Belgium and Sweden with the remaining nations showing mid-level gaps.

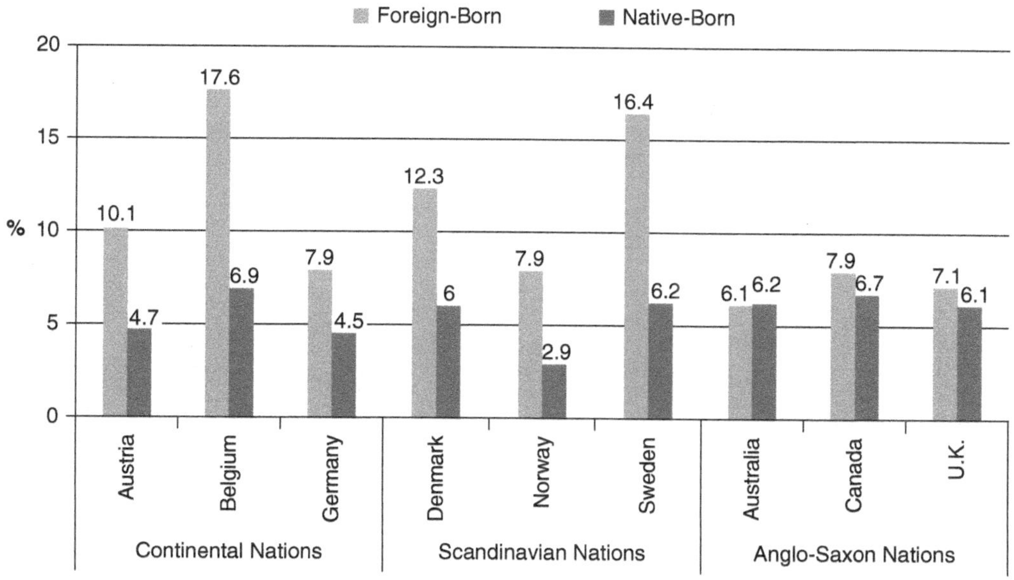

Figure 12.3: Proportion of Unemployed among Native- and Foreign-Born, across Nation Types, 2014

Sources: Organisation for Economic Co-operation and Development. (2016). Native-born unemployment (indicator). doi: 10.1787/0f9d8842-en; Organisation for Economic Co-operation and Development. (2016). Foreign-born unemployment (indicator). doi: 10.1787/ba5d2ce0-en.

It is noteworthy, however, that consistent with what is known about the Liberal welfare state, these unemployment levels are on average higher than those seen in the Continental and Scandinavian nations.

The unemployment levels are rather low for native-born residents in these non–Anglo-Saxon nations, yet it is there that the greatest gap is seen between native- and foreign-born residents. These findings suggest that the main issue being faced in the Continental and Scandinavian nations is having foreign-born residents participate in their generally more supportive labour market. These data, however, say little about the nature of the jobs that native- and foreign-born residents actually have.

Figure 12.4 provides some insight into this by showing the relative poverty rate—set at less than 60 percent of the median income—for employed native- and foreign-born residents. These data suggest that integration into the labour market has differing effects upon income across nations. As an example, Canada showed little difference in unemployment rates between native- and foreign-born residents, but produces the highest levels of relative poverty for those engaged in the workforce with rates rather higher for foreign-born workers. Indeed one-quarter of native-born residents experience relative poverty and this figure rises to a rather significant 30 percent level for working foreign-born residents. In contrast, relative poverty rates are especially low in Germany, Austria, Denmark, Norway, and Sweden for foreign-born residents able to find work.

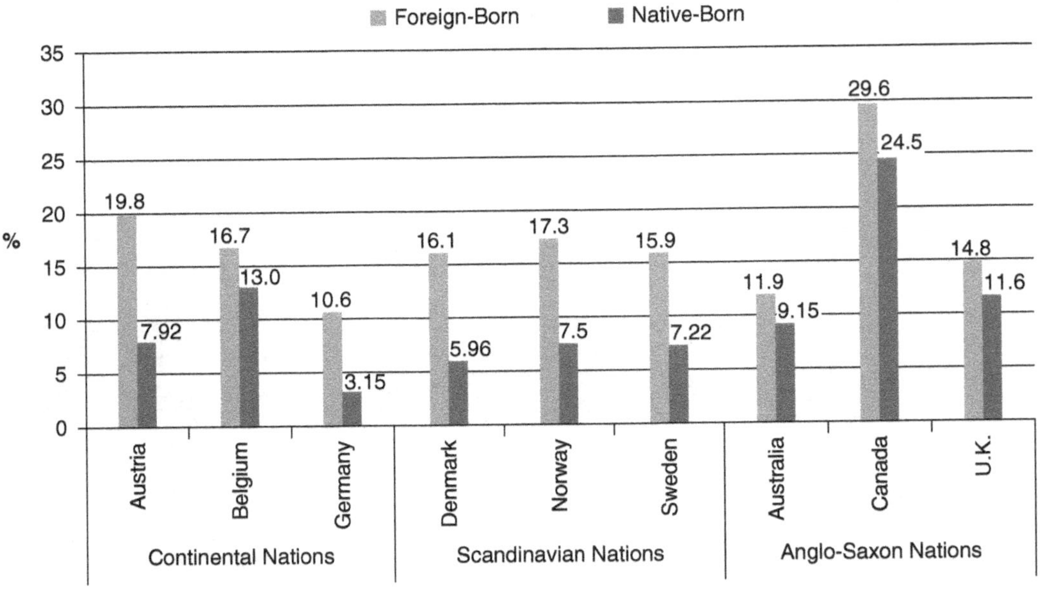

Figure 12.4: In-Work Relative Poverty Rates among Native- and Foreign-Born, across Nation Types, 2012

Source: Organisation for Economic Co-operation and Development. (2015). *Settling in: OECD indicators of immigrant integration 2015*, Table 8.2 (p. 167). Paris: Author.

These figures suggest that the main problem for the Continental and Scandinavian nations is not only integrating foreign-born residents into the workplace, but also working to reduce gaps in incomes produced by these jobs. In contrast, employment differences are less important in Canada with the main issue being the rather large numbers of both native- and foreign-born workers who experience low-waged employment, which leads to high levels of relative poverty.

Figure 12.5 takes into account both employment and unemployment to provide an overall portrait of relative poverty rates among native- and foreign-born residents. These findings suggest in all nations significant proportions of foreign-born residents experience relative poverty as defined by the <60 percent of median indicator. In terms of what we know about the social determinants of health, this provides a pressing public policy issue that needs to be addressed. The most apparent need is providing foreign-born workers with supports for integrating into employment, but a second important need is providing employment that provides workers with the means of avoiding relative poverty. The first need is a challenge for the Scandinavian and Continental nations. And, not surprisingly, the Liberal countries of Australia, Canada, and the United Kingdom face the greatest challenges in meeting the second need.

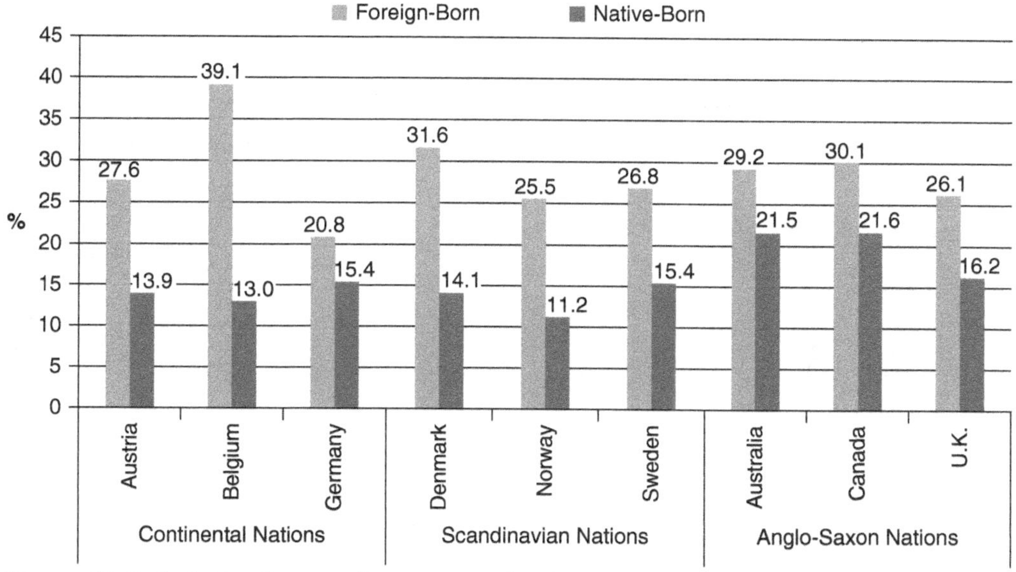

Figure 12.5: Relative Poverty Rate among Native- and Foreign-Born, across Nation Types, 2012

Source: Organisation for Economic Co-operation and Development. (2015). *Settling in: OECD indicators of immigrant integration 2015*, Table 8.1 (p. 165). Paris: Author.

Educational Outcomes

Figure 12.6 provides some compelling evidence about the relative success that each of the nine nations has had in reducing the education gap among 15-year-olds between those with and without immigration backgrounds. Figure 12.6 shows the gap among four groups of 15-year-olds in PISA Reading Scores. These groups are native-born offspring of native-born parents, native-born offspring of parents with a mixed background, native-born offspring of foreign-born parents, and foreign-born children. The most striking finding is that the gap among these four groups is rather smaller among the Anglo-Saxon nations of Australia, Canada, and United Kingdom than the other nations. Particularly striking is the finding that foreign-born 15-year-olds, as well as native-born offspring with either one or both parents being foreign-born, actually outperform native-born children born of native-born parents in Canada. This finding has tremendous implications for the other nations that appear to be struggling to reduce the education gap between children in these groups. Of course an important potential confounder of these findings is that the Liberal nations are English-speaking nations that have increasingly come to restrict immigration to those who possess English-language skills. Such a requirement for immigration may be behind their smaller education gaps.

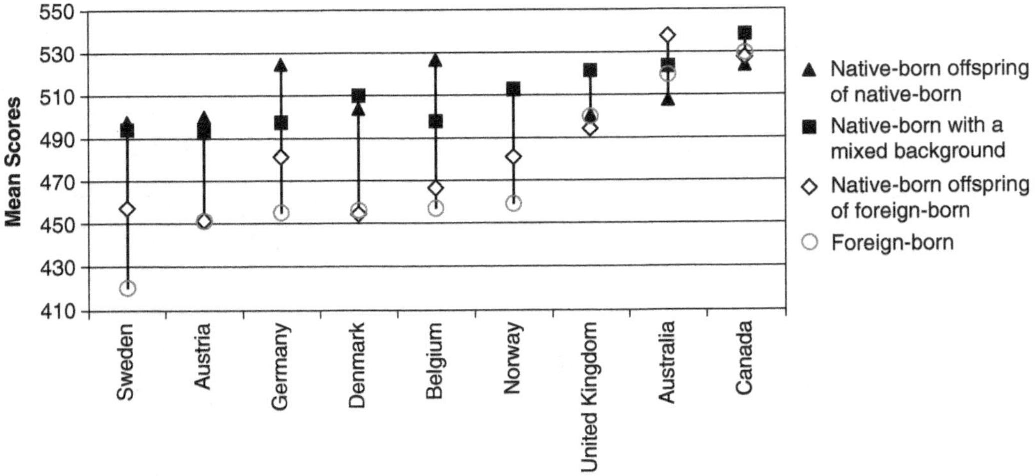

Figure 12.6: Mean PISA Reading Scores of 15-Year-Old Students by Migration Background, 2012

Source: Organisation for Economic Co-operation and Development. (2015). *Settling in: OECD indicators of immigrant integration 2015*, Figure 13.7 (p. 243). Paris: Author.

In contrast, education gaps are greatest in nations where their languages may normally not be taught across the world, i.e., Swedish, German, Danish, French, Dutch, and Norwegian. Further research is needed into identifying the sources of the Liberal nations' superior performance in reducing the education gap. One point worth noting is that a Pearson correlation of .50 is seen between size of the gap and the implementation of multicultural policy activities as measured by the MPI. While not statistically significant, it is suggestive that nations that have embraced multiculturalism as a public policy approach have the smallest gap in educational achievement. Whether this is an actual causal relationship or merely a by-product of the English-language nations having adopted multiculturalism remains to be seen.

Relationship between the Form of the Welfare State and Immigration Policy

There is no clear relationship between the form of the welfare state and immigrants' situations. On broad indicators such as the MIPEX index, there is wide variation among the Social Democratic Scandinavian nations with Sweden scoring first, Norway eighth, and Denmark a rather poor thirteenth. Liberal Anglo-Saxon Canada ranks sixth, Australia eighth, and the United Kingdom fifteenth. Belgium does rather well at seventh, with Germany at tenth and Austria rather less so at twentieth.

Conclusions

The purpose of this volume is to examine the lived experience and health outcomes of immigrants in nine developed nations. An initial hypothesis was that these lived experiences and health outcomes would be related to the specific forms of the welfare state adopted by each nation. There is some evidence in support of this in that immigrants' situations in the Liberal welfare states of Australia and Canada show many similarities, as do immigrants in Norway and Sweden. There are also similarities in the immigrant experiences in Belgium and Germany. However, for each form of the welfare state there is an example that does not conform. Denmark presents a very different profile in how immigrants are integrated, as do Austria and the United Kingdom. In each of these cases immigration policy is more restrictive and the living circumstances of immigrants more difficult.

In all of these cases that deviate in the direction of less favourability, a strong role of politics is apparent. For reasons that are unclear, in these nations anti-immigration parties have been able to have greater influence upon public policy-making than elsewhere. Nevertheless, all nations are dealing with issues of discrimination, in some cases driven by racism. The presence of such attitudes makes integration of immigrants, especially those of colour and from cultures diverse from the dominant culture, more difficult.

Critical Thinking Questions

1. What kinds of data collection could contribute to understanding the immigration experience?
2. What can nations do to combat discrimination and racism toward immigrants, especially immigrants of colour?
3. How can the different kinds of welfare states be modified to facilitate the integration of immigrants into a society?
4. What are the unanticipated effects of placing immigration issues within the broader issue of national security?
5. All in all, which nations seem to be more successful in integrating immigrants into society? Why is this so?

Glossary

Asylum-seekers are people who seek safety from persecution or serious harm in a country other than their own and await a decision on their application for refugee status under relevant international and national instruments. In case of a negative decision, they must leave the country and may be expelled, as may any non-national in an irregular or unlawful situation, unless permission to stay is provided on humanitarian or other related grounds (IOM, 2011).

European Union was founded to enhance political, economic, and social co-operation. The 28 member states of the European Union are: Austria, Belgium, Bulgaria, Croatia, Cyprus, Czech Republic, Denmark, Estonia, Finland, France, Germany, Greece, Hungary, Republic of Ireland, Italy, Latvia, Lithuania, Luxembourg, Malta, The Netherlands, Poland, Portugal, Romania, Slovakia, Slovenia, Spain, Sweden, and the United Kingdom.

Integration can be defined as the process by which migrants become accepted in society, both as individuals and as groups. It generally refers to a two-way process of adaptation by migrants and host societies, while the particular requirements for acceptance by a host society vary from country to country (IOM, 2011).

Refugee claimant is a person who has made a claim for protection as a refugee. This term is more or less equivalent to "asylum-seeker" and is standard in Canada, while "asylum-seeker" is the term more often used internationally (http://ccrweb.ca/sites/ccrweb.ca/files/static-files/glossary.PDF).

Recommended Readings

Brochmann, G., & Jurado, E. (2013). *Europe's immigration challenge: Reconciling work, welfare and mobility.* London: I. B. Taurus.

The view that immigrants compete unfairly for jobs and present an unsustainable burden on the European social model appears to be gathering support in some circles. But at the same time, the "right" type of immigrant has often been perceived as a potential cure for Europe's sluggish labour markets and ailing welfare systems. This book examines this conundrum and argues for a more integrated approach to immigration policy.

International Organization for Migration (IOM). (2011). *Glossary on immigration* (2nd ed.). Geneva: IOM.

This improved edition continues to move the international community toward a common language when discussing migration issues. Uniformity of usage of terms greatly enhances research and statistics gathering, and the exchange of information between and among states.

Kilbride, K. (2014). *Immigrant integration: Research implications for future policy.* Toronto: Canadian Scholars' Press.

This book addresses the growing economic and educational inequality among immigrants and racialized populations in Canada and seeks to guard against further inequities. The authors address policy issues, newcomers' health and well-being, cultural challenges, and resilience in immigrant communities.

Organisation for Economic Co-operation and Development. (2015). *Settling in: OECD indicators of immigrant integration 2015.* Paris: Author.

This publication highlights how immigrants and their children are integrating into OECD societies, judging their progress against key indicators. Many areas are considered, including material living conditions, health, education, labour market, and civic engagement.

Simmons, A. B. (2010). *Immigration and Canada: Global and transnational perspectives.* Toronto: Canadian Scholars' Press.

This volume provides readers with a vital introduction to the field of international migration studies. It presents an integrated critical perspective on Canadian immigration policies, main trends, and social, economic, and cultural impacts.

Related Websites

European Commission: Migration and Home Affairs—http://ec.europa.eu/dgs/home-affairs/what-we-do/policies/index_en.htm

The Directorate-General of the European Commission manages policies that aim at ensuring that all activities necessary and beneficial to the economic, cultural, and social growth of the EU may develop in a stable, lawful, and secure environment. More specifically, they work to build an open and safer Europe.

National Immigration Centre (NIC)—http://www.conferenceboard.ca/nic/default.aspx

The Conference Board of Canada's NIC is a major five-year initiative launched in September 2014. The NIC will develop an evidence-based National Immigration Action Plan to help improve Canada's immigration system. Investors are being invited to support the initiative.

OECD International Migration Policies and Data—http://www.oecd.org/migration/mig/

This website provides access to a range of databases, reports, and analyses concerned with immigration to OECD nations.

Office of the United Nations High Commissioner for Refugees—http://www.unhcr.org/cgi-bin/texis/vtx/home

The Office of the United Nations High Commissioner for Refugees is mandated to lead and coordinate international action to protect refugees and resolve refugee problems worldwide. Its primary purpose is to safeguard the rights and well-being of refugees.

United Nations Human Rights—http://www.ohchr.org/EN/Issues/Migration/Pages/MigrationAndHumanRightsIndex.aspx

This website outlines how a human rights approach to migration places the migrant at the centre of migration policies and management, and pays particular attention to the situation of marginalized and disadvantaged groups of migrants. Migrants should be included in relevant national action plans and strategies, such as for the provision of public housing or national strategies to combat racism and xenophobia.

Notes

1. The Canadian Census has historically collected information on place of birth, time of immigration, and national as well as racial and ethnic background. In Canada, however, government cutbacks on data collection have seriously hampered these activities.

References

Dinca-Panaitescua, S., Dinca-Panaitescu, M., Bryant, T., Daiski, I., Pilkington, B., & Raphael, D. (2011). Diabetes prevalence and income: Results of the Canadian Community Health Survey. *Health Policy, 99*(2), 116–123.

International Organization for Migration (IOM). (2011). *Glossary on immigration* (2nd ed.). Geneva: IOM.

Organisation for Economic Co-operation and Development. (2015). *Settling in: OECD indicators of immigrant integration 2015*. Paris: Author.

CHAPTER 13

Addressing the Social Exclusion of Immigrants through Public Policy Action

Toba Bryant

With the prospect of an ageing and declining population, more immigration into Europe is both likely and necessary in the coming years. More and more, immigration is seen as a necessity in countries with an ageing society and labour shortages in certain areas of the economy and many European countries have had to acknowledge that immigration is here to stay. (Ahokas, 2010, p. 6)

Chapter Objectives

This chapter identifies how the key issues identified in previous chapters can be responded to through action on public policy. The objectives of this chapter are:

- to define the concept of social exclusion and show its relevance for understanding the immigration experience;
- to provide summaries of the nine case studies;
- to identify the role that multiculturalism, racism and discrimination, labour integration, and democratic participation can play in reducing social exclusion of immigrants; and
- to discuss the role that anti-immigration parties are playing in fanning resistance to immigration and the threat they pose to reducing social exclusion.

Introduction

The case studies of immigration policy in these nine developed countries identified a number of themes and issues. Chief among these is the problem of **social exclusion** of immigrants. What can be done to address social exclusion? What public policy measures can help new immigrants settle in and gain acceptance in their new countries? This chapter examines these key immigration issues through the concept of social exclusion and identifies their public policy implications. A particular concern is how the social exclusion of immigrants influences their living and working conditions and ultimately their health. Reducing social exclusion also has important implications for the smooth functioning of societies.

Social Exclusion

Social exclusion is about the societal processes that systematically lead to groups being denied the opportunity to participate in commonly accepted activities of societal membership. As an integrative concept, it provides insights into how and why particular groups experience adverse material and social living and working conditions, and how political, economic, and social conditions contribute to these conditions. In Canada, for example, it has been well documented that social exclusion is especially likely among immigrants of colour coming from non-European nations. The case studies indicate this process is found in other developed nations accepting immigrants. The incidence of social exclusion has implications not only for the health of populations but also for the smooth functioning of societies. The concept emerged out of European concern with the effects of structural changes on social cohesion in general, but the concept has special implications for the issues identified in this volume. Madanipour, Cars, and Allen (1998) define social exclusion as follows:

> Social exclusion is defined as a multi-dimensional process, in which various forms of exclusion are combined: participation in decision-making and political processes, access to employment and material resources, and integration into common cultural processes. When combined they create acute forms of exclusion that find a spatial representation in particular neighbourhoods. (p. 22)

Social exclusion is both a process and an outcome (Galabuzi, 2016). White (1998) identifies four key aspects: (1) exclusion from legal processes; (2) exclusion from acquiring social goods; (3) exclusion from social production; and (4) exclusion from economic activities (see Box 13.1). The origins of social exclusion are seen as being primarily structural and, in the cases of immigrants, exacerbated by racism and discrimination. Social exclusion usually involves a number of social determinants of health such as income, employment and working conditions, and access to health and social services, among others. Galabuzi's (2016) description of social exclusion has particular relevance for the issues identified here.

> Social exclusion can be experienced by individuals and communities, communities of common bond and geographical communities. The characteristics of social exclusion tend to occur in multiple dimensions and are often mutually reinforcing. Groups living in low income areas are likely to also experience inequality in access to employment, substandard housing, insecurity, stigmatization, institutional breakdown, social service deficits, spatial isolation, disconnection from civil society, discrimination and higher health risks. (p. 390)

Box 13.1: The Dimension of Social Exclusion

White (1998) has referred to four aspects of social exclusion. The first is being socially excluded from civil society through legal sanction or other institutional mechanisms, as often experienced by status and non-status migrants. This conception may include substantive disconnection from civil society and political participation due to material and social isolation, which are created through systemic forms of discrimination based on race, ethnicity, gender, disability, sexual orientation, and religion. In the post-9/11 era, racial profiling and new notions of community safety and national security have exacerbated the experience of this form of social exclusion.

Secondly, social exclusion refers to the failure to provide for the needs of particular groups—society's denial of social goods, such as accommodations, income security, language services, and sanctions to deter discrimination, to particular groups, which has intensified in this period of austerity.

Third is exclusion from social production, a denial of opportunity to contribute to or participate actively in society's social and cultural activities as full citizens.

The fourth aspect is economic exclusion from social consumption, that is, unequal access to normal forms of livelihood and economy, and income and social inequality.

Source: Galabuzi, G. E. (2016). Social exclusion. In D. Raphael (Ed.), *Social determinants of health: Canadian perspectives* (3rd ed, pp. 388–418). Toronto: Canadian Scholars' Press.

Summary of Case Studies

The following section provides a summary of some of the distinctive aspects from the case studies. These summaries identify the significant issues that are especially related to the social exclusion of immigrants. This section is followed by identification of means of addressing these issues of social exclusion through public policy action.

Australia

Australia sees itself as a settler nation. Until recently, immigration was restricted to those of European background, with people of colour being excluded. This has now changed and immigrants of colour now constitute a significant proportion of those entering Australia to settle. Australia has incorporated various forms of multiculturalism into its public policy.

The forms of multiculturalism have ebbed and waned, and despite government retreats from such policy beliefs, the concept of multiculturalism remains strong among Australians. Nonetheless, racism and xenophobia are present and appear to have adverse effects on the health and well-being of immigrants of colour. Complicating matters is the recent conflation of immigration with security concerns, which raises significant issues of human rights.

Significant data are available concerning a range of immigrant health and well-being issues, but these data are not systematically collected as part of governmental initiatives. Immigrants of colour compare poorly to the general Australian population in terms of employment rates, quality of employment, type of housing, and poverty rates. Significant issues exist in relation to access to health care and cultural sensitivity. Australia ranks eighth on the MIPEX Integration Index and scores high (8) on the Multicultural Policy Index.

Canada

Canada has experienced profound increase in immigration since the 1970s from non-European nations. Always a settler nation, Canada, like Australia, had until recently limited immigration to Britain, members of the British Commonwealth, or other European nations. At the same time that this discriminatory immigration policy was changed, Canada adopted multiculturalism as a public policy goal and enshrined it in its constitution. Canada uses a points system for immigration that limits entry to well-qualified candidates, and the previous Conservative government had restricted family reunification and refugee asylum claims. Restrictions on access to health care for asylum claimants have been ruled unconstitutional by the courts and have been reversed by the newly elected Liberal government.

The case study documents how multiculturalism has been translated into public policies and community resources that have built social capital and promoted social cohesion among new Canadians. The authors argue that these processes have helped buffer some of the health-threatening experiences that newcomers to Canada experience. Nevertheless they point out that despite higher education credentials and in many cases the ability to speak one of the two official languages of Canada, recent immigrants of colour experience lower employment participation and higher unemployment rates, lower wages, and more threatening social determinants of health.

The authors also point out that newcomers to Canada are subject to the same health-threatening experiences that others experience in Canada as a result of **neoliberal** restructuring of the economy and many government public policies and strategies that weaken the quality of the social determinants of health. The extent to which multiculturalism and its products are able to buffer these potential health threatening living and working conditions remains an area of active inquiry. Canada ranks sixth on the MIPEX Integration Index and scores high (7.5) on the Multicultural Policy Index.

United Kingdom

The United Kingdom provides an interesting example of a nation that has experienced two profoundly different waves of immigration over the past century. Upon the conclusion of the Second World War, the United Kingdom faced a severe labour shortage as many people emigrated from the UK. Immigrants from former British colonies in the Caribbean and India were actively recruited as workers by the United Kingdom. Contrary to what may have been expected, many of these immigrants stayed. Their concentration in some locations stimulated governments to respond to their needs in return for political support from these communities.

While initially these immigrants did well, the decline of industrial production has led to the impoverishment of many of these communities. The same processes that have created economic deindustrialization have also contributed to growing economic and social insecurity that, like elsewhere, has contributed to increasing racism and discrimination. The rise of the anti-immigration UK Independence Party is one such result of this process and has itself fanned anti-immigrant sentiment.

More recently the United Kingdom has come to experience what the authors term *superdiversity* as smaller numbers of immigrants are now coming from each of a greater number of nations. Immigration policy now sees these immigrants being dispersed across the United Kingdom rather than being centred in major urban areas, reducing their political power and voice and making provision of immigration-related services more difficult. In response to growing concerns about immigration, governments have instituted policies of welfarism whereby access to services and resources is restricted. These processes are creating conditions that threaten the health and well-being of immigrants. Not surprisingly, problems of health care access and adverse health outcomes among immigrants are increasing. The United Kingdom ranks fifteenth on the MIPEX Integration Index and scores toward the higher middle range (5.5) on the Multicultural Policy Index.

Austria

Austria is another nation that has come to depend upon immigration to deal with a declining fertility rate and an aging population. The immigration approach is similar to those of other nations in that it has gone through three stages of immigration. The first was focused on the receipt of guest workers, the second was concerned with family unification, and the third was focused on younger workers who were able to work. The grounds for granting of residency are rather strict and granted only upon provision of evidence of adequate means of subsistence, health insurance coverage, and housing.

Public policy takes little note of the diversity of the population and there is a lack of information concerning the day-to-day lived experiences and health outcomes of immigrants. What data are available suggest significant issues of discrimination and adverse health outcomes of foreign-born residents as compared to native-born residents. There are also significant issues related to the quality of interactions with the health care system, mainly related to lack of facility in German. On a more positive note, public policy has recognized the presence of discrimination and there is an Ombudsman for Equal Treatment that has the responsibility of enforcing the right to equality and equal outcomes. It remains to be seen how effective this agency is in dealing with these issues. Austria scores zero on the Multiculturalism Policy Index and there is little effort to have multiculturalism included in public policy. Austria ranks twentieth, the lowest of all the nations in this volume, on the MIPEX Integration Index.

Belgium

Belgium is another nation that that has experienced a wide range of different immigration periods. It has gone through periods of labour immigration, family reunification, and receipt of asylum claimants. Belgium has had unique special conventions with nations such as Morocco and Turkey that have facilitated immigration. More recently, primarily as a result of greater influence of anti-immigration parties, Belgium has come to restrict its immigration practices.

For historical reasons related to experiences during the Second World War, there has been resistance to collecting data on ethnicity and race. Nevertheless, researchers are able to obtain waivers and there is a rich literature developing in Belgium on health outcomes among immigrants as well as inquiries into the day-to-day lived experiences of immigrants. Similar to the other nations in this volume, unemployment rates and greater rates of relative poverty are seen among immigrants. There is also concern about immigrants' interactions with the health care system and special attention is being given the role of intercultural mediators and use of translators in the health care system.

There is also special concern about irregular immigrants, those who do not have legal authorization to stay in the country, and their ability to access health care. Belgium has undertaken processes of regularization, a form of amnesty by which people can come forward and be accepted as residents. Like other countries, it is being faced with increased asylum claims by refugees from conflicts in Northern Africa and the Middle East. Belgium is attempting to balance its humanitarian concerns with the availability of resources. Finally, Belgium has recognized the presence of discrimination and racism and its Center for Equal Opportunities and Opposition to Racism has been divided into the Interfederal Center for Equal Opportunities and the federal Migration Centre. Both of these are concerned with promoting **integration**, reducing discrimination, and promoting the rights of foreigners in Belgium. Belgium ranks seventh on the MIPEX Integration Index and scores a mid-range 5.5 on the Multiculturalism Policy Index.

Germany

Germany has made identifying how different groups of immigrants differ in health status an active area of inquiry. Significant attention has been directed toward collecting information on the backgrounds of individuals who are part of these health-related surveys. Findings are similar to other nations in that the health status of immigrants tends to fall behind those of native-born residents. Germany also shows a healthy immigrant effect by which the health of immigrants is initially better than those of natives, but over time comes to resemble them and in many cases falls behind.

Even though immigrants in Germany are a very diverse group, researchers have been able to identify health outcomes among first-, second-, and third-generation immigrants as well as the causes behind these adverse health profiles. The case study identifies greater rates of poverty and lower quality of employment as implicated in these findings. Research has also identified significant anti-immigration attitudes among Germans toward particular immigrant groups. This situation has not been assisted by systematic reforms to social and labour policy that has led to a reconstruction of the German welfare state in ways that are not favourable to health. Growing rates of poverty and income inequality have affected the social determinants of health of Germans in general with particular impact on immigrants, especially those of diverse backgrounds.

Significant attention has also been focused on the interactions of immigrants with the health care system. The importance of facilitating positive interactions with the health care system requires reducing barriers such as language difficulties, difficulties in communication between cultures, and access to information. Immigrants are less likely to use preventive and health promotion measures, make use of nursing services, and use rehabilitation services. Germany ranks tenth on the MIPEX Integration Index and scores a low 2.5 on the Multiculturalism Policy Index.

Denmark

Denmark is one of the Nordic Social Democratic countries. It has a large immigrant community. A significant proportion of these immigrants come from non-European countries. Statistics Denmark reported that at the end of 2014 the immigrant population was 653,041 people. Of these, 233,484 were from Western countries and 419,557 were from non-Western nations. The immigrant population represents 11.5 percent of the total Danish population. Most arrive as labour immigrants, asylum-seekers, or for family reunification. All of these immigrant categories have increased over the last 50 years.

The authors identify immigrant integration as a key issue in Denmark, especially with the emergence of gaps in a number of important indicators of societal participation between immigrants from non-European countries and native Danes. Immigrants' participation in the labour market is considerably lower compared to that of natives, and employment rates for Danish natives are higher than that for non-Western immigrants. Immigrant women are more likely to have lower educational achievement compared to male immigrants and women with Danish citizenship.

Immigrant populations tend to have higher poverty rates. Poverty rates for non-Western immigrants have grown from 30 percent to 50 percent since the mid-1980s and remained at this high level from the mid-1990s to the present. This has led to a significant increase in immigrants' dependence on welfare benefits.

Significant political opposition to immigrants has led to regulations that restrict immigrants' access to welfare benefits and reduce opportunities for them to enter Denmark. Immigrant health has been of rather less concern compared to employment, culture, and national security. Denmark ranks thirteenth on the MIPEX Integration Index and scores zero on the Multicultural Policy Index.

Norway

In Norway, a key issue is immigrant health and well-being. Non-Western immigrants (NWIs) tend to face the greatest challenges in terms of social exclusion and health. The NWI category comprises individuals with parents from Asia, Africa, Latin America, Oceania (except Australia and New Zealand), and Europe (not the European Union/ European Economic area). Immigration to Norway includes labour migrants, family, and asylum-seekers.

In the early 1960s, the main source of immigrants to Norway was labour migrants from Turkey and Morocco. Since roughly 1975, immigration from non-Western countries has been primarily family and asylum-seekers. NWIs are young with 57 percent between the ages of 20 to 44 years. The proportion of the Norwegian-born population in this age range is 15 percent. Schou and Fosse argue that this has implications for health promotion policy since aging immigrant populations' health needs tend to differ from younger immigrant populations.

One of the Nordic Social Democratic welfare states, Norway has initiated a number of efforts to welcome immigrants and help them integrate in Norwegian society. The focus is on individual integration as opposed to group integration. The authors characterize Norwegian immigrant policy as "combined socialist and individualist integration." It is multicultural since it maintains and encourages immigrants' cultural heritage. This is particularly the case for the government's policy toward the Sami people compared to government policy toward immigrants.

Norway ranks fourth on the MIPEX Integration Index and toward the low end on the Multiculturalism Policy Index at 3.5. However, the policy on immigrants supports ethnic group organizations and heritage language instruction, but not affirmative action. There is no formal recognition of dual citizenship, non-Christian holidays, religious instruction, or languages other than Norwegian and Sami. The policy promotes integration of immigrants into the host culture.

Sweden

Sweden has a rather significant proportion of its population that is either foreign-born or children born in Sweden to immigrant parents. Until recently, much of this immigration consisted of immigrants from other Nordic nations accepted primarily for labour. More recently, Sweden has admitted many asylum-seekers from non-European nations. Significant public policy attention has been directed toward immigration integration and, like other nations, Sweden has gone through various phases of immigration policy.

Immigrants have access to the same significant welfare state resources provided to the native-born. The idea of multiculturalism is seen as having an innate contradiction to the strong sense of community and solidarity that underlies the Swedish welfare state, yet Sweden scores high on the Multicultural Policy Index. Significant support is provided to immigrants that include language training, employment training, and instruction in children's first language if it is not Swedish. While Sweden scores the best among nations at integrating immigrants on the MIPEX Integration Index, it is struggling with higher unemployment and relative poverty rates among immigrants as compared to the native-born population.

This focus on integration has led to neglect of data collection related to racial and ethnic differences that might be related to health outcomes. The available data on such issues are primarily focused on the senior population, and these data suggest that foreign-born elderly Swedes do not fare as well as native-born Swedes on a variety of health outcomes. While, like other nations, Sweden exhibits profound differences between the employment- and income-related outcomes of foreign-born to native-born, it expends significant effort to create public policy that can reduce these differences. Sweden ranks first on the MIPEX Integration Index and scores high at 7 on the Multicultural Policy Index.

Multiculturalism, Racism and Discrimination, Labour Integration, and Democratic Participation

Multiculturalism, racism/discrimination, labour integration, and democratic participation all have implications for successful integration of immigrants and reducing social exclusion. Reducing social exclusion has important implications for health.

Multiculturalism

Multiculturalism refers to policies that promote respect and acceptance of immigrant populations in an effort to promote successful settlement and integration by reducing social exclusion. The Canadian and Australian case studies provide detailed examinations of the rationale behind and goals of multicultural policy. The Australian case in particular illustrates how the concept of multiculturalism is subject to differing interpretations and means of implementation.

Frequently, there is tension between assimilation and the extent to which immigrants are encouraged to retain their cultural heritage and practices. Some immigrant populations may meet resistance to their cultural practices, which reflects resistance to ethnocultural/ethno-racial diversity more generally. This has especially been the case for Muslim immigrants in recent years with post–September 11, 2001, tensions. Indeed, some governing authorities or political parties are specifically fanning these issues for electoral gain. For example, policies that proposed restricting Muslim women from wearing the niqab during citizenship ceremonies and while employed by the public service in Canada was used as an electoral ploy during the last political election by the ruling Conservative Party. This ploy came to be associated with Muslim women being subjected to violent hate-related incidents during the federal election campaign in October 2015.

Considering that immigration has the strong potential to fan racist and xenophobic attitudes in the dominant culture toward those of differing cultural and ethnic backgrounds, it seems obvious that multiculturalism policy can provide a means of countering these adverse attitudes. It probably is not a coincidence that the nations that do worse according to the MIPEX Integration Index are those scoring lower on the Multiculturalism Policy Index. Among the Anglo-Saxon nations, the United Kingdom scores lowest on both integration and multiculturalism. Among the Conservative countries, Austria scores lowest on both integration and multiculturalism, and among the Scandinavian countries, Denmark also scores lowest on both indicators.

An important dimension of the term is *accommodation*. This does not mean assimilation, but rather acceptance and acknowledgement of diverse cultural heritages of immigrants. Research is needed into the specific aspects of multicultural policy that are associated with specific aspects of integration policy. Both the MIPEX and

Multiculturalism Policy Index consist of eight dimensions. It is beyond the scope of the present inquiry to examine the complex interrelationships between these dimensions, but such inquiry seems worthwhile.

Racism and Discrimination

Underscoring many aspects of social exclusion and resultant adverse health profiles is the experience of immigrants of discriminatory practices frequently fanned by racism. This is a particular concern for immigrants coming from low-income countries of the developing world (Organisation for Economic Co-operation and Development, 2015). Austria and Australia had high reported rates of discrimination at 34 percent and 24 percent, respectively, for immigrants 15 to 64 years from low-income countries. Since these nations differ on their Multicultural Index Scores, yet both report relatively higher discrimination scores, adoption of such policies does not appear to be the sole means of managing such discrimination. What may be of more importance than multiculturalism policies themselves is the extent to which anti-immigration sentiments are allowed to shape both the immigration policies of ruling mainstream parties as well as the popularity of anti-immigration parties.

Anti-immigration political parties have emerged across many European countries (see Appendix). In Denmark, the anti-immigration party has had influence on the political process since the 1970s. This is now happening in Belgium. These parties fuel anti-immigrant sentiments among the population, which results in growing discrimination and racism toward immigrant populations. Additional anti-immigrant sentiment toward Muslims has grown since the events of September 11, 2001, and Muslims have become targets of policy measures ostensibly aimed at strengthening national security. This is especially the case in Denmark and Austria, but is apparent across nations. And it also has the potential to stop governments in their tracks from implementing progressive immigration policy (see Box 13.2).

Box 13.2: Angela Merkel Wants to "Drastically Decrease" Number of Refugees Coming to Germany

Chancellor Angela Merkel said on Sunday she wanted to "drastically decrease" the number of refugees coming to Germany, signalling a compromise to critics of her open-door policy from within her conservatives on the eve of a party congress.

Merkel has resisted pressure from allies within her Christian Democratic Union (CDU) to put a cap on the number of refugees entering Germany, which is expected to top 1 million this year.

"At the same time we took on board the concerns of the people, who are worried about the future, and this means we want to reduce, we want to drastically decrease the number of people coming to us," Merkel told broadcaster ARD.

Merkel, whose popularity has fallen over her handling of the refugee crisis, said the word "limit" did not feature in the CDU's main resolution which will be debated at the two-day party congress starting on Monday in the southern city of Karlsruhe.

> The chancellor added there was broad support in the CDU for her strategy to reduce the numbers. This included working with Turkey to fight traffickers, improving the situation at Syrian refugee camps in Turkey, Lebanon, and Jordan, and strengthening control of the European Union's outer borders.
>
> Merkel's conservative critics want her to get the number of arrivals down before three state elections in March and say her hopes of running for a fourth term in 2017 would be in danger.

Source: Rinke, A., Nasr, J., & Williams, A. (2015, December 13). Angela Merkel wants to "drastically decrease" number of refugees coming to Germany. *Thompson Reuters*. Retrieved from www.cbc.ca/news/world/merkel-refugees-germany-1.3363453.

Not surprisingly, during the last 10 to 15 years, there has been increasing concern about how well Muslim—as well as other groups—in European nations have integrated in their host countries (Modood, 2013). This has been fostered by fears that terrorist activities will result from the mere presence of Muslim youth in nations. A more useful approach would be to express concern with the social exclusion of Muslim and other visible-minority populations in European and other countries. The means for reducing social exclusion would involve reducing discrimination and racism, promoting integration into labour markets, and increasing democratic participation.

Promoting Labour Integration

Integration is defined in a number of ways but many such policies are often tied to employment. Some countries require immigrants to have employment as a prerequisite for admission and all consider it a prima facie indicator of successful integration. It should not be surprising that immigrant integration is equated with employment success, considering the strong role employment plays in providing income security and avoiding poverty, thereby reducing the need for governmental social assistance. And from a health perspective, employment is certainly an important social determinant of health that enables access to other social determinants of health such as food and housing security.

There is rather less attention paid to the types of jobs that immigrants may have. This is especially important when nations report small gaps in unemployment between native-born and immigrant populations, yet the poverty rates between employed native- and foreign-born residents loom large, as is the case in Canada. In all nations, precarious employment has increased and recent immigrants are among the groups most at risk of having precarious employment. Employment is important for integration, but quality of employment is as or more important.

A preoccupation with labour market participation of immigrants may preclude consideration of their health and well-being. Having access to the social determinants of health requires high-quality employment. Such employment will support food and housing security, among others (Raphael, 2016).

Democratic Participation

Democratic participation refers to the extent to which immigrants are integrated into the political process such that they can contribute to policy development to meet their needs. Few nations are making efforts to consult immigrants concerning their health and well-being. Norway funds the activities of ethnic groups and is ensuring that municipal authorities are promoting the social determinants of immigrant health, hopefully in participatory ways.

All the authors in this volume call for greater efforts to integrate immigrants in society. A useful tool would be to use the social determinants of health as a direct focus for integration activities and to assess their quality as an indicator of successful immigrants' integration. Indeed, integration policies and health promotion policies are related (Schou & Fosse, this volume) and the implications of such an approach deserve attention. Immigration policy is ultimately nation building and requires the input of immigrants to develop public policies and programs that will be responsive to the needs of immigrants. This will enable them to make positive contributions to their host countries.

Health Policy as a Key Component of Integration Policy

An important theme in this book is the relationship between integration and health policy.

It is notable that immigrants eventually have poorer health outcomes compared to the native-born in most countries (OECD, 2015). These poorer outcomes have been attributed to their less favourable socio-demographic characteristics as compared to the larger native-born population. These characteristics may include the race, cultural backgrounds, and even the religions of recent immigrants. These characteristics may trump the effects of education, which is supported by findings that in many nations, immigrants have higher educational achievement compared to the native-born, yet poorer health outcomes. Higher education of immigrants may therefore not be protective against disadvantage for this group, as it is for the native-born.

Accessing the health care system is an important part of this analysis. Every case study identified such concerns, and examples of means of reducing problems with access and quality of interaction were provided. Access issues may be especially important for undocumented residents, creating critical ethical and public issues for health providers.

Instituting Public Policy Change

How can public policy improve the health and well-being of immigrant populations? Much has been said in this volume about policy changes that will improve the health and well-being of immigrants. An important challenge in all nations and especially in a number of European countries is overcoming the power and influence of anti-immigrant political parties, thereby allowing room for promoting the social and political rights of immigrants.

The social determinants perspective highlights living and working conditions of immigrants, and takes into account their health and social well-being. It can also draw attention to means to identify and address the health and social needs of immigrant populations. This would involve consulting these populations directly to identify appropriate means to help them integrate, find employment, and meet their social determinants of health.

There is a need for laws that designate the national government in each country responsible for collecting data on social and health indicators for immigrant populations. This would ensure systematic tools for gathering information on immigrants and developing appropriate policies and programs to meet their needs.

As noted, welfare states vary in their capacity to address the needs of immigrant populations. Consultative mechanisms by which immigrants can contribute to policy development are an essential component of such a strategy (Sainsbury, 2012). These mechanisms are also consistent with principles of health promotion (WHO, 1986) and democratic participation (Fischer, 2003).

> The political participation of immigrants is one dimension of the integration process: the greater the political participation, the greater the integration in the democratic domain. Although traditionally integration policies tend to focus on socio-economic topics, governments are increasingly concerned with the importance of the socio-cultural sphere, participation, the personal dimensions of integration, and the frequency and intensity of social interactions. This approach stipulates the need for integrating immigrants into all aspects of society, including the civic, cultural and political fields. (Ahokas, 2010, p. 1)

These processes include allowing all residents to vote, and developing ongoing consultative processes to allow immigrants' voices to be heard. In short, their political inclusion can help shift the balance of political forces advocating inclusive and exclusionary measures. Other potential measures identified to help move immigrant health and well-being onto the political agenda is shifting from intercultural to equity care (Dauvrin, this volume). *Equity care* provides a broader perspective that can highlight the multiple social locations—or vulnerabilities—of immigrant populations.

All the case studies identified the need for responsive public policy that meets the general health and health care needs of immigrant populations. Responsive health policy recognizes that immigrant populations have particular needs associated with settlement and adjusting to a new culture. Responsive health care recognizes that timely and effective care must meet the needs of all individuals. Both approaches require public policy that provides affordable housing, employment, schools for their children, and the finding of and access to health and social services.

Conclusion

The evidence contained in this volume indicates that developed nations must identify means to recognize and measure diversity and then address the specific needs of these diverse groups. Yet, nations must balance addressing particular group needs with the needs of the entire society. Diversity and solidarity need not be in opposition but frequently are. Too much emphasis on solidarity can lead to neglect of the issues identified in this volume. Too much emphasis on diversity can weaken solidarity and promote conflict. Nations need to strike a balance between these two seemingly polar opposites.

It is clear that developed nations must accept that their populations will become increasingly more racially and ethnically diverse. Nations also have no choice but to face the fact that xenophobic and racist attitudes toward these diverse groups are present and there are forces that will attempt to benefit from such attitudes. Anti-immigration parties must be actively resisted (Bershidsky, 2015). Nations therefore have to respond to both the needs of diverse groups as well as the forces that will resist such efforts.

Multiculturalism as a public policy recognizes these needs and problematic issues and is an approach with promise. The most important issue, however, is to implement public policy for both native- and foreign-born that provides the economic and social security necessary for health. The Anglo-Saxon (Liberal) nations' acceptance of multiculturalism as a public policy provides a lesson all nations should consider. At the same time, the Continental (Conservative) and Scandinavian (Social Democratic) nations' public policies that provide economic and social security is a worthy goal to which all nations should aspire. The important task is to assure that economic and social security promoting public policies are available and applied to all citizens regardless of where they were born and their racial and ethnic backgrounds.

Critical Thinking Questions

1. How useful is the concept of social exclusion for understanding and promoting the integration of immigrants into a nation?
2. What are some of the forces that make it difficult to reduce social exclusion and promote integration of immigrants of differing cultural traditions in the receiving nation?

3. What are some of the key points that would be part of a public education program to promote the acceptance of immigrants into a nation?
4. What are some of the aspects of differing forms of the welfare state that both support and make difficult the reduction of social exclusion and the integration of immigrants into a nation?
5. What can be done to reduce the attractiveness of anti-immigration parties to the average person?

Glossary

Democratic participation is the degree to which immigrants are integrated into and participate in the political process, and contribute to policy development by identifying issues and means to address their needs.

Integration is the process by which newcomers to a country are helped to settle in the host country through the provision of services and programs to assist in finding housing, employment, and community amenities.

Neo-liberalism is a political ideology that emphasizes the market as the most important institution for resource allocation, stimulating economic growth, and meeting the needs of citizens.

Social exclusion is the process by which individuals or groups are prevented from participating in societal activities such as voting and employment.

Recommended Readings

Ahokas, L. (2010). *Promoting immigrants' democratic participation and integration. Exchanging good practices for the promotion of active citizenship in the EU.* Tampere, Finland: Tampere University Press. Retrieved from http://tinyurl.com/j9u8ch6

This publication is geared toward the promotion of immigrant integration and especially the issues of enhancing immigrant democratic participation. The practical aim of the publication is to present some good practices and reflect lessons learned from recent research.

Bryant, T. (2016). *Health policy* in canada (2nd ed.). Toronto: Canadian Scholars' Press.

This volume examines how public policy is developed and implemented by providing various models of the policy-development and implementation process. It outlines key themes in public policy in general and health policy in particular and directs attention to the forces that shape health policy in Canada and in other Western nations.

Galabuzi, G. E. (2016). Social exclusion. In D. Raphael (Ed.), *Social determinants of health: Canadian perspectives* (3rd ed, pp. 388–418). Toronto: Canadian Scholars' Press.

Galabuzi carefully outlines the components of social exclusion and the political, economic, and social forces that are driving this process in Canada. The origins of social exclusion experienced by recent immigrants are primarily structural and complicated by racism and discrimination within Canadian society.

Modood, T. (2013). *Multiculturalism*. Oxford: Polity Press.

Modood assesses the relationship between multiculturalism, cosmopolitanism, and assimilation. He sees multiculturalism as posing a significant challenge to existing forms of secularism, but also demonstrates that multiculturalism is crucial for successful integration.

Organisation for Economic Co-operation and Development. (2015). *Settling in: OECD indicators of immigrant integration 2015*. Paris: Author.

This publication highlights how immigrants and their children are integrating into OECD societies, judging their progress against key indicators. Many areas are considered, including material living conditions, health, education, labour market, and civic engagement.

Raphael, D., & Bryant, T. (2015). Power, intersectionality, and the life course: Identifying the political and economic structures of welfare states that support or threaten health. *Social Theory & Health, 13*(3–4), 245–266.

This article builds on Esping-Andersen's insights into different forms of the welfare state to theorize how forms of welfare states can shape the resources and supports available to those occupying various social locations during important periods of the life course. It also specifies the specific health outcomes of special relevance to those situated in vulnerable social locations across the life course.

Related Websites

Amnesty International. Fight Discrimination in Europe—http://www.amnesty.eu/en/campaigns/fight-discrimination-in-europe/#.VpFXqU9I4Wo

Discrimination is one of Europe's most pressing human rights concerns, affecting the lives of millions of people across the continent. Amnesty International's Fight Discrimination campaign aims to ensure that all individuals in Europe enjoy effective protection against discrimination.

European Commission. Poverty and Social Exclusion—http://ec.europa.eu/social/main.jsp?catId=751

With more than 120 million people in the EU at risk of poverty or social exclusion, EU leaders have pledged to bring at least 20 million people out of poverty and social exclusion by 2020. The fight against poverty and social exclusion is at the heart of the Europe 2020 strategy for smart, sustainable and inclusive growth.

European Commission. Tackling Discrimination—http://ec.europa.eu/justice/disination/index_en.htm

This website provides information and links on how the EU acts on behalf of EU citizens to prevent them being discriminated against on grounds of racial or ethnic origin, religion or belief, disability, age, or sexual orientation and sex.

European Union External Action. Commission Combating Racism, Xenophobia and Discrimination—http://eeas.europa.eu/human_rights/discrimination/index_en.htm

The EU works actively with the UN, the Organisation for Security and Co-operation in Europe (OSCE), and the Council of Europe. The work of the European Commission against Racism and Intolerance (ECRI) is used by the European Commission in the framework of EU enlargement. The EU combats racism, xenophobia, and discrimination also within its borders.

References

Ahokas, L. (2010). *Promoting immigrants' democratic participation and integration. Exchange for good practices for the promotion of active citizenship in the EU.* Tampere, Finland: Tampere University Press. Retrieved from http://tinyurl.com/j9u8ch6

Bershidsky, L. (2015, July 19). Ignorance fuels Europe's anti-immigration victories. *Bloomberg View.* Retrieved from http://www.bloombergview.com/articles/2015-06-19/ignorance-fuels-europe-s-anti-immigration-victories

Fischer, F. (2003). *Reframing public policy: Discursive politics and deliberative practices.* New York: Oxford University Press.

Galabuzi, G. E. (2016). Social exclusion. In D. Raphael (Ed.), *Social determinants of health: Canadian perspectives* (3rd ed.) (pp. 388–418). Toronto: Canadian Scholars' Press.

Madanipour, A., Cars, G., & Allen, J. (1998). *Social exclusion in European cities.* London: Jessica Kingsley.

Modood, T. (2013). *Multiculturalism.* Oxford: Polity Press.

Organisation for Economic Co-operation and Development (OECD). (2015). *Settling in: OECD indicators of immigrant integration 2015.* Paris: Author.

Raphael, D. (Ed.). (2016). *Social determinants of health: Canadian perspectives* (3rd ed.). Toronto: Canadian Scholars' Press.

Sainsbury, D. (2012). *Welfare states and immigrant rights.* London: Oxford University Press.

White, P. (1998). Ideologies, social exclusion, and spatial segregation in Paris. In S. Mursterd & W. Ostendorf (Eds.), *Urban desegregation and the welfare state: Inequality and exclusion in Western cities* (pp. 148–167). London: Routledge.

World Health Organization (WHO). (1986). *Ottawa Charter for Health Promotion.* Retrieved from http://www.who.int/hpr/NPH/docs/ottawa_charter_hp.pdf

Appendix: Strength of Nationalist Parties in Europe

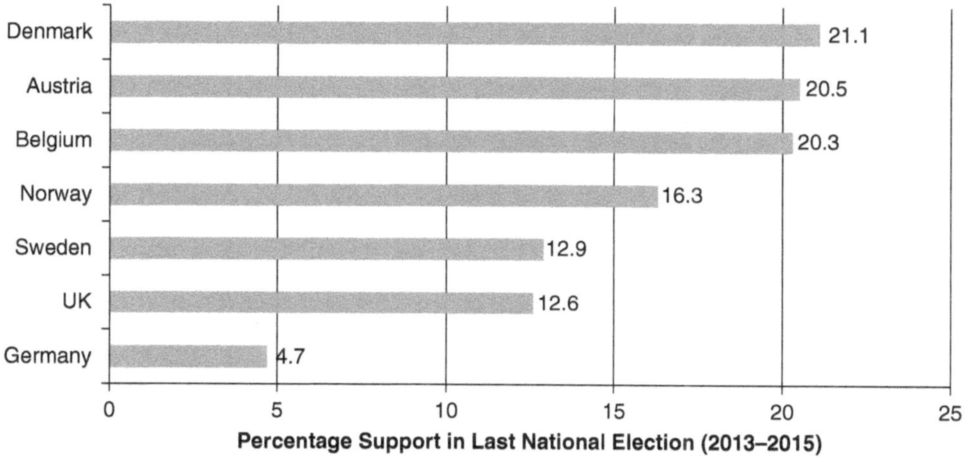

Figure 13.1: Strength of Nationalist Parties in Europe

Source: List of active nationalist parties in Europe. (2016). Retrieved from https://en.wikipedia.org/wiki/List_of_active_nationalist_parties_in_Europe

Author Biographies

Hurriyet Babacan is a Professor and Pro Vice-Chancellor (Academic and Research) at Torrens University in Australia. Dr. Babacan has been responsible for development and implementation of multicultural, gender, and social development policies at federal and state government levels. She was one of the authors of the Cultural Responsiveness Framework for the Victorian Department of Health and has been a Commissioner with the inaugural Victorian Ethnic Affairs Commission. She has published extensively on cultural diversity, multiculturalism, gender, health, public policy, human rights, social justice, and social development. Dr. Babacan has been recognized for her work by a number of awards, including the Multicultural Services Award 1999, Bi-Centennial Medal by the Prime Minister of Australia 2002, the Telstra Businesswomen's Award 2003, and the prestigious Order of Australia Award 2014 for her contribution as an academic to community affairs and policy development.

Heinrich Bollinger is a Professor of Sociology at the Fulda University of Applied Sciences, where he has been Dean of the Social and Cultural Studies Faculty since 2003. His research and teaching interests include the sociology of organizations, project management and occupational health and safety, knowledge logistics in supply networks, and trends in health care professions.

Hannah Bradby is a Professor in the Department of Sociology at Uppsala University, having previously been employed at the universities of Warwick and Glasgow. Her research addresses the sociology of health and how this relates to the social construction of racialized and ethnic categories. The challenge of researching cultural, religious, and ethnic diversity both as a positive and as an imposed identity has been an ongoing interest. Her latest paper is "International medical migration: A critical conceptual review of the global movements of doctors and nurses," in *Health: An Interdisciplinary Journal, 18*(6), 580–596. A special issue on medical mobilities is forthcoming in the journal *Ethnicity & Health.*

Toba Bryant is an Assistant Professor in the Faculty of Health Sciences at the University of Ontario Institute of Technology. She is author of *Health Policy in Canada* (2016) and co-editor of *Staying Alive: Critical Perspectives on Health, Illness, and Health Care* (2010). Dr. Bryant is also the author of several journal articles and book chapters, including recent publications in *Health Policy, Social Theory and Health,* and the *Canadian Journal of Public Policy.* Her research interests centre on the areas of health and social policy, globalization and the health of Canadians, social determinants of health, and urban health.

Romana Careja is an Assistant Professor at the Political Science Department, University of Southern Denmark. Her academic interest is immigration in a comparative perspective. In a number articles and book chapters, she has studied immigration both on an individual level and a macro level. Her publications include *Policy Coherence and Economic Reforms in Central and Eastern Europe* (2010) as well as articles in journals such as *International Migration Review, Comparative Political Studies, International Political Science Review*, and *European Journal of Political Research.*

Marie Dauvrin is a Guest Lecturer at the Université catholique de Louvain, Professor in Nursing Sciences at the Parnasse-ISEI, and post-doctoral researcher at the Institute of Health and Society. Dr. Dauvrin worked as a registered community health nurse for several years before moving to academia, and she continues to work as a volunteer nurse with homeless people and irregular migrants. Her teaching and research interests include access and quality of health care for vulnerable populations, including migrants and ethnic minorities, homeless people, irregular migrants, asylum-seekers and refugees, and people living in poverty, with a focus on organizational, political, and institutional levels. Since 2007, she has been involved in several projects around migrant and health at national and international levels. She was a contributor to the Belgian ETHEALTH project, aimed at providing recommendations for intercultural care for migrants and ethnic minorities, and in charge of the MIPEX health strand for Belgium.

Elisabeth Fosse, PhD, is a Professor of Health Promotion and Head of the Department of Health Promotion and Development, University of Bergen, Norway. She also holds a position as Professor at Buskerud and Vestfold University College. She is a political scientist and her area of specialization is in the formation and implementation of health promotion policies in European countries. Over the last years she has particularly studied European policies to reduce social inequalities in health. She has participated in several EU-funded projects in the area of health promotion. Currently she is involved as project leader in one and researcher in another national project studying Norwegian policies to reduce social inequalities in health in municipalities.

Narayan Gopalkrishnan is Course Coordinator for the Bachelor of Social Work and Master of Social Work degree programs in the College of Arts, Society and Education at James Cook University, Australia. Dr. Gopalkrishnan's teaching and research interests relate to diversity, cross-cultural and community development, diaspora studies, racism, immigrant integration, cultural diversity in health, alternative health systems, mental health multiculturalism, human rights, globalization, international aid and human development, policy and program and service development, leadership and organizational change. Dr. Gopalkrishnan has convened a number of international conferences, including the International Conference on Racisms in the New

World Order, Multicultural Families Conference, and Discrimination and Mental Health Symposium. Dr. Gopalkrishnan was the Founding Director of the Centre for Multicultural and Community Development, an academic research centre of the University of the Sunshine Coast, which focused on research and development relating to multiculturalism and community development.

Gudrun Hentges is Chair of Political Science, Education Policy, and Civic Education in the Faculty of Humanities at the University of Cologne. She was previously a Professor of Political Science focusing on migration and integration (2004–2016) and Vice-Dean of the department of Social and Cultural Studies (2009–2016) at the Fulda University. She is also a Member of the Centre for Intercultural and European Studies (CINTEUS). Her teaching and research focuses on racism and anti-Semitism, migration and integration, right-wing populism and extremism in Germany and Europe, and institutions and methods of civic education. On these topics she has published numerous contributions in German, English, and Turkish. Her latest monograph, "State and Civic Education" (2013), is considered "pioneering work" among scholars of political science and civic education. She was involved in the development of the innovative study program Social Sciences on Intercultural Relations, and in 2007 this program was honoured by the state government of Hesse with the Hessian Integration Award.

Ilene Hyman earned a PhD in Epidemiology, a Master of Health Science in Community Health and Epidemiology, and a Bachelor of Science in Physical Therapy. Dr. Hyman is a Social Epidemiologist, Research Consultant, and Professor in the Dalla Lana School of Public Health at the University of Toronto. Much of her research explores health and social equity among newcomer and racialized populations in Canada. She has led several research projects exploring mental health, family violence, and chronic disease within new immigrant communities in Canada. She is also a frequent author and contributor to government and organizational reports on immigration, racialization, and health, including *Racism as a Determinant of Immigrant Health, Racialization and Health Inequalities*, and *The Role of Multiculturalism Policy in Addressing Social Inclusion Processes in Canada*. Dr. Hyman was recently the Project Coordinator and POD Lead for a project called Immigrant Integration and Inclusion: Investigating the Canadian Partnership Model from a Complex-System Perspective.

Heidi Vad Jønsson is an Assistant Professor at the Institute of History and Centre for Welfare State Research, University of Southern Denmark. She holds a PhD in political history and has specialized her research in immigration and integration policy in Scandinavia. Her main research areas, in addition to migration research, welfare state history, party politics, as well as health policy and public health policy. Recent publications include *I velfærdsstatens randområde, Socialdemokratiets integrationspolitik*

1960'erne til 2000'erne (forthcoming) and three chapters of which two are co-authored with Klaus Petersen: "Immigration og integrationspolitik" in the six-volume publication on the history of the Danish welfare state *Dansk Velfærdshistorie.*

Agnes Meinhard is an Associate Professor of Organizational Behaviour and Theory, and the founding and current Director of the Centre for Voluntary Sector Studies (CVSS) in the Ted Rogers School of Management at Ryerson University. She was instrumental in establishing Canada's first undergraduate interdisciplinary curriculum in non-profit and voluntary sector management at Ryerson. Her research interests include the formation, growth, and demise of voluntary organizations, the emergence of hybrid organizational forms, intersector collaborations for food security, volunteer behaviour and development, corporate social responsibility, employer-supported volunteering, and service learning. Her more recent projects include: Immigrant Integration and Inclusion; Effective Governance of Social Enterprises; Diverse Nonprofit Organizations for Diverse Communities; Social Return on Investment in a Work Integration Social Enterprise; and Social Businesses and Marginalized Social Groups. Dr. Meinhard has been a three-time recipient of Best Paper awards from the Administrative Sciences Association of Canada and a semi-finalist in TVO's Best Lecturer competition.

Jenny Phillimore is Professor of Migration and Superdiversity and Director of the Institute for Research into Superdiversity (IRiS) at the University of Birmingham. Dr. Phillimore's research interests include migrants' access to welfare in superdiverse areas and migrant integration with a particular focus on migrant health and social capital. She has published extensively on these subjects and on qualitative research methods with recent texts, including *Community Research for Community Participation* and *New Migrants in the UK.* She has worked as an adviser to local, regional, national, and EU governments and is a Fellow of the Royal Society of Arts. She is currently leading two EU projects on migrant integration and access to health in superdiverse neighbourhoods.

Dennis Raphael, PhD, is a Professor of Health Policy and Management at York University in Toronto. He is editor of *Social Determinants of Health: Canadian Perspectives* and *Tackling Health Inequalities: Lessons from International Experiences*, co-editor of *Staying Alive: Critical Perspectives on Health, Illness, and Health Care*, and author of *Poverty in Canada: Implications for Health and Quality of Life*, all published by Canadian Scholars' Press. Dr. Raphael is also co-author of *Social Determinants of Health: The Canadian Facts*, a primer for the Canadian public that has been downloaded over 350,000 times from http://thecanadianfacts.org.

Arild Schou, PhD, is a Professor in Public Administration and Politics at the School of Business and Social Science, Buskerud and Vestfold University College. His area of specialization is ethnopolitics, local government reform, municipal governance, and public health. His research is globally oriented. He has been working for the

World Bank and OECD (DAC) and has done research on implementation of HIV/AIDS programs in Africa, particularly in Malawi. Currently he is involved as a project leader for a research evaluation of the Norwegian Coordination Reform (coordination between central and local government), which focuses on the reform's effect on health prevention and health promotion at municipal level.

Abiola Sulaiman is a public policy professional who has studied Health Policy and Management at York University in Toronto as well as Public Policy at the University of Toronto. Abiola began his Canadian journey as an immigrant to Canada, and was raised in a middle-class family under hard-working parents. Abiola's policy interests include urban planning and development, and foreign affairs.

Sandra Torres is a Professor of Sociology and Chair in Social Gerontology at Uppsala University, Sweden. Her research problematizes old age–related constructs (e.g., successful aging, diminished everyday competence, autonomy, dependence, and independence), sheds critical light on commonly used methods in health and social care (e.g., standardized testing, need assessment practice, and case file documentation), and deconstructs some of the taken-for-granted assumptions that guide policy and practice for the older segments of our populations (through policy and media analyses). Her latest paper is published in *Ageing & Society*, "Expanding the gerontological imagination on ethnicity: Conceptual and theoretical perspectives." An edited book (together with U. Karl) titled *Aging in Context of Migration* is forthcoming with Routledge.

Ursula Trummer received her PhD in the Sociology of Health and Medicine, MSc in Organisational Development and Counselling, and Master degree in Socioeconomic Sciences. Dr. Trummer is co-founder and head of the Center for Health and Migration (C-HM), Vienna (www.c-hm.com). C-HM works on the development of a theoretical and empirical knowledge base in terms of the complex interplay of health, migration, and social inclusion. She works as Senior Scientist at the Vienna University of Economics and Business, Lecturer at the Medical University of Vienna (Diversity and Medicine, Gender Medicine) and the Medical University of Graz (Public Health). Dr. Trummer acted as Project Director of various European and international projects and co-authored the Amsterdam Declaration "Towards Migrant Friendly Hospitals in an Ethno-Culturally Diverse Europe."

Ina Wilczewska obtained an MA in Psychology at the University of Social Sciences and Humanities in Warsaw, where she also provided culture competence workshops for international students. Currently, she is a PhD candidate at the Department of Sociology of the University of Vienna. Her research focuses on the acculturation of migrants in Austria and the consequences for their health and well-being. She works as a Junior Researcher at the Center for Health and Migration (C-HM), Vienna (www.c-hm.com).

Copyright Acknowledgements

Figure 1.1: *Facts and figures 2013—Immigration overview: Permanent residents.* (2015, April 23). Retrieved from www.cic.gc.ca/english/resources/statistics/facts2013/permanent/10.asp. Copyright © Government of Canada. Reprinted with permission.

Box 1.1: Canadian Citizenship & Immigration Resource Center. (2014). Express Entry Immigration Program to launch in 2015. Retrieved from www.immigration.ca/en/2014/152-canada-immigration-news-articles/2014/april/738-express-entryimmigration-program-to-launch-in-2015.html. Copyright © Canadian Citizenship & Immigration Resource Center.

Box 1.2: O'Neil, P. (2015, October 13). Stephen Harper takes aim at temporary foreign worker program. Retrieved from www.vancouversun.com/news/Stephen+Harper+takes+temporary+foreign+worker+program/9396893/story.html. Copyright © Vancouver Sun.

Figure 1.2: Fertility Rates as Measured by Average Number of Children Per Woman (1970–2013). Fertility rates (indicator). doi: 10.1787/8272fb01-en. Copyright © Organisation for Economic Co-operation and Development, 2016.

Figure 1.3: Share of the Population That Is Aged 65 and Over (1970–2013). Elderly population (indicator). doi: 10.1787/8d805ea1-en. Copyright © Organisation for Economic Co-operation and Development, 2016.

Figure 1.4: Brunner, E., & Marmot, M. G. (2006). Social Organization, Stress, and Health. In M. G. Marmot & R. G. Wilkinson (Eds.), *Social Determinants of Health* (p. 9). Copyright © Oxford University Press.

Table 1.1: Adapted from the Migrant Integration Policy Index. (2015). Results infograph. Retrieved from www.mipex.eu/download-pdf#/add-selection. Copyright © the Migrant Integration Policy Index (MIPEX).

Table 1.2: Multiculturalism Policies in Contemporary Democracies. (2015). Multiculturalism policies for immigrant minorities, summary scores, 1980, 2000, 2010. Kingston, ON. Retrieved from www.queensu.ca/mcp/immigrant-minorities/results. Copyright © Multiculturalism Policy Index.

Figure 2.1: Saint-Arnaud, S., & Bernard, P. (2003). Convergence or resilience? A hierarchical cluster analysis of the welfare regimes in advanced countries. *Current Sociology*, 51(5), 499–527, Figure 2, 503. Copyright © Sage Publications.

Table 3.1: Adapted from Australian Bureau of Statistics. (2012). *Cultural diversity in Australia: Reflecting nation-stories from the 2011 census.* Retrieved from www.abs.gov.au/ausstats/abs@.nsf/lookup/2071.0main+features902012-2013. Copyright © Australian Bureau of Statistics.

Figure 4.1: Statistics Canada. (2008). *Canada's ethnocultural mosaic, 2006.* Catalogue no. 97-562-X. Retrieved from www12.statcan.gc.ca/english/census06/analysis/ethnicorigin/pdf/97-562-XIE2006001.pdf. Copyright © Statistics Canada.

Figure 4.2: Ng, E., Wilkins, R., Gendron, F., & Berthelot, J. M. (2005). Dynamics of immigrants' health in Canada: Evidence from the National Population Health Survey. *Healthy today, healthy tomorrow? Findings from the National Population Health Survey*, 2. Catalogue no. 82-618-MWE2005002. Retrieved from www.statcan.gc.ca/pub/82-618-m/2005002/pdf/4193621-eng.pdf. Copyright © Statistics Canada.

Figure 9.1: Adapted from Ministry of Children, Gender Equality, Integration and Social Affairs, Fact Sheet: Immigrants and Descendants. Retrieved from https://ec.europa.eu/migrant-integration/librarydoc/fact-sheet-immigrants-and-descendants. The Immigration Database of the Ministry of Social Affairs and Integration, managed by Statistics Denmark, IMUDD06. Copyright © Statistics Denmark.

Figure 9.2: Calculation based on data from Ankestyrelsen (2015) *Integration: Status Og Udvikling 2014.* For further statistical information, see also Ministry of Children, Gender Equality, Integration and Social Affairs, *Fact sheet: Immigrants and descendants.* Retrieved from https://ec.europa.eu/migrant-integration/librarydoc/fact-sheet-immigrants-and-descendants.

Figure 12.1: Adapted from Organisation for Economic Co-operation and Development. (2015). *Settling in: OECD indicators of immigrant integration 2015*, Figure 1.1 (p. 17). Copyright © Organisation for Economic Co-operation and Development.

Figure 12.2: Adapted from Organisation for Economic Co-operation and Development. (2015). *Settling in: OECD indicators of immigrant integration 2015*, Figure 1.5 (p. 25). Copyright © Organisation for Economic Co-operation and Development.

Index